CANCER PAIN MANAGEMENT

CANCER PAIN MANAGEMENT

Edited by

Deborah B. McGuire, Ph.D., R.N.
Instructor
The Johns Hopkins University
School of Nursing
Coordinator, Nursing Research
The Johns Hopkins Oncology Center
Department of Nursing
Baltimore, Maryland

and

Connie Henke Yarbro, B.S.N., R.N.
Editor
Seminars in Oncology Nursing
Clinical Assistant Professor
Department of Medicine
University of Missouri–Columbia
Columbia, Missouri

Grune & Stratton, Inc.
Harcourt Brace Jovanovich, Publishers
Orlando   New York   San Diego   London
San Francisco   Tokyo   Sydney   Toronto

Library of Congress Cataloging-in-Publication Data

Cancer pain management.

    Includes bibliographies and index.
    1. Cancer—Complications and sequelae. 2. Intractable
pain. 3. Analgesia. I. McGuire, Deborah B.
II. Yarbro, Connie Henke. [DNLM: 1. Neoplasms.
2. Pain—therapy. QZ 200 C2153635]
RC262.C29119   1987   616.99'406   87-279
ISBN 0-8089-1868-0
    Chapters 1, 2, 3, 5, 7, and 10 are updated and expanded
    from SEMINARS IN ONCOLOGY NURSING,
    Vol. 1, No. 2, May 1985.

Grune & Stratton, Inc.
Orlando, Florida 32887

Distributed in the United Kingdom by
Grune & Stratton, Ltd.
24/28 Oval Road, London NW 1

Library of Congress Catalog Number 87-279
International Standard Book Number 0-8089-1868-0
Printed in the United States of America
87 88 89 90   10 9 8 7 6 5 4 3 2 1

CONTENTS

PREFACE

Over the past several decades, long-term survival from cancer has increased. In the 1930s less than 20 percent of cancer patients lived five years after diagnosis, but now half live five years or longer.[1] Morbidity from cancer and its treatment, however, remains common. We must deal with both the unpleasant and often devastating physical and emotional side effects of major treatment modalities and the disease-related processes such as pain, fatigue, anorexia, and immobility.

Pain probably has a greater impact than any other aspect of cancer on the individual, those close to him, and health workers. Often, pain is unfortunately viewed by the lay public as synonymous with cancer.[7,15] One survey of knowledge about cancer revealed that pain was incorrectly listed by many respondents as one of the American Cancer Society's seven warning signals of cancer.[9] Equally unfortunate is the extent to which many health care workers have misconceptions about and inadequate knowledge of cancer pain and its management.[3,4,6,11,13] Cancer is not always accompanied by pain, nor do all patients with advanced cancer develop pain. However, some of those who do develop cancer-related pain may receive inadequate or inappropriate treatment, even as their lives are prolonged by our therapeutic and technological advances.

A number of ethical and moral problems arise in the management of cancer-related pain. Vaux wrote that personal perception and professional treatment of pain become moral issues because they reflect moral values and dispositions.[16] The implication of this statement is that such values and dispositions influence both how people with pain react to it and how they are perceived and treated by care givers. There is much data demonstrating that many people in pain, cancer patients and others, are woefully undertreated and/or mismanaged.[2,4,5,10,17] The major ethical and moral problem related to cancer pain is the appalling, and unfortunately all too common, lack of adequate relief of pain, which occurs for a variety of reasons including ignorance, timidity, insecurity, overcaution, misconceptions, values, and attitudes. Both Vaux[16] and Levine[8] urged the need for an ethical approach to pain management that included reciprocity, responsibility, and involvement in care on the part of the care giver and the patient. Such an approach calls for mutual respect of values, autonomy, and dignity, as well as the safeguarding of rights and the meeting of needs.

Twycross[14] described several principles inherent in the management of patients with advanced cancer, particularly those with disease-related pain: (1) care is given with the knowledge that eventually all patients will die; (2) there is no duty to preserve life at all costs; (3) an individual does not have to accept medical treatment if he does not wish to, even though his refusal may result in an earlier death; and (4) all treatment has some inherent risk. Although Twycross's major focus was the terminally ill and the differences between euthanasia and "letting Nature take its course," he described the need for a broad-based approach to the assessment and management of pain in cancer patients, regardless of whether or not they are "terminal."

The major purpose of this book is to present a broadbased, multidisciplinary approach to the management of cancer pain. With this in mind, we have assembled chapters dealing with many aspects of the pain problem: prevalence, pain syndromes, etiology, assessment, measurement, pharmacologic management (including new methods of delivery), neurosurgical management, and psychological management. Of great importance is an analysis of how we as health professionals can improve pain management by developing an understanding of and an appropriate attitude toward the patient in pain. The management of cancer pain is inherently a multidisciplinary challenge requiring the closest cooperation between health professionals, all of whom must be aware of how much progress has been made in understanding the complex phenomenon of pain. The most recent Consensus Development Conference Statement on pain, published by the National Institutes of Health,[12] notes the progress we have made in just the last few years and emphasizes the importance of the "integrated approach" to pain management. Integration in this context describes an approach to the most effective combination of pharmacological and nonpharmacological techniques and our chapters have been constructed to emphasize this theme, including a description of the unique problems posed by the pediatric patient with cancer.

We view pain as a multidimensional phenomenon with a multidisciplinary solution. Although much remains to be learned, as indicated by several authors who discuss directions for future research, our greatest need now is to fully utilize what we have already learned. We hope this volume will help all health care professionals understand their unique roles and the roles of their colleagues in an integrated approach to the cancer patient with pain.

REFERENCES

1. American Cancer Society: 1986 Cancer Facts and Figures. New York, American Cancer Society, 1986
2. Bonica JJ: Cancer pain: A major national health problem. Cancer Nurs 1: 313–316, 1978
3. Bonica JJ: Management of cancer pain. Acta Anaesth Scand (suppl 74) 26: 75–82, 1982
4. Charap AD: The knowledge, attitudes, and experience of medical personnel treating pain in the terminally ill. Mt. Sinai J Med 45; 561–580, 1978
5. Cohen FL: Postsurgical pain relief: Patients' status and nurses' medication choices. Pain 9: 265–274, 1980
6. Grossman SA, Sheidler VR: Skills of medical students and house officers in prescribing narcotic medications. J Med Educ 60: 552–557, 1985
7. Levin DN, Cleeland CS, Darr R: Public attitudes toward cancer pain. Cancer 56: 2337–2339, 1985
8. Levine ME: Bioethics of cancer nursing. J Enterostom Ther 9: 11–13, 1982
9. Luther SL, Price JH, Rose CA: The public's knowledge about cancer. Cancer Nurs 5: 109–116, 1982
10. Marks RM, Sachar EJ: Undertreatment of medical inpatients with narcotic analgesics. Ann Int Med 78: 173–181, 1973
11. Myers JS: Cancer pain: Assessment of nurses' knowledge and attitudes. Oncol Nurs Forum 12 (4): 62–66, 1985
12. National Institutes of Health Consensus Development Conference Statement: The integrated approach to the management of pain. Vol 6, No 3 (NIH Publication 1986-491-292:41148). Washington, DC, U.S. Government Printing Office, 1986
13. Rankin MA, Snider B: Nurses' perceptions of cancer patients' pain. Cancer Nurs 7: 149–155, 1984
14. Twycross RG: Ethical and clinical aspects of pain treatment in cancer patients. Acta Anaesth Scand (suppl 74) 26: 83–90, 1982
15. Twycross RG, Lack SA: Symptom Control in Far Advanced Cancer: Pain Relief. London, Pitman, 1983
16. Vaux KL: Pain: The moral dimensions. Cancer Bull Univ Texas MD Anderson Hosp Tum Insti 33: 86–87, 1981
17. Weis OF, Sriwatanakul K, Alloza JL, et al: Attitudes of patients, housestaff, and nurses toward postoperative analgesic care. Anesth Analg 62: 70–74, 1983

ACKNOWLEDGMENTS

We would first like to thank the contributors for their excellent and informative chapters, since without them this book could not have been produced. Second, we would like to acknowledge and thank Tim Ahles, Ph.D.; Marilee Donovan, Ph.D., R.N.; Stuart Grossman, M.D.; and Vivian Sheidler, M.S., R.N., for their reviews of selected manuscripts. And finally, we would especially like to thank our husbands, William P. McGuire and John W. Yarbro, for their understanding, support, and assistance during the preparation of the book.

Deborah B. McGuire
Connie H. Yarbro
Editors

CONTRIBUTORS

Tim A. Ahles, Ph.D *Assistant Professor, Behavioral Medicine Section, Department of Psychiatry, Dartmouth Medical School, Hanover, New Hampshire*

Benjamin S. Carson, M.D. *Assistant Professor of Neurosurgery, Assistant Professor of Oncology, Director of Pediatric Neurosurgery, Department of Neurological Surgery, The Johns Hopkins Hospital, Baltimore, Maryland*

Robert B. Catalano, Pharm. D. *Coordinator of Clinical Investigations, Fox Chase Cancer Center, Associate Professor of Clinical Pharmacy, Department of Pharmacy Practice, Philadelphia College of Pharmacy and Science, Philadelphia, Pennsylvania*

C. Richard Chapman, Ph.D. *Director, Pain and Toxicity Research Program, Fred Hutchinson Cancer Research Center; Professor, Departments of Anesthesiology and Psychiatry and Behavioral Sciences, University of Washington, School of Medicine, Seattle, Washington*

Nessa Coyle, M.S., R.N. *Nurse Clinician, Director, Supportive Care Program, Department of Neurology, Pain Service, Memorial Sloan-Kettering Cancer Center, New York, New York*

Marilee Ivers Donovan, Ph.D., R.N.   *Chairperson, Department of Medical Nursing, Rush-Presbyterian St. Luke's Medical Center, Chicago, Illinois*

Kathleen Foley, M.D.   *Associate Professor of Neurology and Pharmacology, Cornell University Medical College; Chief, Pain Service, Department of Neurology, Memorial Sloan-Kettering Cancer Center, New York, New York*

Josie Howard-Ruben, M.S., R.N.   *Doctoral Student, University of Illinois; Formerly, Oncology Clinical Nurse Specialist, Rush-Presbyterian-St. Luke's Medical Center, Chicago, Illinois*

Patricia M. Klopovich, M.N., R.N.   *Clinical Nurse Specialist, University of Kansas Medical Center, Department of Pediatrics, Division of Hematology/Oncology, Kansas City, Kansas*

Judith Kornell, M.S., R.N., O.C.N.   *Clinical Nurse Specialist Oncology Nursing Care, Pain and Toxicity Research Program, Fred Hutchinson Cancer Research Center, Seattle, Washington*

Deborah B. McGuire, Ph.D., R.N.   *Instructor, The Johns Hopkins University, School of Nursing; Coordinator, Nursing Research, The Johns Hopkins Oncology Center, Department of Nursing, Baltimore, Maryland*

Katherine L. Patterson, B.S.N., R.N.   *Nurse Clinician, University of Kansas Medical Center, Department of Pediatrics, Division of Hematology/Oncology, Kansas City, Kansas*

Vivian R. Sheidler, M.S., R.N.   *Clinical Specialist, The Johns Hopkins Oncology Center, Baltimore, Maryland*

Karen L. Syrjala, Ph.D.   *Associate in Clinical Research, Pain and Toxicity Research Program, Fred Hutchinson Cancer Research Center; Acting Assistant Professor, Psychiatry and Behavioral Sciences, and Multidisciplinary Pain Center, University of Washington, Seattle, Washington*

Connie Henke Yarbro, B.S.N., R.N.   *Editor, Seminars in Oncology Nursing; Clinical Assistant Professor, Department of Medicine, University of Missouri-Columbia, Columbia, Missouri*

CANCER PAIN MANAGEMENT

Deborah B. McGuire, Ph.D., R.N.

1

The Multidimensional Phenomenon of Cancer Pain

Cancer-related pain is a multidimensional experience consisting of physiologic, sensory, affective, cognitive, behavioral, and sociocultural components. Pain is also highly subjective and unique to the individual experiencing it. In this chapter, definitions and theories of pain and the various factors that influence an individual's perception of and response to pain are presented.

DEFINITIONS OF PAIN

As Livingston[32] wrote over 40 years ago, "The chief difficulty encountered in a search for a satisfactory definition for pain, is the fact that it can be considered from either a physiologic or psychologic approach. Any consideration of pain, by one approach alone, without due regard to the other, is incomplete" (p. 62). Melzack and Wall[40] commented, "Pain is such a common experience that we rarely pause to define it in ordinary conversation. Yet no one who has worked on the problem of pain has ever been able to give it a definition which is satisfactory to all of his colleagues" (p. 9). They view "pain" as representing "a *category* of experiences, signifying a multitude of different, unique experiences having different causes, and characterized by different qualities varying along a number of sensory and affective dimensions" (p. 71).

Although a number of authors have proposed definitions of pain,[38,42,50] the most widely accepted definition is that of the International Association for the Study of Pain (IASP),[24] which has developed standard definitions of pain terms, descriptions of chronic pain syndromes, and a classification and coding schema for these syndromes for members of different disciplines who work in the field of pain. Pain is defined as "an unpleasant sensory and emotional experience associated with actual or potential tissue damage, or described in terms of such damage." This definition encompasses not only pain of pathophysiologic origin but also pain of psychologic origin. It accounts for the sensory, affective, and motivational aspects of the experience described by Melzack and Casey.[38] Finally, it provides a nontheoretical, relatively complete, and valid taxonomy that is extremely useful for clinicians and researchers alike.[11]

THEORIES OF PAIN

Through the years, a number of theories have been proposed to explain what pain is and how it occurs. In 1664, Descartes proposed "that pain is like a bell-ringing alarm system whose sole purpose is to signal injury of the body" (p. 10).[40] This notion governed much of the subsequent thought and research on pain until the past few decades.

There have been two traditional and opposing schools of thought on the nature of pain. The *specificity theory* proposed that pain was a specific entity, similar to sight or smell, with its own peripheral and central components. Specific pain receptors in the skin were thought to project to a specific pain center in the brain. The *pattern theory*, on the other hand, proposed that there were no specific fibers or endings. Rather, the nerve impulse pattern for pain was produced by stimulation of nonspecific receptors. Several versions of the pattern theory were developed. Some versions stressed the intensity of the painful stimulation as the critical determinant of pain, while others emphasized a central summation mechanism.

A few individuals in the mid-20th century struggled to develop a new concept of pain in which the perception of pain was determined by factors other than the injury itself; for example, culture, individual personality and experience, and other activities of the nervous system. Livingston[32] discussed individual sensory perception, and associated ideas, apperceptions, and fears that a patient may have. These notions influenced researchers to espouse the view that pain was an experience consisting of a sensory (input) component and a reaction (processing) component.[3,4,23] This concept enabled clinicians and researchers to recognize that stimulation of sensory nerve endings caused pain and the perceived experience of pain depended upon the emotional state of the individual.

In 1965, Melzack and Wall[39] challenged the adequacy of the specificity and pattern theories of pain to provide a satisfactory physiologic and psychologic explanation of the phenomenon of pain. In their opinion, neither theory explained the diverse theoretical mechanisms of pain, and neither had received substantial experimental verification. They proposed, instead, the now classic *Gate Control Theory of Pain*. This theory postulated that pain phenomena were determined by the interactions among three spinal cord systems. First, peripheral stimulation sent nerve impulses to the substantia gelatinosa in the dorsal horn of the spinal cord, where these cells modulated the afferent impulses (the "gate control" mechanism). Second, the afferent patterns in the fibers of the dorsal column acted as a central control trigger that activated selective brain processes. These processes in turn influenced the modulating gate control properties of the substantia gelatinosa. Third, central transmission cells in the dorsal horn activated neural mechanisms, comprising an action system that was believed to be responsible for the perception of and response to pain.

The concepts of the Gate Control Theory of Pain explained many observed phenomena of pain. More than any previous theory of pain, the theory emphasized the different aspects of pain perception, including both sensory and emotional components. The Gate Control Theory was based on experimental neurophysiologic evidence in cats, and some of the proposed mechanisms and components of the theory have never been adequately documented in the research arena.[44] Nevertheless, Weisenberg[56] voiced a common opinion:

the gate-control theory of pain has been the most influential and important current theory of pain perception. It ties together many of the puzzling aspects of pain perception and control. It has had profound influence on pain research and the clinical control of pain. It has generated new interest in pain perception, stimulating a multidisciplinary view of pain for research and treatment. It has been able to demonstrate the tremendous importance of psychologic variables. Still, there is little doubt that research will produce changes in the original gate-control conceptions (p. 1012).

In a discussion of the Gate Control Theory, Melzack and Wall[40] commented, "Clearly, we do not imply that the gate theory is the final 'truth' about pain. However, a satisfactory alternative to the theory has not yet been proposed" (p. 235). In view of this widely acknowledged fact, the Gate Control Theory still serves as the most important vehicle for understanding the causes and nature of pain.

SUBJECTIVITY OF THE PAIN EXPERIENCE

The IASP and numerous authors have noted the importance of viewing pain from the subjective vantage point of the individual experiencing it.[5,6,24,28,32,34,40,42,51,56] Indeed, "the first and overriding rule is that the patient's valid experiences are data from which the doctor or the health professional commences his work."[41]

Viewing pain from the patient's subjective experience is fraught with problems that affect assessment, measurement, and management of pain.[14,16,53] It is not possible to compare cancer patients who are experiencing pain, even when they have the same type and extent of disease. Although pathophysiologic causes may be identified in many individuals who report pain, in others they may not be found. However, the lack of an organic mechanism to explain the pain should not lead to the conclusion that pain does not exist or that it is of psychogenic origin. Any complaint of pain in a patient with cancer must be thoroughly investigated to ascertain its etiology if possible and implement appropriate interventions.[14]

The unique aspects of an individual's experience of pain are due to the multidimensional components that comprise the experience. It is of utmost importance in the management of cancer-related pain that health workers be cognizant of these various components and the impact they may have on an individual's perception of and response to pain.

MULTIDIMENSIONAL COMPONENTS OF PAIN

Melzack and Casey[38] proposed a new conceptual model of pain using the basic concepts of the Gate Control Theory. They described three determinants of the pain experience. First, the selection and modulation of incoming pain sensations in the neospinothalamic projection system serve as a neural basis for the sensory/discriminative component of pain. Second, the brain reticular formation and limbic system become involved in aversive drive and affective reactions to pain, i.e., the motivational/affective component of pain. Third, higher central nervous system or central control (cognitive) activities are involved in the pain experience and response. These activities are primarily cognitive functions that act selectively on sensory processes and/or motivational mechanisms. The influences of present and past experiences are integral to the cognitive activities as well. Melzack and Casey believed pain to be a "function of the interactions of all three determinants, and cannot be ascribed to any one of them" (p. 434).[38] Thus, the complex sequences of behavior observed in individuals with pain " are determined by sensory, motivational, and cognitive processes acting on motor mechanisms" (p. 434).[38]

Ahles and his colleagues[1] expanded these ideas into a multidimensional conceptualization of cancer-related pain. They viewed the patient's interpretation of the pain experience as having five separate components: (1) physiologic (organic cause of pain); (2) sensory (intensity, location, quality); (3) affective (anxiety, depression); (4) cognitive (thought processes and views of one's self); and (5) behavioral (physical activity, medication intake). Ahles et al. were the first to examine cancer-related pain from a multidimensional view by assessing each component of their model.

This multidimensional conceptualization of cancer-related pain can be further expanded into a broad framework for understanding not only the patient's interpretations of the pain experience, but for delineating and understanding the plethora of other factors that may affect an individual's perception and interpretation of pain. In the following sections, each dimension of Ahles et al.'s original model will be expanded and discussed, with particular emphasis on the various factors that comprise the dimension. Additionally, a sixth dimension, sociocultural, will be added to present a more complete picture of factors affecting the perception and interpretation of pain (Table 1-1).

Table 1-1
Multidimensional Components of the Experience of Pain

1. Physiologic
   A. Etiology/organic origin of pain
   B. Type of pain
   C. Endorphins/enkephalins
   D. Other
2. Sensory
   A. Location
   B. Intensity
   C. Quality
3. Affective
   A. Neuroticism/extroversion
   B. Hypochondriasis
   C. Depression/anxiety
   D. Mood states
   E. Locus of control
   F. Health self-concept
   G. Ego strength/repression-sensitization
4. Cognitive
   A. Thought processes
   B. Views of self
   C. Meaning of pain
   D. Other
5. Behavioral
   A. Communication of pain
   B. Use of medications
   C. Activity level
   D. Other
6. Sociocultural
   A. Ethnic background
   B. Demographic variables
   C. Other

Adapted from Ahles TA, Blanchard EB, Ruckdeschel JC: The multidimensional nature of cancer-related pain. Pain 17:277–288, 1983.

Physiologic Component

Ahles et al.[1] described the physiologic component of cancer-related pain as the organic etiology of the pain, including bone metastases, nerve compression, and infiltration of a hollow viscus. Foley[20] described three separate pain syndromes seen in people with cancer: (1) pain associated with direct tumor involvement, (2) pain associated with cancer therapy, and (3) pain unrelated to cancer or cancer therapy, and she thoroughly delineated the many specific causes of pain related to both tumor and treatment. Coyle and Foley[14] explore common etiologies of pain in more detail, with emphasis on the impact etiology has on the individual's perception of and response to pain. For example, a patient who presents with pain at the time of diagnosis may always associate subsequent pain with recurrent cancer and respond with uncertainty and fear, regardless of the cause, while a patient whose pain is due to side effects of treatment will not experience the same feelings.

A second aspect of the physiologic component of pain is the type of pain a patient has. The generally accepted classification is the dichotomy of acute and chronic pain, each having various subdivisions depending on the authors one reads. Acute pain is due to tissue damage, has a definite pattern of onset, and lasts only a limited amount of time. Hyperactivity of the autonomic nervous system may be present. Healing of the damaged tissue usually results in resumption of normal tissue function. Chronic pain, on the other hand, may or may not be associated with tissue damage, persists three months or more,[24] and is usually accompanied by adaptation of the autonomic nervous system. There is not always a clear pattern of onset nor of cessation. Cancer-related pain can be dichotomized into acute and chronic types, with subdivisions based on specific etiologies.[14] As with the organic etiology of pain, these etiologies will also influence the individual's response to pain.

The role of endogenous opioids in people's responses to pain has only recently been explored. The major types of these morphine-like peptides are endorphins and enkephalins,[13] and both have opiate agonist properties. Like morphine, they can bind to opiate receptors in the periacqueductal gray areas of the brain. These substances may influence the amount of pain relief an individual receives from an analgesic and thus may help to account for the various differences individuals exhibit in response to narcotic therapy.[15] Additionally, endorphins are neurotransmitters at many synaptic relay points in the pain pathway. Because of this fact, they appear to influence transmission of pain impulses at multiple levels of the nervous system,[15] thus modulating perception of and response to pain.

A variety of other factors may be involved in an individual's reaction to pain and are being arbitrarily placed within the physiologic component by the author. Fatigue, lack of sleep, and insomnia may increase sensitivity to pain.[55] Adequate rest and sleep, on the other hand, may help an individual cope with pain more easily, even if the pain has the same severity.[55] Obviously, these factors may affect the sensory, affective, cognitive, and behavioral components as well.

Sensory Component

The sensory component of pain is related to where pain is located and how it feels. The location of pain will affect an individual's physical and emotional response to pain. A single site of pain that is not aggravated by physical movement may be easier for a patient to bear than multiple sites of pain that are affected by movement. Likewise, a single site of pain may not cause the same degree of anxiety or depression that multiple sites might. There is evidence that many patients with advanced cancer have more than one site of pain, which clearly could affect their responses to pain.[54]

The perceived intensity of pain, or how strong it feels, is a second aspect of the sensory component. Intensity is the most commonly assessed parameter of pain, and a number of methods exist for such assessment.[16,53] Intensity is an extremely subjective phenomenon that may be affected by individual pain threshold (the least stimulus intensity at which a person perceives pain), which in turn is influenced by a number of factors such as mood, physical comfort, social environment, and medications.[55] These factors can be put into the general multidimensional framework of pain and will affect not only response to intensity of pain, but sensitivity to pain in general (Table 1-2). The intensity of an individual's pain, however, will have a direct effect on perception and response. For example, higher intensity undoubtedly stimulates increased perception and response.

Another major aspect of the sensory component of pain is how the pain actually feels, or its quality. The McGill Pain Questionnaire (MPQ)[37] has been extremely useful in helping patients describe exactly how their pain feels by selecting specific adjectives from lists of sensory words on the MPQ. For example, one person might choose sharp, stabbing, and cutting, while another selects dull, heavy, and tender. Investigators have accumulated conflicting evidence about whether pain due to different disease processes (e.g., arthritis, cancer) can be characterized by different sets of adjectives on the MPQ.[17,37,45]

Several investigators reported that patients with cancer-related pain chose specific words to describe their pain.[12,17,22,33] Sensory words selected from the MPQ by 30 percent or more of cancer patients in one study were stabbing, heavy, shooting, and tender[33]; and in two others were shooting, sharp, gnawing, and burning.[17,22] In a fourth study, where cancer patients with pain were asked to volunteer descriptive adjectives, the words most often given were grouped into aching/sore/tender (40 percent) and sharp/knifelike (33 percent) sensations.[12] It is clear that shooting, sharp, and tender are consistently used to describe cancer-related pain. The overall

Table 1-2
Multidimensional Factors Affecting Pain Threshold and Pain Sensitivity in Individuals with Cancer-related Pain

Lowered threshold/more sensitivity		Elevated threshold/less sensitivity	
Factor	Dimension	Factor	Dimension
Insomnia/fatigue Discomfort	Physiologic Sensory	Sleep/rest Relief of symptoms	Physiologic, sensory
Anger Anxiety	Affective	Reduction in anxiety/ elevation of mood	Affective
Depression Fear Introversion Sadness		Diversional activities	Cognitive, behavioral
Boredom Mental isolation	Cognitive, behavioral	Medications (analgesics, anxiolytics, antidepressants)	Physiologic, affective, behavioral
Social abandonment	Sociocultural	Companionship/sympathy/ understanding	Sociocultural

Adapted from Ahles TA, Blanchard EB, Ruckdeschel JC: The Multidimensional nature of cancer-related pain. Pain 7:277–288, 1983, and from Twycross RG, Lack SA: Symptom Control in Far Advanced Cancer: Pain Relief. London, Pitman, 1983.

impact that these sensations, and others described by fewer patients, have on an individual's response to pain is unclear as yet, but it is likely that sensations influence sensitivity to pain and responses to it. An individual who describes pain as heavy and tender may be less uncomfortable and therefore less anxious and/or depressed than an individual who describes pain as sharp, stabbing, and knifelike.

In summary, the sensory component of pain includes location, intensity, and quality. All three of these parameters interact within each individual to influence the individual's perception of and response to pain. The nature of such interactions remains to be elucidated, particularly in relation to the other major components of the pain experience.

Affective Component

The affective component of the pain experience consists of anxiety, depression, and many other psychological reactions to pain. This component of pain has received the most attention from researchers. A fairly large body of literature exists that addresses the relationships between a variety of psychological factors (depression, hypochondriasis, neuroticism, perceptual style, etc.) of individuals and their responses to pain. A review of these studies is beyond the scope of this chapter, but can be found elsewhere.[35]

A number of researchers, however, have investigated various psychological aspects of the cancer pain experience (Table 1-3). Differences in samples, instruments, and procedures make direct comparisons impossible, but results can be examined with respect to the general psychological constructs studied.

In general, cancer patients both with and without pain appear to have higher neuroticism (N) scores and lower extroversion (E) scores on the Eysenck Personality Inventory than normal populations,[8,9,25] although in one study N scores were lower and E scores were equivalent.[21] Jacox and Stewart[25] found that higher N and E scores were negatively correlated with pain intensity. Lower E scores (i.e., more introversion) were correlated with higher pain intensity. Bond[8] observed that N scores were positively correlated with pain intensity. Additionally, he found that N scores became lower and E scores became higher after patients with severe pain were treated with cervical percutaneous cordotomy. Higher N and E scores have also been found to correlate with greater use of analgesic medication.[9]

Hypochondriasis is another personality characteristic apparently associated with cancer pain,[7,36,58] although Bond[7] was the only researcher who used an instrument designed specifically to measure hypochondriasis. Increased somatization and hostility scores on the Symptom Checklist-90 have also been related to cancer pain.[1]

Depression in patients with cancer-related pain has been studied by several investigators,[1,7,27,36,58] with higher levels of depression in samples of

Table 1-3 (*continued*)
Studies of Psychological Aspects of Cancer-related Pain

Authors/Sample	Instruments	Major Results
Bond & Pearson.[9] 52 cervical cancer pts (39 with pain, 13 without); 24 hospitalized pts without pain	Eysenck Personality Inventory (EPI)	All cancer pts had higher Neuroticism(N)/lower Extroversion(E) scores than controls; both correlated with medication use; cancer pts with pain had higher N scores than pain-free cancer pts
Woodforde & Fielding.[58] 54 cancer pts referred to pain clinic; 55 cancer pts not referred to pain clinic	Cornell Medical Index (CMI)	Referred pts had higher CMI total score and higher depression and hypochondriasis scores than unreferred; no correlation between CMI total score and response to treatment in referred pts
Bond.[7] 39 cervical cancer pts with pain; 13 cervical cancer pts without pain	CMI; Whiteley Index of Hypochondriasis	Pts with pain scored higher on both
Bond.[8] 30 cancer pts with severe pain	EPI	N scores increased prior to percutaneous cervical cordotomy and decreased after; E scores decreased before and increased after; pts with higher N scores before also had increased pain level
Jacox & Stewart.[25] 31 pts with acute postoperative pain; 31 pts with chronic rheumatoid arthritis pain; 40 pts with progressive cancer pain	EPI; Health Self-Concept (HSC)	All groups had increased N compared to normals and all had decreased HSC; in cancer pts N had a negative correlation with pain intensity, E had a negative correlation with assessment of problems, N had a negative correlation with E, E had a negative correlation with pain intensity

(*continued*)

Table 1-3 *(continued)*

Authors/Sample	Instruments	Major Results
Fotopoulos et al.[21] 17 advanced cancer pts with pain	Ego-Strength Scale (ESS); EPI; Repression– Sensitization Scale (RSS); Rotter Locus-of- Control (LOC)	When compared to normals and/or hospitalized tuberculosis pts, cancer pts had lower ESS, lower N scores, more internal LOC than external (males only), and no differences on E scores or RSS
McKegney et al.[36] 101 cancer pts with prognosis of 3–12 mos, divided into high–low CMI and high–low LOC	CMI; Rotter LOC	240 days before death no differences between groups; 60 days before death high CMI had more pain; 180–60 days before death high LOC had more pain
Ahles et al.[1] 40 cancer pts with pain; 37 cancer pts without	Beck Depression Inventory(BDI); Spielberger State-Trait Anxiety Scale (STAI); Symptom Checklist- 90(SCL-90) Visual Analogue Scales-anxiety and depression (VASA/ VASD)	Pain pts elevated on BDI; no differences on STAI; pain pts elevated on SCL-90 depression, somatization, and hostility scales; pain pts elevated on VASA and VASD
Spiegel & Bloom.[48,49] 86 breast cancer pts (48 with pain, 38 without)	Profile of Mood States (POMS)	Scores on POMS scales and total mood disturbance(TMD) not given; TMD had a positive correlation with increased pain, as did the scales for depression, anxiety, and fatigue
Lansky et al.[27] 505 female cancer pts	Hamilton Rating Scale for Depression(HRSD); Zung Self-rating Depression Scale(SDS)	Women with elevated HRSD and SDS scores (n = 27) reported more pain than nondepressed women (n = 478)

Adapted from McGuire DB: Cancer-related Pain: A Multidimensional Approach. Unpublished
doctoral dissertation, University of Illnois at Chicago, 1987.

such patients found by all of them. Anxiety has been less well-studied. Only Ahles et al.[1,2] have attempted to measure anxiety in cancer patients with pain; they found no differences in anxiety between such individuals and pain-free cancer patients.

Spiegel and Bloom[48,49] assessed the mood states of cancer patients using the Profile of Mood States (POMS). Although they did not give actual scores on any of the separate mood states measured by the POMS, they reported that breast cancer patients with pain had elevated scores on anxiety, depression, and fatigue scales, as well as elevated total mood disturbance (TMD) scores. They also found elevated TMD scores to be positively correlated with increased pain intensity.

Locus of control is a construct that has been explored by two groups of investigators. Male cancer patients with severe pain had more internal expectations of control than normative samples.[21] In a sample of 55 terminal cancer patients, McKegney et al.[36] reported that 34 had high internal–external (I–E) scores, and 21 had low I–E scores. Although the two groups had no demographic or disease differences, when they were followed over time the high I–E scoring group had higher mean pain scores from 180 to 60 days prior to death.

Several other psychological variables have been studied in cancer patients with pain. Jacox and Stewart[25] found that such patients had a decreased health self-concept. Fotopoulos et al.[21] observed that advanced cancer patients with severe pain had significantly lower ego strength scores than either normative samples or hospitalized tuberculosis patients. Additionally, the same patients did not differ from normals in repression-sensitization.

All of these studies clearly indicate that many psychological factors are involved in the cancer pain experience. An unresolved issue in the affective dimension of pain is related to whether affective disturbances play a causal role in the perception of and response to cancer-related pain. A distinction must be made between individuals with major affective disorders versus those who simply have elevated scores on standard psychological measures that may be due to situational factors such as diagnosis of cancer and the presence of pain. It is not clear, for example, whether individuals who are already depressed are more likely to report higher levels of pain than those who are not depressed, or whether individuals with more pain are simply more depressed *because* of their pain. Clearly, the etiologic interdependencies among personality traits (neuroticism, hypochondriasis), psychological factors (depression, anxiety), and the perception of and response to pain are at best muddy and need further clarification. More important from the clinical standpoint is the careful identification of psychological variables in each individual's cancer pain experience that might be amenable to therapeutic interventions.

Cognitive Component

The cognitive component of the pain experience consists basically of the manner in which pain influences the individual's thought processes and/or the way in which he views himself.[1] Several researchers have addressed aspects of this component. Ahles and his colleagues[1] examined it in their study by assessing the meaning of pain to patients. Those with cancer-related pain were asked whether they believed its presence to be an indicator of progressive disease. Sixty-one percent of the patients reported that they were afraid pain indicated a deteriorating condition; these individuals had significantly elevated scores on standard measures of anxiety and depression as compared to patients with pain who had not considered the possibility of pain as an indicator of progressive disease. Spiegel and Bloom[48] also assessed the meaning of pain in their sample of patients with metastatic breast cancer. The belief that pain was indicative of worsening illness was significantly correlated with reports of more pain and also with more mood disturbance (more depression and anxiety). There are certainly other cognitive factors involved in responses to pain, but research is needed to identify them and assess their impact. As indicated in Table 1-2, such factors might include boredom, feelings of mental isolation from others, and diversional activities. Other factors not listed in Table 1-2 could include health self-concept or locus of control.

Behavioral Component

The behavioral component of pain is described by Ahles et al.[1] as consisting of behaviors related to pain, such as level of activity or intake of analgesics. Such behaviors may be related to the cognitive component of pain in that individuals' thought processes or interpretation of the meaning of their pain could influence their observable behaviors.

As with the cognitive component, little research exists on the behavioral component of cancer-related pain. Bond and Pilowsky[10] studied the relationships between advanced cancer patients' subjective assessments of pain, their communication of pain, and the reactions of nursing staff. Of the 71 percent of their sample who had pain, 28 percent did not communicate it to staff, and their self-reported pain scores were significantly lower than 53 percent who had pain and either reported it to staff or were offered drugs by the staff. Additionally, the researchers found a low correlation between pain intensity and the strength of administered analgesics. In another study, Pilowsky and Bond[46] found that patients who considered themselves as ''ill'' reported considerable pain and requested medication frequently.

Ahles et al.[1] found that patients in pain spent significantly less time walking or standing than those who were not in pain. Additionally, a majority (77 percent) of patients with cancer-related pain reported that significant others in their environment could tell when they were in pain because of facial expression, changes in mood, going to bed, or making verbal complaints of pain. Such specific and observable behaviors related to perception of and response to pain are beginning to receive more attention from researchers.[26,29]

Sociocultural Component

The sociocultural component of pain includes demographic characteristics (age, race, sex, religion), ethnic background, and other factors. There is a paucity of research examining the relationship between such factors and the experience of pain. The bulk of published studies, well-reviewed by Wolff and Langley,[57] are 20–40 years old, had very small samples, and often used experimentally induced pain in the laboratory setting. Racial, age, religious, and ethnic differences in pain threshold and tolerance were studied.

None of the studies allows definitive conclusions about the existence of differences in pain response because of age, ethnic, racial, or religious characteristics.[57] However, the evidence in many studies supports the strong role of culturally determined attitudinal factors in pain perception and response. Since the investigators used experimentally induced pain, it is not clear whether their general conclusions can be extrapolated to individuals with clinical pain, particularly those with cancer-related pain.

A few individuals have investigated relationships between ethnic and demographic variables and the interpretation of and response to pain. The most widely cited study is that of Zborowski,[59] who studied the pain reactions of four ethnic groups: Irish, Italian, Jewish, and Old American (White Anglo-Saxon Protestants). The generalizability of his findings is limited because of a small, nonrandom sample and other methodologic flaws. Zborowski's results can be summarized as follows: (1) Jews and Italians had low pain tolerance and exhibited emotional and uninhibited responses to pain; Jews, however, were more likely to complain to family and health workers than Italians. (2) Old Americans were nonexpressive about pain except when asked by health workers to describe it, and generally tended to be withdrawn. (3) Irish patients were reluctant to discuss their pain, and often withdrew from family and friends.

Zborowski's study unfortunately led to unfair stereotyping of ethnic groups with respect to pain reactions. More recently, however, Zborowski[60] described a continuum of expression and behavior within particular cultural groups, and emphasized the necessity of exploring the meaning of pain to each individual, regardless of ethnic origin.

Lipton and Marbach[31] conducted a study to examine interethnic differences and similarities in the reported pain experience of Black, Irish, Italian, Jewish, and Puerto Rican patients with facial pain. They found that all five ethnic groups were similar in their reported responses to pain; however, each group was very different with respect to the factors that influenced their responses to pain. The response of Italians, for example, was most influenced by the duration of pain, while for Jews and Puerto Ricans the level of psychological distress was most important. Lipton and Marbach concluded that the relationship between ethnicity and pain experience is very subtle, and may best be viewed as a continuum of behaviors, attitudes, and feelings that actually comprise the pain experience.

Demographic and ethnic differences have been studied in relation to the expression of pain. In two studies, females and older individuals had increased verbal expressions of pain.[43,52] Blacks used more moderate words than Whites in describing both the presence and intensity of pain.[43] Flannery et al.,[19] however, were unable to demonstrate any significant differences in pain expression in Black, Italian, Irish, Jewish, and White Anglo-Saxon Protestant patients. In one study of cancer inpatients,[33] females and nonwhites had significantly lower scores on the Pain Rating Index-Total of the McGill Pain Questionnaire than males or whites.

Very few reported studies have addressed the relationship between the factors discussed above and patients' perception of and response to cancer-related pain. Other factors in the sociocultural component of pain that may be related to individuals' perception and expression of, and response to pain are social support,[47] familial pain models,[18] and patterns of interpersonal communication.[16] Although it is clear that sociocultural variables affect the pain experience, their roles are unclear and require further investigation.

CONCLUSION AND IMPLICATIONS

The concept of the multidimensional nature of pain, based on the work of Ahles,[1] Beecher,[3,4] Melzack, Wall, Casey, and others[38–40] provides an extremely appropriate framework for the assessment, management, and study of cancer-related pain. Although pain has many individual components, it must be viewed as an interrelated and interactive whole. In writing about holistic nursing, Levine[30] urged that the "individual must be recognized in his wholeness, and the powerful influence of adaptation recognized as a dynamic and ever-present factor in evaluating his care" (p. 257). This notion can be extended to the assessment and management of the patient with cancer-related pain, yielding a sensitive and careful identification of the individual's responses to pain and his adaptive processes.

Clinical Practice

Although it is clear that pain is an extremely complicated phenomenon, its complexity should not deter clinicians from assessment and management. It may be tempting to throw one's hands up and claim powerlessness and inability to deal with such a convoluted and challenging problem. An example of this attitude occurs when the clinician is faced with a patient in severe pain whose projected lifespan is so short that interventions beyond the prescription of narcotics (and suboptimally at that) seem unwarranted and a waste of time. Indeed, this attitude may even be inappropriately extended to individuals with cancer-related pain who will live many months or even years before ultimately dying of their cancer.

The current advances in therapeutic and palliative technologies are producing a population of cancer patients who must live with their disease-related pain for extended (but unknown) periods of time. As a result, both cancer and cancer-related pain have become chronic processes requiring continuous and prolonged strategies for management. Recognition of this trend by all health professionals, with the subsequent development of plans of care that address the chronicity of the situation, will result in improved care and higher quality of life for patients with cancer-related pain.

The complexity of the experience of pain *can* be simplified in the clinical arena. Specific components or factors related to perception of and response to pain, as discussed previously, can be assessed in a brief and relevant fashion by clinicians. In this monograph, both Donovan[16] and Syrjala[53] discuss approaches that can be effectively used on a day-to-day basis in clinical practice. Additionally, specific components or factors related to perception of and response to pain can be managed by clinicians. A multidisciplinary, multimodal approach to managing pain, as described by several other authors in this monograph, is an efficient and logical means of dealing with cancer-related pain.

A major issue related to assessment and management of cancer pain is the fact that although the experience is comprised of multiple components, not all of them will be present in every individual with pain, nor will they all be relevant to individual health care workers. For example, a patient with minor cancer-related pain relieved by nonnarcotic analgesics may be reasonably comfortable, capable of functioning relatively normally, and thus pose little or no management problem for the primary health care worker. On the other hand, a patient with severe, intractable cancer-related pain that interferes with multiple aspects of daily life poses a challenge to the primary caretaker and requires the involvement of multiple health workers because of the complex care issues involved.

Management of such individuals requires a multidisciplinary approach, as no one health care professional possesses the skills and knowledge to provide truly comprehensive care. Each member of the health care team can make specific contributions, the nature of which should be prescribed based on educational and experiential qualifications, collaborative and cooperative clinical practice, individual patient preferences, and institutional organization and support. Thus, as challenging and overwhelming as the assessment and management of cancer-related pain may seem, it is a phenomenon for which clinicians can do something to improve the well-being of their patients.

Various facets of assessment and management, handled by various health care workers, can be conceptualized within the multidimensional model described by Ahles et al.[1] and expanded in this chapter. The *physiologic component* of pain can be addressed with therapeutic interventions such as radiotherapy, chemotherapy, analgesics, and surgical procedures that are aimed at the organic cause(s) of pain. The *sensory dimension* of pain can be modulated through the use of analgesics, surgical procedures, psychological approaches, and other treatment modalities. *Affective aspects* of the pain experience such as depression or anxiety may be alleviated by teaching the individual more about his pain and how to control it, by identifying and developing coping strategies, by providing individual or group therapy, or by simply reducing the amount of pain. The *cognitive component* of pain can be influenced by providing information and education about cancer, prognosis, treatment, pain, the "normal" course of events, expected sensations or experiences, and methods available to manage problems related to pain. A variety of interventions can be aimed at the *behavioral component* of pain, including careful planning and moderation of physical activity, development of an effective analgesic regimen, and construction of problem-solving strategies for the management of pain. Finally, the *sociocultural component* of pain may best be handled by a careful exploration and assessment of the factors that seem to influence each individual's response to pain, including ethnic background, demographic variables, and family and social support. The influence of these factors on the experience of pain and on the success of interventions for pain cannot be underestimated or ignored.

Research

The multidimensional nature of cancer-related pain has clear implications for research. The factors comprising the dimensions of pain need to be further delineated, and the interactions among them elucidated if possible. The complexity of the phenomenon of pain requires a creative approach for study, including the use of multivariate statistics.[35] Adequate assessment and measurement of cancer-related pain in the research and clinical arenas must encompass these multiple dimensions.[1,16,40,53] Additionally, the development and testing of therapeutic interventions must include the various components of the pain experience if the interventions are to be successful in alleviating pain.

In conclusion, the evolution of our understanding of the phenomenon of pain from Descartes' simple bell-ringing alarm system to a comprehensive, multidimensional, and holistic conceptualization has opened entirely new vistas in the assessment, management, and study of pain. As a result, our potential to successfully alleviate the suffering of individuals with cancer-related pain may be greater than ever before. Our task as health care providers is to accept and meet this challenge.

REFERENCES

1. Ahles TA, Blanchard EB, Ruckdeschel JC: The multidimensional nature of cancer-related pain. Pain 17:277–288, 1983
2. Ahles TA, Ruckdeschel JC, Blanchard EB: Cancer-related pain — II. Assessment with visual analogue scales. J Psychosom Res 28:121–124, 1984
3. Beecher HK: Pain in men wounded in battle. Ann Surg 123:96–105, 1946
4. Beecher HK: Relationship of significance of wound to the pain experienced. JAMA 161:1609–1613, 1956.
5. Beecher HK: Measurement of Subjective Response. Quantitative Effects of Drugs. New York, Oxford University Press, 1959
6. Benoliel JQ, Crowley DM: The Patient in Pain: New Concepts. Proceedings of the National Conference of Cancer Nurses. New York, American Cancer Society, 1973, pp 70–78
7. Bond MR: The relation of pain to the Eysenck Personality Inventory, Cornell Medical Index, and Whiteley Index of Hypochondriasis. Br J Psych 119:671–678, 1971
8. Bond MR: Personality studies in patients with pain secondary to organic disease. J Psychosom Res 17:257–263, 1973
9. Bond MR, Pearson IB: Psychological aspects of pain in women with advanced cancer of the cervix. J Psychosom Res 13:13–19, 1969
10. Bond MR, Pilowsky I: Subjective assessment of pain and its relationship to the administration of analgesics in patients with advanced cancer. J Psychosom Res 10:203–208, 1966
11. Bouckoms AJ: Recent developments in the classification of pain. Psychosomatics 26:637–642, 645, 1985
12. Bressler LR, Hange PA, McGuire DB: Characterization of the pain experience in cancer outpatients. Oncol Nurs Forum 13:51–55, 1986
13. Chapman CR: New directions in the understanding and management of pain. Soc Sci Med 19:1261–1277, 1984
14. Coyle N, Foley K: Prevalence and profile of pain syndromes in cancer patients, in McGuire DB, Yarbro CH (eds): Cancer Pain Management. Orlando, FL, Grune & Stratton, 1987, pp 21–46
15. Davis GC: Endorphins and pain. Psychiatr Clin North Am 6:473–487, 1983
16. Donovan MI: Clinical assessment of cancer pain, in McGuire DB, Yarbro CH (Eds): Cancer Pain Management. Orlando, FL, Grune & Stratton, 1987, pp 105–131
17. Dubuisson D, Melzack R: Classification of clinical pain descriptions by multiple group discriminant analysis. Exp Neurol 51:480–487, 1976
18. Edwards PW, Zeichner A, Kuczmierczyk AR, et al.: Familial pain models: The relationship between family history of pain and current pain experience. Pain 21:379–384, 1985
19. Flannery RB, Sos J, McGovern P: Ethnicity as a factor in the expression of pain. Psychosomatics 22:39–40, 1981
20. Foley KM: Pain syndromes in patients with cancer, in Bonica JJ, Ventafridda V (Eds): Advances in Pain Research and Therapy, Vol 2. New York, Raven Press, 1979, pp 59–75
21. Fotopoulos SS, Graham C, Cook MR: Psychophysiologic control of cancer pain, in Bonica JJ, Ventafridda V (Eds): Advances in Pain Research and Therapy, Vol 2. New York, Raven Press, 1979, pp 231–243
22. Graham C, Bond SS, Gerkovich MM, et al.: Use of the McGill Pain Questionnaire in the assessment of cancer pain: Replicability and consistency. Pain 8:377–387, 1980

23. Hardy JD, Wolff HG, Goodell H: Pain Sensations and Reactions. Baltimore, Williams & Wilkins, 1952
24. International Association for the Study of Pain: Pain terms: A current list with definitions and notes on usage. Pain 3:S216–S221, 1986
25. Jacox A, Stewart M: Psychosocial Contingencies of the Pain Experience. Iowa City, IA, University of Iowa Press, 1973
26. Keefe FJ, Brantley A, Manuel G, Crisson JE: Behavioral assessment of head and neck cancer pain. Pain 23:327–336, 1985
27. Lansky SB, List MA, Hermann CA, et al.: Absence of major depressive disorder in female cancer patients. J Clin Oncol 3:1553–1560, 1985
28. Lasagna L: The clinical measurement of pain. Ann NY Acad Sci 86:28–37, 1960
29. LeResche L, Dworkin SF: Facial expression accompanying pain. Soc Sci Med 19:1325–1330, 1984
30. Levine ME: Holistic nursing. Nurs Clin North Am 6:253–264, 1971
31. Lipton JA, Marbach JJ: Ethnicity and the pain experience. Soc Sci Med 19:1279–1298, 1984
32. Livingston WK: Pain Mechanisms: A Physiologic Interpretation of Causalgia and its Related States. New York, MacMillan, 1943
33. McGuire DB: Assessment of pain in cancer inpatients using the McGill Pain Questionnaire. Oncol Nurs Forum 11:32–37, 1984
34. McGuire DB: The perception and experience of pain. Semin Oncol Nurs 1:83–86, 1985
35. McGuire DB: Cancer-related Pain: A Multidimensional Approach. Unpublished doctoral dissertation, University of Illinois at Chicago, 1987
36. McKegney FP, Bailey LR, Yates JW: Prediction and management of pain in patients with advanced cancer. Gen Hosp Psychiatry 3:95–101, 1981
37. Melzack R: The McGill Pain Questionnaire: Major properties and scoring methods. Pain 1:277–299, 1975
38. Melzack R, Casey KL: Sensory, motivational, and central control determinants of pain: A new conceptual model, in Kenshalo D (Ed): The Skin Senses. Springfield, IL, Charles C. Thomas, 1968, pp 423–439
39. Melzack R, Wall PD: Pain mechanisms: A new theory. Science 150:971–979, 1965
40. Melzack R, Wall PD: The Challenge of Pain. New York, Basic Books, 1982
41. Merskey H: The nature of pain, in Smith WL, Merskey H, Gross SC (Eds): Pain: Meaning and Management. New York, SP Medical and Scientific Books, 1980, pp 71–74
42. Merskey H, Spear FG: Pain: Psychological and Psychiatric Aspects. London, Balliere, Tindall, and Cassell, 1967
43. Miller JF, Shuter R: Age, sex, race affect pain expression. Am J Nurs 84:981, 1984
44. Nathan PW: The Gate-Control Theory of Pain: A critical review. Brain 99:123–158, 1976
45. Nehemkis AM, Charter RA: Comparison of arthritis and cancer pain patients: Are distinct clinical syndromes definable using the McGill Pain Questionnaire? Percept Mot Skills 58:126, 1984
46. Pilowsky I, Bond MR: Pain and its management in malignant disease: Elucidation of staff–patient transactions. Psychosom Med 31:400–404, 1969
47. Revenson TA, Wollman CA, Felton BJ: Social supports as stress buffers for adult cancer patients. Psychosom Med 45:321–331, 1983
48. Spiegel D, Bloom J: Pain in metastatic breast cancer. Cancer 52:341–345, 1983
49. Spiegel D, Bloom JR: Group therapy and hypnosis reduce metastatic breast carcinoma pain. Psychosom Med 45:333–339, 1983
50. Sternbach RA: Pain: A Psychophysiological Analysis. New York, Academic Press, 1968
51. Sternbach RA: Pain Patients: Traits and Treatment. New York, Academic Press, 1974
52. Swanson DW, Maruta T: Patients complaining of extreme pain. Mayo Clin Proc 55:563–566, 1980

53. Syrjala KL: The measurement of pain, in McGuire DB, Yarbro CH (eds): Cancer Pain Management. Orlando, FL, Grune & Stratton, 1987, pp 133–150
54. Twycross RG, Fairfield S: Pain in far-advanced cancer. Pain 14:303–310, 1982
55. Twycross RG, Lack SA: Symptom Control in Far Advanced Cancer: Pain Relief. London, Pitman, 1983
56. Weisenberg M: Pain and pain control. Psychol Bull 84:1008–1044, 1977
57. Wolff BB, Langley L: Cultural factors and the response to pain: A review, in Weisenberg W (Ed): Pain: Clinical and Experimental Perspectives. St. Louis, MO, Mosby, pp 144–151
58. Woodforde JM, Fielding JR: Pain and cancer. J Psychosom Res 14:365–370, 1970
59. Zborowski M: Cultural components in responses to pain. J Soc Issues 8:16–30, 1952
60. Zborowski M: People in Pain. San Francisco, CA, Jossey-Bass, 1969

Nessa Coyle, M.S., R.N. and
Kathleen Foley, M.D.

2

Prevalence and Profile of Pain Syndromes in Cancer Patients

Fear of pain associated with cancer may play a major role in an individual's quality of life from time of diagnosis. National and international studies on the incidence, prevalence, and severity of cancer pain are lacking.

Bonica,[2] in an attempt to understand the magnitude of the problem, summarized the data from 32 reports on the prevalence of cancer-related pain. He then used the mean figures from these reports to estimate the total number of Americans with advanced disease who experienced pain in 1983. By extrapolation from the 1983 American Cancer Society mortality data, he estimated that of the 440,000 people who died from cancer in that year, 297,000 or 68 percent had significant pain requiring the use of narcotic analgesics. Of the remaining 1.51 million Americans with less advanced disease, 730,000 or 50 percent were estimated to have pain. Bonica then looked at the prevalence of pain world-wide using the same mean figures for advanced and intermediate cancer as were used for the American population, and extrapolating using World Health Organization cancer figures for 1983. These computations suggest that, worldwide, approximately 19 million cancer patients experience pain each year.

Lack of systematic data on the incidence, prevalence, and severity of cancer pain reflects the traditional lack of importance attached to the pain experience. The interpretation of existing data is difficult. Methods of measuring pain vary, as do the means of data collection. Different types of cancer are frequently grouped together. Primary tumors may be identified but the nature and site of the pain not specified. Sometimes the extent of disease is documented, at other times not. Much of the information collected on cancer-related pain comes from major medical or cancer research centers. The extent of the problem for patients being cared for at home or in small community hospitals is not known. Some surveys suggest the problem may be even greater. Foley and Sundaresan[13] summarized available epidemiological data on cancer pain from a variety of medical settings in different countries. Patient population, stage of disease, medical care setting, and survey method were all included (Table 2-1). The highest prevalence of pain was in Cartwright et al.'s[3] study, where reports of surviving spouses were used to determine prevalence. This finding raises the question of a component of suffering experienced not only by the patient, but by family or friends, and how this may be expressed in the language of pain.

In considering cancer-related pain, not only is consistency of measurement a problem, but also that not all pain is directly related to tumor involvement. The pain may be associated with cancer treatment, with the immobilization so frequently seen with advanced disease, or with other chronic disease processes unrelated to cancer; for example, rheumatoid arthritis or osteoarthritis. In an attempt to sort out this lack of specificity, Foley[10] classified cancer pain according to a series of common pain syndromes and their pathophysiology. One category of pain syndromes is that associated with cancer therapy. This group accounted for 19 percent of pain problems in an inpatient population and for 25 percent among outpatients. Pain occurring as a result of surgery, chemotherapy, or radiation therapy was included. Another category of pain syndromes involves those unrelated to cancer or its treatment. In inpatients, 3 percent of pain problems fell within this category, while the number increased to 10 percent when outpatients were surveyed.

Pain Related to Cancer

Pain associated with direct tumor involvement accounted for 78 percent of the pain problems found in a survey of inpatients at Memorial Sloan-Kettering Cancer Center.[10] In an outpatient survey by Daut and Cleeland,[9] tumor-associated pain accounted for 62 percent of problems. The most common causes of pain from direct tumor involvement were metastatic bone disease, nerve compression or infiltration, and hollow viscus involvement. In Foley's survey,[10] where analgesic requirement was taken as the measure of pain, site of disease was found to be important. Eighty-five percent of patients with primary bone tumors, 52 percent of patients with breast disease, and 45 percent of patients with lung cancer had significant pain. Patients with genitourinary cancer also had a high prevalence of pain, varying from 70 to 75 percent, as did those with oral cavity cancer where the prevalence was 80 percent. Certain cancers were found to be associated with

Table 2-1
Epidemiology of Cancer Pain

Author	Patient population	Stage of Disease	Medical Care System	Survey Method	Prevalence of Pain (%)
Cartwright et al.[3]	215 adults	Far advanced cancer	Inpatients & outpatients, England	Reports of surviving spouses	87
Foley[10]	156 adults and children	Early & advanced cancer	Cancer hospital, USA	Chart review of analgesic use	29
Foley[10]	397 adults				
	358	Early & advanced cancer	Cancer hospital, USA	Patient interview	38
	39	Far advanced cancer	Cancer hospital, USA	Patient interview	60
Haram[20]	607 adults	Far advanced cancer	Hospice, England	Patient interview	66
Molinari[31]		Far advanced head & neck cancer	NCI, Milan, Italy	Patient interview	50
Norton & Lack[33]	100 adults	Far advanced cancer	Hospice, USA	Patient interview	75
Pannuti et al.[37]	284 adults	Far advanced cancer	Oncology service, Italy	Patient interview & follow-up	64
Rubin et al.[45]	53 children	All stages	Inpatient cancer hospital, USA	Patient interview	47
Trotter et al.[50]	237 adults	Far advanced cancer	Outpatient oncology service, England	Patient interview	72
Twycross[51]	500 adults	Far advanced cancer	Hospice, England	Analgesic use	80
Wilkes[53]	300 adults	Far advanced cancer	Hospice, England	Patient interview	58

Adapted from Foley KM, Sundaresan N: Management of cancer pain, in DeVita VT, Hellman S, Rosenberg SA (Eds): Cancer Principles and Practice of Oncology, Vol. 2 (2nd ed). Philadelphia, J. B. Lippincott Company, 1985, p 1941.

less pain—lymphomas, 20 percent, and leukemias, 5 percent.[10] In a second study by Foley,[10] stage of disease was examined as a variable in the prevalence of cancer pain. Patients were asked directly about their pain. Although, overall, 38 percent of the patients reported significant pain, the prevalence increased to 60 percent in patients identified as having end-stage disease, thus revealing that stage of disease was an important variable in the prevalence of pain.

Daut and Cleeland[9] surveyed a group of 667 inpatients and outpatients at a comprehensive cancer center in order to estimate the prevalence and severity of pain in this population. Only patients with breast, prostate, colorectal, and three gynecologic cancers were included in the sample. Patients with metastatic disease were found more likely to report pain than those without it, except for those patients with cervical cancer. Site of disease, as reflected in other surveys, was also found to be important. Patients with breast and prostate cancer reported more pain than those with cervical or uterine disease. Chart reviews were used to classify the pain as cancer-related, treatment-related, or related to neither the disease or its treatment. Six percent of patients with nonmetastatic disease and 33 percent of patients with metastatic disease were found to have pain associated with their disease.

Multiple Sites of Pain in an Individual Patient

Another problem with pain in the advanced cancer patient is that there are often multiple sites of pain. Twycross and Fairfield[52] examined the different sites of pain experienced by the cancer patient. One hundred patients were interviewed within a few days of admission to a special care unit for patients with advanced disease. Each anatomically distinct pain was recorded, and classified within four possible categories: (1) pain caused by the cancer itself; (2) pain related to the treatment; (3) pain associated with the cancer but not directly caused by it, for example, pain associated with chronic disease and debility, or postherpetic neuralgia; and (4) pain unrelated to the cancer or its treatment (Table 2-2). Eighty patients (80%) were found to have more than one pain, with 34 (34%) with four or more different pains. Ninety-one patients (91%) had pain caused by the cancer itself; bone involvement and nerve compression were found to be the most common causes of this pain. Twelve patients had treatment-related pain, and 19 patients had pain associated with chronic disease. Thirty-nine patients (39%) had pain unrelated to cancer or its treatment; myofacial pain was the most frequently identified cause. In only 41 patients (41%) was all the pain caused by the disease alone.

The results of this survey are extremely useful, as they indicate the importance of identifying each source of pain so that appropriate management can be employed by physicians and nurses.

Table 2-2
Causes of Pain in 100 Cancer Patients

	Number of Pains		
	Male	Female	Total
Caused by Cancer (67%)			
Bone	30 (16)	28 (15)	58 (31)
Nerve compression	24 (16)	32 (15)	56 (31)
Soft tissue infiltration	21 (19)	14 (12)	35 (31)
Visceral involvement	15 (15)	18 (16)	33 (31)
Muscle spasm	9 (7)	5 (4)	14 (11)
Lymphedema	—	4 (3)	4 (3)
Raised intracranial pressure	—	2 (2)	2 (2)
Myopathy	—	2 (1)	2 (1)
	99 (42)	105 (49)	204 (91)
Related to treatment (5%)			
Postoperative	1 (1)	7 (6)	8 (7)
Colostomy	1 (1)	1 (1)	2 (2)
Nerve block	—	2 (1)	2 (1)
Postoperative adhesions	1 (1)	—	1 (1)
Post-radiation fibrosis	—	1 (1)	1 (1)
Esophageal	—	1 (1)	1 (1)
	3 (3)	12 (9)	15 (12)
Associated pains (6%)			
Constipation	6 (6)	5 (5)	11 (11)
Capsulitis of shoulder	1 (1)	3 (3)	4 (4)
Bedsore	—	1 (1)	1 (1)
Post-herpetic neuralgia	—	1 (1)	1 (1)
Pulmonary embolus	1 (1)	—	1 (1)
Penile spasm (catheter)	1 (1)	—	1 (1)
	9 (9)	10 (10)	19 (19)
Unrelated pains (22%)			
Musculoskeletal	19 (10)	24 (17)	43 (27)
Osteoarthritis	2 (1)	2 (2)	4 (3)
Migraine	1 (1)	1 (1)	2 (2)
Miscellaneous	6 (5)	10 (8)	16 (13)
	28 (15)	37 (24)	65 (39)
Total:	138	165	303 100

Figures in parentheses indicate number of patients in this category, as distinct from number of pains.
Adapted from Twycross RG, Fairfield S: Pain in far-advanced cancer. Pain 14:303–310, 1982.

Pain in the Patient who Dies of Cancer versus
Death from Other Causes

In response to the question of whether terminally ill cancer patients experience more pain than patients dying from other causes, Osler et al.[35] addressed the question by examining the narcotic requirements and nurses' records of 90 terminally ill patients, approximately half of whom had cancer. Patients dying of cancer were found to have a significantly higher prevalence of pain than those dying from other diseases, 72 percent versus 45 percent. Daut and Cleeland,[9] when comparing the mean pain severity ratings of patients with metastatic cancer and those with rheumatoid arthritis who were not terminal, found them to be similar. A comparison group of patients with chronic orthopedic pain had a higher mean pain severity rating than both the rheumatoid arthritis and metastatic cancer groups. From this study, the severity of the pain experienced by patients with terminal pain is unclear, although the prevalence is high.

In summary, pain is a significant factor in some but not all patients with cancer. The type of cancer, site(s) of disease, and stage of disease are all important variables in the incidence and prevalence of pain. Furthermore, patients with cancer can have pain unrelated to either the disease or its treatment. The wide variety of study methodologies used to examine the incidence and prevalence of cancer pain underline the need for consistency in approach to, and measurement of, pain.

Definition of Pain

In order for pain to be effectively managed, it is necessary for the clinician to have an understanding of the different types of pain, the profile of patients with pain, and the common pain syndromes seen in the cancer population.

Pain is defined by the International Association for the Study of Pain as "an unpleasant sensory and emotional experience associated with actual or potential tissue damage or described in terms of such damage (p. 249)."[21] Pain is described in subjective terms and may be either acute or chronic. The signs of acute pain frequently parallel those of anxiety, with hyperactivity of the autonomic nervous system. There is a well-defined pattern of onset, evidence of tissue damage, and resolution of pain with restoration of normal tissue function. Suffering is not usually a major component in this situation. In chronic pain (i.e., pain persisting for six months or longer), the autonomic system adapts, and the objective signs seen in acute pain (hyperactivity of the central nervous system) are no longer present. The signs of chronic pain frequently parallel those of depression and the patient's report of pain is the only measure of its existence.

PROFILE OF PATIENTS WITH CANCER PAIN

Patients with cancer pain can be subdivided into five groups as shown in Table 2-3.[14] The first group encompasses those patients with acute cancer-related pain. It can be further subdivided into those patients with tumor-associated pain and those patients whose pain is associated with cancer therapy. Patients with acute tumor-related pain may have first sought medical attention because of a complaint of pain. That is, pain was the harbinger of their cancer. For this group of patients, future pain episodes immediately imply recurrence of cancer. Defining the etiology of the pain and treating the cause, for example, radiation therapy to bony metastasis, is usually associated with dramatic relief. Adequate pain management for this group of patients is usually the rule, although uncertainty and fear color any recurrent pain symptoms, even if they have been cured of their disease.

Those patients whose acute pain is associated with cancer therapy (e.g., postoperative pain or pain secondary to mouth ulcerations from chemotherapy) do not have the same uncertainty and fear. The cause of the pain is known, the potential for pain associated with the treatment modality may have been discussed with them, and the duration of the pain is limited. These patients will frequently withstand a considerable amount of discomfort and pain, and some may view the pain as a necessary part of getting well. At times they will endure significant pain for the chance of a cure.

The second group includes patients with chronic cancer-related pain, that is, pain persisting for six months or longer. As with the acute pain group, these patients can be further subdivided into those with chronic pain from tumor progression and those with chronic pain related to cancer

Table 2-3
Types of Patients with Pain from Cancer

A. Acute cancer-related pain
   1. Associated with the diagnosis of cancer
   2. Associated with cancer therapy
B. Chronic cancer-related pain
   1. Associated with tumor progression
   2. Associated with cancer therapy
C. Pre-existing chronic pain and cancer-related pain
D. A history of drug addiction and cancer-related pain
   1. Actively involved in illicit drug use
   2. In methadone maintenance program
   3. With history of past drug abuse
E. Dying patients with cancer-related pain

Adapted from Foley KM, Sundaresan N: Management of cancer pain, in DeVita VT, Hellman S, Rosenberg SA (Eds): Cancer Principles and Practice of Oncology, Vol. 2 (2nd ed). Philadelphia, J. B. Lippincott Company, 1985, p 1941.

treatment. In patients with chronic pain associated with tumor progression, the escalating pain is associated with tumor infiltration of pain-sensitive structures such as bone, nerve, or soft tissue. Suffering plays a major role in the "total pain" these patients experience. Anxiety, depression, anger, and a sense of helplessness and despair surface as the patients' pain becomes a constant reminder of both the presence of cancer and the immediacy of death. Physiologic and psychologic fatigue occur in the patients and their families. These factors must be addressed if therapy is to be adequately managed. An interdisciplinary and multimodal approach is necessary, using such measures as antitumor therapy, analgesics, anesthetic blocks, and behavioral and psychological approaches.

Cancer treatment may also be associated with chronic pain (e.g., postmastectomy, postthoracotomy, and phantom limb pain). The cause of the pain is secondary to nerve injury and the development of a traumatic neuroma. Because of the difficulty in removing the cause of the pain, treatment is often directed toward the pain itself. It is of prime importance that the etiology of the pain is identified to the patient and family as being unrelated to the tumor, since this has major implications for the patient's psychological state. Methods of treatment concentrate on alternative methods of therapy rather than analgesics, with an emphasis on maintaining or improving the patient's functional level. As patients with cancer are living longer, the incidence of treatment-related pain is increasing. The pain is a constant reminder of the diagnosis of cancer, and may influence the patient's psychological state.

The third group includes patients with a history of chronic pain, from any cause, who develop cancer and pain. These patients and their families may already have a compromised psychologic and functional state because of their chronic pain. With the added stress of cancer and pain of a different significance, they are at high risk for further psychologic and functional deterioration. Early identification of this group of patients enables appropriate support mechanisms to be implemented.[7]

The fourth group includes patients with a history of drug abuse who develop cancer-related pain. Within this group are patients who are actively using street drugs, patients who are in methadone maintenance programs, and patients who have not used drugs for many years. These patients are most vulnerable for having their pain poorly managed. The first subgroup strain the resources of the most sophisticated pain management team, and tight controls on the way their analgesics are dispensed, especially when discharged home, are required. The second and third subgroups do not present a management problem. However, it must also be recognized that these patients are at risk for recidivism because of the high stress associated with cancer and pain is necessary. It must also be recognized that patients who are in methadone maintenance programs are tolerant to narcotics because of previous narcotic use. A larger amount of the drug than is normally anticipated may be required to control their pain. Multidisciplinary staff conferences are essential at a unit level so that the nurses and physicians understand the multiple factors involved in the care for these patients and have an opportunity to explore their own attitudes and concerns. Unless this is done, these patients may be discriminated against, both consciously and unconsciously, and their pain may be poorly managed.

Patients with cancer and pain who are dying are included in the fifth group. Treatment for these patients is no longer directed toward the disease; rather, comfort is the primary goal. Pain, unless well-controlled, interferes with the patients' and families' ability to communicate, to be with each other, and to come to terms with present and future losses and the pending separation. At no time is pain more destructive than as the patient draws closer to death. The family and care givers harbor enormous guilt and anger that not only must this person whom they love and care about die, but also die in pain. Feelings of vulnerability and impotence frequently surface. Rapid escalation of analgesic therapy may be necessary for these patients, as well as the provision of consistent and competent support for the patient and family in dealing with issues surrounding the dying process.

The different profiles of patients with cancer pain illustrate the necessity of understanding the psychological needs of the patient and family, as well as the temporal factors, in order to assess the pain and manage it appropriately.[7]

COMMON PAIN SYNDROMES

Cancer pain has also been classified according to a series of common pain syndromes. Because knowledge of the etiology of the pain mandates its treatment, each pain needs to be carefully delineated. The pattern of pain is frequently characteristic of a specific pain syndrome. Pain may result from tumor infiltration of pain-sensitive structures, or from injury to nerves, bone, and soft tissue as a result of chemotherapy, radiation therapy, or surgery.[14] There are three major types of cancer pain, somatic or nociceptive pain, visceral pain, and deafferentation pain.[38]

Somatic pain occurs as a result of activation of nociceptors in cutaneous and deep tissues without disruption of neuronal pathways. The pain may be acute or chronic, is usually constant and well localized, and is described as aching and gnawing. Tumor metastatic to the bone is an example of this type of pain. It is the most common type of pain experienced by the cancer patient.

Visceral pain results from stretching or distention of the thoracic or abdominal viscera, usually as a result of primary or metastatic tumors (e.g., pancreatic cancer or liver metastasis). This type of pain is usually poorly localized, often described as "deep," "squeezing," and "pressure," and may be associated with nausea, vomiting, and diaphoresis, especially when acute. Often visceral pain is referred to cutaneous sites that may be remote from the site of the lesion (e.g., shoulder pain from diaphragmatic irritation), and may be associated with tenderness in the referred cutaneous site).

Deafferentation pain results from injury to the peripheral and/or central nervous systems as a result of tumor compression or infiltration of peripheral nerve or the spinal cord, or injury to the peripheral nerve as a result of surgery or chemotherapy.[14] Examples of deafferentation pain include pain from brachial or lumbosacral plexopathies, and postsurgical pain syndromes.[14,48] Pain resulting from the neural injury is often severe, and is typically described as a constant dull ache, with superimposed paroxysms of burning and/or electric shock-like sensations. These paroxysms involve spontaneous and ectopic firing of damaged peripheral nerve structures.[8] Peripheral nerve injury also induces "epileptiform" activity in the medial thalamus, in the area of projection of the paleospinothalamic tract.[1]

Because specific pain syndromes in cancer patients can be associated with direct tumor involvement, as described in Table 2-4, or with cancer treatment, as described in Table 2-5, a differential diagnosis must be made to establish whether the syndrome is disease-related or treatment-related. The etiology of the pain guides its subsequent management. With this in mind, characteristic features of the more commonly seen disease-related and treatment-related pain syndromes are reviewed below.

Pain Associated with Direct Tumor Involvement

Pain associated with direct tumor involvement includes a variety of syndromes caused by tumor infiltration of the bone, peripheral nerves, and spinal cord. Bone metastasis, brachial plexopathy, lumbosacral plexopathy, and epidural cord compression are frequently associated with significant pain and are discussed in turn. The effect of tumor infiltration of the hollow viscus is also reviewed.

Bone Metastasis

Bone metastasis represents the most common cause of pain in patients with cancer.[10] The lesions are most frequently seen in certain parts of the skeleton: the vertebral bodies of the spine, the skull, and the pelvis, ribs, and the proximal ends of long bones, especially the femur and humerus. Bone lesions may be primarily osteolytic (as with all cancers), or osteoblastic (seen most frequently in cancer of the breast or prostate).[32] Elements of both processes may be found in the same lesion.

The metastatic process in bony tumors is associated with active bone destruction (osteolytic), and the formation of new bone (osteoblastic).[12] Most bony metastases arise from within the bone marrow and spread to contiguous bone.[32] Although the underlying neurophysiologic and neuro-

Table 2-4
Pain Associated with Direct Tumor Involvement

Direct Tumor Involvement	Signs and Symptoms
I. Tumor infiltration of bone a. Base of skull syndrome[19]	Pain may precede neurologic signs and symptoms by weeks or months.
1. Jugular foramen metastases	Occipital pain, referred to vertex of head. Pain exacerbated by movement. Tenderness over the occipital condyle. Depending on nerves involved, may include hoarseness, dysarthria, dysphagia, neck and shoulder weakness, ptosis.
2. Clivus metastases	Vertex headache exacerbated by neck flexion. Lower cranial nerve dysfunction begins unilaterally, progresses to bilateral dysfunction.
3. Sphenoid sinus	Severe bifrontal headache (radiates to both temples). Intermittent retroorbital pain. Nasal stuffiness, fullness in head.
b. Vertebral body syndromes	Pain is an early symptom.
1. Odontoid process[19] C1 involvement may result in pathologic fracture, subluxation, and spinal cord or brain stem compression.	Severe neck pain radiating over posterior aspect of the skull and vertex. Pain exacerbated by flexion. Progressive sensory and motor signs begin in upper extremities. Pain localized to adjacent paraspinal area.

(continued)

Table 2-4 (*continued*)
Pain Associated with Direct Tumor Involvement

Direct Tumor Involvement	Signs and Symptoms
2. C7-T1[4,26,29] Tumor spread may be hematogenous, or along nerves from tumor originating in brachial plexus or paravertebral space to contiguous vertebral body and epidural space.	Constant dull ache, radiating to both shoulders. Tenderness on percussion over spinous process at this level. Radicular pain, usually unilateral in posterior arm, elbow, and ulnar aspect of hand. Ptosis and miosis (Horner's syndrome).
3. L1[19]	Dull, aching, mid-back pain. Exacerbated by lying or sitting, relieved by standing. Pain-radiating, girdle-like band anteriorly or to both paraspinal, lumbosacral area. May be referred to sacroiliac joint and/or superior iliac crest.
c. Sacral syndrome[23] Most frequent in patients with gynecologic, genitourinary, or colon cancers.	Aching pain in low back or coccygeal area. Insidious onset. Exacerbated by lying/sitting, relieved by walking. Increasing pain with perianal sensory loss. Bowel, bladder dysfunction. Impotence.
II. Tumor infiltration of nerve[17,42]	
a. Epidural spinal cord compression. Neurologic symptoms vary with site of disease. Considered a medical emergency.	Severe neck and back pain is initial symptom in 96% of patients. Motor weakness-paraplegia. Sensory loss with level. Loss of bowel/bladder function.
b. Peripheral nerve proximal infiltration occurs from paravertebral or retroperitoneal tumor.	Constant burning pain. Hypoesthesia and dysesthesia in area of sensory loss, early symptom.

(*continued*)

Table 2-4 (*continued*)
Pain Associated with Direct Tumor Involvement

Direct Tumor Involvement	Signs and Symptoms
c. Plexus	
1. Brachial plexopathy[4,26,29] Associated with lung (Pancoast), breast and lymphoma.	Pain radiating to ipsilateral shoulder and posterior aspect of arm and elbow (C8-T1 distribution). Pain and paresthesias in 4th and 5th fingers, may precede objective clinical signs by weeks or months. Paresthesias progress to numbness, weakness, C7-T1 distribution.
2. Lumbar plexopathy[23] Result of extension of genitourinary, gynecologic and colon cancer.	Pain in L1-L3 distribution radiates to anterior portion of thigh or groin. Pain in L5-S1 distribution radiates down posterior aspect of leg to the heel. Paresthesias followed by numbness and dysesthesias. Progressive motor and sensory loss in plexus distribution.
3. Sacral plexopathy[23] Occurs most frequently in patients with colon, genitourinary and gynecologic cancers.	Pain dull, aching, midline. Sensory loss beginning in perianal area. Sensory findings are at first unilateral. Progression to bilateral sacral sensory loss and autonomic dysfunction. Impotence, bowel and bladder dysfunction. Patient unable to lie or sit down.
d. Root	
1. Leptomeningeal metastases.[34] Result of tumor infiltration of the leptomeninges with or without invasion of the parenchyma of the nervous system.	Pain occurs in 40% of patients. May be constant headache with or without stiff neck. May be localized low back and buttock pain.

Table 2-5
Pain Syndromes Associated with Cancer Therapy

Syndromes	Signs and Symptoms
1. Postsurgical syndromes	
a. Post-thoracotomy.[15,27,28] Caused by injury to intercostal nerves.	Constant pain in distribution of intercostal nerve. Occurs 1–2 months postsurgery. Pain, band-like in area of sensory loss. Occasional intermittent shock-like pains. Dysesthesias in the scar area with hyperesthesias in the surrounding area. Pain worse with movement. May develop frozen shoulder.
b. Postmastectomy.[15,18,28] Caused by interruption of intercosto-brachial nerve (T1-T2).	Pain in posterior aspect of arm, axilla, radiates to anterior part of chest wall. Pain starts 1–2 months after surgery. Pain tight and constricting. No associated lymphedema. Pain worse on movement. May result in frozen shoulder.
c. Radical neck dissection.[15] Caused by injury or interruption of cervical nerves.	Constant burning sensation in area of sensory loss. May be dysesthesias and intermittent shock-like pain (unpleasant tingling and stinging).
d. Phantom limb syndrome[15,46]	Two types: 1. Phantom pain identical in nature to preoperative pain. 2. Stump pain from traumatic neuroma.
2. Postchemotherapy syndromes[15,30,54] a. Peripheral neuropathy associated with symmetric polyneuropathy from vinca alkaloid treatment.	Painful dysesthesias. Localized to feet and hands. Pain increased by superficial stimuli. Resolves with reduction in chemotherapy.

(*continued*)

34

Table 2-5 (*continued*)
Pain Syndromes Associated with Cancer Therapy

Syndromes	Signs and Symptoms
b. Steroid pseudorheumatism[15,42,44] caused by steroid withdrawal.	Diffuse myalgias and arthralgias. Muscle and joint tenderness. No inflammatory signs. Generalized malaise and fatigue. Disappears if steroids resumed.
c. Aseptic necrosis[22] of the femoral head and less frequently of humeral head (complication of steroid therapy—more common in patients with Hodgkin's disease).	Shoulder or hip pain.
d. Postherpetic neuralgia[43] Herpes zoster infection occurs in areas of tumor or of RT—more common in patients who develop the infection after age 50.	Pain with three distinct components: either all three or only one may be present. Continuous burning in area of sensory loss. Intermittent and shock-like pain. Painful dysesthesias.
3. Postradiation syndromes[15,16,29] a. Radiation fibrosis of brachial and lumbar plexus (may occur 6 months to 20 years after RT).	Numbness or paresthesias of the hand. Lymphedema in arm. Radiation skin changes. Induration of supraclavicular and axillary areas. Motor weakness, deltoid and bicep muscles; C5, C6 distribution. Progression of signs leading to painful, swollen, useless arm.
b. Radiation myelopathy[24,36,47] (Pain early symptom in 15% of patients.)	Pain may be localized to area of spinal cord damage, or referred to distant site. Dysesthesias below level of cord lesion.
c. Radiation-induced secondary tumors[11] occurring 4–20 years after radiation.	Painful enlarging mass in previously irradiated area.

pharmacologic mechanism of bone pain is not clearly understood, the role of prostaglandins in the metastatic process is the current hypothesis for the origin of bone pain. From a clinical perspective, Foley[12] identified the occurrence of bone pain in two ways: by direct tumor involvement of the bone and activation of nociceptors locally; or, by compression of adjacent nerves, soft tissue, or vascular structures.

Pain may be the first complaint, as in patients with multiple myeloma, or it may represent the first sign of metastatic spread, as in patients with breast cancer, sometimes surfacing many years after the primary tumor has been treated. The pain may occur at the site of the lesion (e.g., rib pain), or may be referred to a distant area of the body (e.g., knee pain associated with metastatic hip disease). Pathologic fractures and hypercalcemia may occur. The initial approach to pain management in these patients is directed toward treatment of the primary tumor using radiation therapy, chemotherapy, or hormonal manipulation. Relief may be only transient or partial, however. Analgesics play a major role in the management of this frequently multifocal pain. Bony metastases are clearly an important cause of morbidity in the cancer patient and require aggressive treatment.

Nerve Compression or Infiltration

Nerve compression or infiltration by tumor may result in deafferentation pain. Deafferentation pain is associated with damage to the peripheral or central nervous system. A series of syndromes are associated with pain of this description.

Brachial plexopathy. This is a common example where metastatic infiltration by tumor or radiation fibrosis may be the cause. Less frequent etiologies of a brachial plexopathy in a cancer patient include acute brachial neuritis, trauma to the plexus during surgery, or a radiation-induced plexus tumor.

An accurate diagnosis of the etiology of the plexopathy is important, as it determines prognosis and treatment. There are certain clinical signs that help differentiate between metastatic plexopathy and radiation injury.[16] With tumor infiltration of the brachial plexus, the lower cord of the plexus is most commonly involved. This is seen most commonly in patients with carcinoma of the lung, and specifically, the Pancoast syndrome.

The Pancoast syndrome or pulmonary sulcus tumor, is an anatomical diagnosis, as both primary and metastatic tumors in the apex of the lung produce the characteristic symptoms. In a review of 30 patients diagnosed as having tumors of the superior sulcus at Memorial Sloan-Kettering Cancer Center between 1975 and 1979,[25] 28 had pain as the initial symptom. Typical of the pain is an aching sensation in the shoulder and paraspinal region, localized, in some patients, with painful paresthesias in the fourth and fifth fingers of the hand. In patients with Pancoast syndrome, brachial plexopathy is characterized by involvement of the lower plexus, with weakness in the distribution of the C8, T1 nerves and atrophy of the hand, usually with a Horner's syndrome. The pain initially results from compression and or infiltration of the plexus, and evolves to a form of deafferentation pain characterized by burning dysesthetic pain in the distribution of the nerve injury.

Tumor infiltration involving all levels of the brachial plexus can be seen in patients with breast cancer or other primary tumors. Pain is the most common presenting symptom. The distribution of the pain and accompanying neurologic findings depend on the site of tumor infiltration. For example, in patients with carcinoma of the breast, tumor infiltration can occur with the first symptom as pain in the shoulder, biceps area, elbow, or hand. Burning dysesthetic sensations in the index finger or thumb are common in patients who develop tumor in the supraclavicular region, while pain in the shoulder, elbow, and fourth and fifth fingers are common in patients with tumor infiltration of the lower end of the plexus. Patients who have not undergone radiation therapy to the brachial plexus, who present with pain and neurologic symptoms in the arm, raise a strong index of suspicion of tumor infiltration of the plexus.

Patients who have already received radiation therapy to the plexus present a more difficult diagnostic problem, however. A study by Kori et al.[29] addressed this problem by reviewing the pain patterns of 100 patients with brachial plexus lesions. Some of these lesions were related to tumor infiltration and others to radiation injury. Pain was the most common presenting symptom in the patients with tumor infiltration of the plexus, occurring in 75 percent of patients who had not received radiation to the area, and 89 percent of patients who had been previously radiated. The pain was described as moderate to severe in intensity, beginning in the shoulder girdle and radiating to the elbow and medial side of the forearm and fourth and fifth fingers. Movement of the shoulder led to an increase in pain. In some patients, pain was localized to the posterior aspect of the arm or the elbow. Other patients complained of burning or freezing sensation and hypersensitivity of the skin along the outer aspect of the hand.

In contrast to the frequency with which pain was the presenting symptom of tumor infiltrating the plexus, only 18 percent of patients with radiation injury to the plexus initially presented with pain. Sixty-five percent of patients had some pain later, but in only 35 percent of patients was pain a major problem. The more common presenting symptoms were paresthesias of the whole hand, often starting in the thumb and forefinger before spreading to the whole hand, swelling and heaviness of the arm, and proximal weakness of the arm.

A summary of the clinical signs to differentiate between metastatic plexopathy and radiation injury concludes that metastatic plexopathy is suggested if there is early and severe pain and weakness (C8–T1) and a

Horner's Syndrome, whereas radiation plexopathy is suggested if there is weakness of shoulder abduction and arm flexors with progressive lymphedema. Radiation damage to the brachial plexus was found to be unusual if the radiation dose was less than 6000 rads. If more than 6000 rads were given, and if the neurologic symptoms occurred within a year, radiation damage was likely. If the symptoms appeared after a year, the diagnosis could be either radiation damage or tumor recurrence.

Lumbosacral plexopathy.   In patients with cancer, this may result in major incapacitating pain and leg weakness, so that the patient becomes immobilized. The plexopathy can be caused by intra-abdominal tumors or by metastases from extra-abdominal tumors. In a study of 85 patients with lumbosacral plexopathy,[23] 73 percent had direct lumbosacral tumor invasion by intra-abdominal extension, while 27 percent had metastases from extra-abdominal tumors.

Seventy percent of patients had pain as the presenting symptom, followed weeks to months later by paresthesias and weakness. In one-third of the patients, there was a lag time of at least three months between the complaint of pain and the onset of symptoms. Although pain was experienced by all the patients, it was the only symptom in 20 of the 85 patients. Pain was usually aching and pressure-like in quality. The pain was of three different types: local in 72 of the 85 patients (85%), radicular in 72 of the 85 patients (85%), or referred in 37 of the 85 patients (43%). Almost all of the patients with lymphoma, breast cancer, colorectal cancer, and sarcoma complained of posteriorly located focal pain. Many patients complained of pain in more than one distribution. Only two-thirds of patients with bilateral plexus involvement complained of bilateral pain.

Epidural spinal cord compression.   This is a neuro-oncologic complication in which pain is the presenting complaint in 96 percent of patients and can result in paraplegia if not recognized early and treated appropriately. It occurs in 5 to 10 percent of patients with cancer, is more commonly seen in patients with breast, lung, and prostate disease, and although more common in the advanced cancer patient, can be associated with any stage of the disease.[42] Spinal cord damage results from compression by tumor in the epidural space or by direct invasion of the cord. The former is more common. Metastatic tumor reaches the epidural space in one of two ways. The most frequent is when a vertebral body metastasis spreads to the epidural space. Less commonly, but characteristic of lymphomas, is when a paravertebral tumor grows into the spinal canal through an intervertebral foramen.[42] Metastatic epidural spinal cord compression damages the cord by direct compression, with demyelination and axonal damage, and by secondary vascular compromise causing ischemia, edema, and infarction.

Back pain is the presenting symptom in more than 90 percent of patients with epidural cord compression.[42] Pain is usually present for days or weeks before other neurological signs and symptoms appear. There are two kinds of pain. Local pain is present in the midline or slightly to the side of the neck or back, near the site of the involved vertebral body. This pain is usually dull, aching, steady and gradually increases over time. It is often made worse by lying down, and may be relieved by sitting or standing. Radicular pain usually develops later, and is more common when the cervical or lumbosacral spine is involved. Cervical and lumbosacral pain is usually unilateral, while thoracic radicular pain is usually bilateral, and may be described as a band-like constricting pain radiating around to the chest or abdomen. After weeks of pain, the patient, if untreated, then progresses to neurological signs and symptoms including weakness, sensory changes, and bowel and bladder dysfunction. Once neurological symptoms other than pain develop, the patient may progress very rapidly over a matter of hours or days to complete paraplegia. The prognosis depends on the neurological status of the patient when treatment is started. Patients who are ambulatory when they start treatment usually remain so, while those who are not ambulatory when treatment starts, do not regain function after treatment. Therefore, early diagnosis of the cause of the pain is imperative to prevent irreversible neurological damage.

Infiltration of Hollow Viscus

Tumor infiltration or compression of the intestinal tract or viscera are a source of both acute and chronic pain in the cancer patient. Although the intestines are not in themselves sensitive to pain, the surrounding peritoneum is pain sensitive. Distortion, stretching, or inflammation of the peritoneum may result in severe pain. Such pain may be local or referred. For example, the pain associated with pancreatic cancer may be referred to the back or to the top of the left scapula, while the capsular pain from expanding intrahepatic metastasis may be referred to the right subscapular region. In addition, any obstruction to the normal peristaltic flow of the gut will result in a compensatory hyperperistalsis and cramping colicky pain, which can be severe. Episodic bowel obstruction associated with colon cancer is a familiar cause. Abdominal pain requires prompt diagnosis and treatment. Associated symptoms need to be evaluated and referral sites of pain assessed. The management approach is selected within the framework of the patient's extent of disease.[5]

Pain Syndromes Associated with Cancer Therapy

Pain syndromes associated with cancer therapy involve the three major treatment modalities: surgery, chemotherapy, and radiation therapy. The most commonly seen pain syndromes within each class are reviewed by Chapman in Chapter 3 of the present volume.

Postsurgical Pain Syndromes

Chronic postsurgical pain starts either at the time of surgery or evolves shortly thereafter, increasing in intensity from the time of the surgery. In contrast, acute postoperative pain is initially intense and then slowly decreases as tissue healing takes place. The characteristics of a postsurgical pain syndrome are persistent pain, or recurrent pain after the initial postoperative pain has cleared.[28] Postmastectomy pain syndrome, postthoracotomy pain syndrome, postradical neck dissection pain, and phantom limb and stump pain are the most frequently seen painful sequelae of cancer surgery.

Postmastectomy pain syndrome. This occurs in 4–10 percent of women following any surgical procedure on the breast from lumpectomy to mastectomy. The pain may occur immediately after the surgery or several months later.[15] The etiology of postmastectomy pain is the development of a traumatic neuroma from interruption of the intercostal brachial nerve at the time of surgery. Treatment is directed toward identifying the cause of the pain to the patient, physical therapy to prevent disuse atrophy and a frozen shoulder, nerve blocks with local anesthetics to the trigger point, counterirritation, and low doses of amitriptyline.[15]

Postthoracotomy pain syndrome. This occurs in the distribution of any of the intercostal nerves following disruption. The pain is of two types.[15] The first occurs in the immediate postoperative period and is associated with sensory loss in the immediate site of the scar. The pain clears in 75 percent of patients within three months, although the sensory loss persists. The second type of pain is postoperative pain, which persists for three months or longer, or reoccurs after an initial resolution in the acute postoperative phase. Kanner et al.[27] suggest that the latter type of pain is more characteristic of recurrent tumor or infiltration of the chest wall, paraspinal or epidural space. Treatment of the pain is determined by its cause. Tumor-related pain requires treatment focused on the tumor. When the pain is caused by nerve injury alone, the treatment is similar to that of postmastectomy pain syndrome.

Postradical neck dissection pain. This pain occurs from surgical injury or interruption of the cervical nerves. The pain is described as a constant burning sensation in the area of sensory loss. Intermittent shock-like pain and dysesthesias may be present. The pain becomes dominant as the acute postoperative pain fades. Carbamazepine is useful in dealing with the dysesthetic quality of the pain. A second type of pain following radical neck dissection may occur as a result of surgical injury to motor nerves that innervate the shoulder and upper arm, or following surgical removal of neck muscles. Musculoskeletal imbalance occurs and the patient complains of an aching sensation in the shoulder and neck made worse by sitting up and walking around, and relieved by lying down. Local nerve blocks and a supportive sling can be of help to these patients.[15]

Phantom limb and stump pain. This pain may occur after the amputation of a limb. This differs from phantom limb sensation, which is experienced by all patients following the amputation of a limb. Phantom limb pain and stump pain are two different entities. Phantom limb pain usually occurs in patients with pain in the same site prior to surgery. Amputation may initially make the pain worse. The pain may be described as a cramping, burning sensation in the phantom limb, and is often identical in nature and location to the preoperative pain. This pain usually clears within two months of the surgical procedure. Its recurrence may be the first sign of recurrent disease.[15] Stump pain is pain that occurs at the site of the surgical scar several months to years following amputation.[28] The pain is frequently described as having a sharp, shooting, electric shock-like character. The pain results from the development of a traumatic neuroma. In contrast to phantom limb pain, stump pain is exacerbated by movement and relieved by rest. Carbamazepine is helpful for the sharp shooting quality of the pain, and amitriptyline for the burning component. Local transcutaneous nerve stimulation can also be helpful.

Postchemotherapy Pain Syndromes

Postchemotherapy pain syndromes result from the use of agents that are toxic to peripheral nerves (e.g., the vinca alkaloids, corticosteroids that may cause inflammation or necrosis of bone or soft tissue). These syndromes are being seen with increased frequency as patients survive longer with more effective chemotherapy. Peripheral neuropathy, steroid pseudorheumatism, aseptic necrosis of bone, and postherpetic neuralgia, as the more common of these syndromes, are reviewed below.

Peripheral neuropathy. This is seen most frequently following the use of the vinca alkaloid drugs such as vincristine, cisplatin, and procarbazine.[30,54] The painful dysesthesias are usually part of a symmetric polyneuropathy.[15] The dysesthesias are localized to the hands and feet, and have a burning quality made worse by superficial stimulation. Relief of pain may occur with the use of amitriptyline. Transcutaneous nerve stimulation is also helpful in some people.

Steroid pseudorheumatism. This occurs in patients being withdrawn from corticosteroids. This syndrome may occur regardless of whether the withdrawal is rapid or slow[44] and whether the steroids have been taken for a long or short period of time. The patient complains of diffuse myalgias and arthralgias with muscle and joint tenderness. Malaise and fatigue are also frequent complaints. Treatment consists of reinstituting the steroids at a higher level and withdrawing more slowly.[39] Steroid reduction often results in a marked exacerbation of pain in patients with bony metastases or epidural cord compression.[15]

Aseptic necrosis of bone. This is sometimes seen in patients on chronic steroid therapy. Sites of necrosis are the femoral or humeral head.[22] Pain in the shoulder or knee and leg are the most common presenting complaints. X-ray changes may not be seen for several weeks or months following the first complaint of pain.[15] Progressive inability to use the affected hip or arm functionally occurs. The syndrome is most commonly seen in patients with Hodgkin's disease, but can occur in any patient on chronic steroid therapy.[15] Early treatment consists of decreasing or stopping the steroids and using both non-narcotic and narcotic analgesics for pain.[39] When progressive bone destruction has occurred, replacement of the diseased area may dramatically eliminate the pain.[15]

Postherpetic neuralgia. This occurs with increased frequency in patients with cancer and those receiving immunosuppressive drugs.[39] The syndrome occurs more frequently in patients who develop acute herpes zoster after the age of 50, and in the cancer patient, in the area of the tumor or radiation port.[15] The quality of the pain in postherpetic neuralgia is of three types: continuous burning pain in the area of sensory loss, intermittent shock-like pain, and painful dysesthesias. Itching may also be a prominent component of the pain. Because the involved dermatome is hyperesthetic, the patient may splint the area to avoid precipitating the pain. This may lead to secondary musculoskeletal pain.[41] The current management for postherpetic pain syndrome includes mild analgesics, amitriptyline in low doses, and carbamazepine for the intermittent shock-like pain.[43] Transcutaneous nerve stimulation may also be helpful for some patients. Secondary musculoskeletal pain is treated with physical therapy.

Postradiation Pain Syndromes

Pain as a sequela to radiation therapy is seen less frequently than pain associated with chemotherapy. The three most common pain syndromes following radiation therapy are radiation fibrosis of the brachial or lumbar plexus, radiation myelopathy, and radiation-induced peripheral nerve tumors.[40]

Radiation fibrosis of the brachial plexus. This is associated with fibrosis of the surrounding connective tissue and secondary injury to nerve. It may occur from 6 months to 20 years following radiation treatment.[47] This is an extremely difficult pain syndrome to treat.

Radiation fibrosis of the lumbosacral plexus. This occurs less frequently than radiation fibrosis of the brachial plexus.[49] Foley[15] suggests this may be associated with tumor type and the long survival more commonly seen in patients with breast cancer. Pain in the leg and perineum may progress with loss of sensory and motor function and eventual paraplegia. The differential diagnosis of radiation fibrosis versus recurrent disease is helped by a history of radiation therapy, with local skin changes and lymphedema of the leg.[15]

Radiation myelopathy. This occurs as either a transient myelopathy or a chronic progressive myelopathy. The transient myelopathy is seen most frequently about four months following radiation therapy to the upper respiratory tract where the cervical spinal cord is included in the radiation port.[40] The patient complains typically of electric shock-like sensations brought on by neck flexion and made worse by exercise. This is known as the Lhermitte's sign. These symptoms gradually disappear over 2 to 36 weeks.

Chronic progressive myelopathy may develop following radiation therapy to the head and neck area, mediastinum, and cervical/supraclavicular and axillary nodes.[36] The spinal cord may be unavoidably included in the radiation port. The incidence of myelopathy increases with increasing radiation exposure to the cord. The prognosis is poor, with signs and symptoms progressing over months. Pain can be severe, and is usually localized to the area of the spinal cord damage, with dysesthesias below the level of the injury. Pain management is difficult and may include amitriptyline, non-narcotic and narcotic analgesics, transcutaneous nerve stimulation, and physical therapy. Supportive consistent care is of major importance to these patients and their families.

Radiation-induced peripheral nerve tumors. These are a rare complication of radiation therapy and may occur 4 to 20 years following radiation therapy.[11] The patient presents with a painful enlarging mass in an area of previous irradiation.

SUMMARY

Pain in the patient with cancer may be associated with a variety of factors. It may be the presenting complaint leading to a diagnosis of the primary tumor, it may be the first sign of recurrent disease, it may be related to treatment, or it may be unrelated to the cancer or its treatment. The etiology of each pain and its meaning to the patient are key factors in the management approach.

REFERENCES

1. Albe-Fessard D, Condes-Lara M, Sanderson P, et al.: Tentative explanation of the special role played by the areas of paleospinothalamic projection in patients with deafferentation pain syndromes, in Kruger L, Liebskind J (Eds): Neural Mechanisms of Pain (Advances in Pain Research and Therapy, Vol. 6). New York, Raven Press, 1984, pp 167–182
2. Bonica JJ: Treatment of cancer pain: current status and future needs, in Fields HL, Dubner R, Cervero F (Eds): Advances in Pain Research and Therapy, Vol. 9. New York, Raven Press, 1985, pp 589–599
3. Cartwright A, Hockey L, Anderson ABM: Life Before Death. London, Routledge and Kegan Paul, 1973
4. Cascino TL, Kori SH, Krol G, et al.: CT scanning of the brachial plexus in patients with cancer. Neurology 35:8–14, 1985
5. Cope Z: The Early Diagnosis of the Acute Abdomen (15th ed). New York, Oxford University Press, 1979
6. Coyle N, Foley KM: Pain in patients with cancer: profile of patients and common pain syndromes. Semin Oncol Nurs 1:93–99, 1985
7. Coyle N, Monzillo E, Loscalzo M, et al.: A model of continuity of care for cancer patients with pain and neuro-oncologic complications. Cancer Nurs 8:111–119, 1985
8. Culp WJ, Ochoa J: Abnormal nerves and muscles as impulse generators. New York, Oxford University Press, 1982
9. Daut RL, Cleeland CS: The prevalence and severity of pain in cancer. Cancer 50:1913–1918, 1982
10. Foley KM: Pain syndromes in patients with cancer, in Bonica JJ, Ventafridda V (Eds): Advances in Pain Research and Therapy, Vol. 2. New York, Raven Press, 1979, pp 59–75
11. Foley KM, Woodruff J, Ellis F, et al.: Radiation-induced malignant and atypical schwannomas. Ann Neurol 7:311–318, 1979
12. Foley KM: The analgesic management of bone pain, in Weiss L, Gilbert HA (Eds): Bone Metastasis. Boston, G.K. Hall Medical Publishing, 1981, pp 348–350
13. Foley KM, Sundaresan N: Management of cancer pain, in DeVita VT, Hellman S, Rosenberg SA (Eds): Cancer: Principles and Practice of Oncology, Vol. 2 (2nd ed). Philadelphia, J.B. Lippincott Company, 1985, pp 1941–1962
14. Foley KM: The treatment of cancer pain. N Engl J Med 313:84–95, 1985
15. Foley KM: Control of pain in cancer, in Calabresi P, Schein P, Rosenberg S (Eds): Medical Oncology: Basic Principles and Clinical Management of Cancer. New York, McMillan Publishing Co., 1985, pp 1385–1405
16. Foley KM: Overview of cancer pain and brachial and lumbosacral plexopathy, in Management of Cancer Pain—Syllabus of the Postgraduate Course, Memorial Sloan-Kettering Cancer Center, November 14–16, 1985, New York City, pp 31–39
17. Gilbert RW, Kim JH, Posner JB: Epidural spinal cord compression from metastatic tumor: diagnosis and treatment. Ann Neurol 5:40–51, 1978
18. Granek I, Ashikari R, Foley KM: The post-mastectomy pain syndrome. Proc Am Soc Clin Oncol 3:122, 1984 (Abstr)
19. Greenberg JS, Deck MDF, Vikram B, et al.: Metastases to the base of the skull: clinical findings in 43 patients. Neurology 31:350–357, 1981
20. Haram BJ: Facts and Figures in Management of Terminal Disease. London, Edward Arnold, 1978, pp 12–18
21. IASP Subcommittee on Taxonomy: Pain terms: a list with definitions and notes on usage. Pain 6:249–252, 1979
22. Ihde DC, DeVita V: Osteonecrosis of the femoral head in patients with lymphoma treated with intermittent combination chemotherapy (including corticosteroids). Cancer 36:1585–1588, 1975

23. Jackel KA, Young DF, Foley KM: The natural history of lumbosacral plexopathy in cancer. Neurology 35:8–15, 1985
24. Jellinger K, Sturm KW: Delayed radiation myelopathy in man. J Neurol Sci 14:389–408, 1971
25. Kanner RW, Martini N, Foley KM: Epidural spinal cord compression in pancoast syndrome (superior pulmonary sulcus tumor): clinical presentation and outcome. Ann Neurol 10:77, 1981
26. Kanner RM, Martini N, Foley KM: Incidence of pain and other clinical manifestations of superior pulmonary sulcus (Pancoast tumors), in Bonica JJ, Ventafridda V (Eds): Advances in Pain Research and Therapy, Vol. 4. New York, Raven Press, 1982, pp 27–38
27. Kanner RM, Martini N, Foley KM: Nature and incidence of post-thoracotomy pain. Proceedings of the American Society of Clinical Oncology 1:152, 1982 (Abstr)
28. Kanner R: Post-surgical pain syndromes, in Management of Cancer Pain—Syllabus of the Postgraduate Course, Memorial Sloan-Kettering Cancer Center, November 14–16, 1985, New York City, pp 65–69
29. Kori S, Foley KM, Posner JB: Brachial plexus lesions in patients with cancer: clinical findings in 100 cases. Neurology 31:45–50, 1981
30. LeQuesne PM: Neuropathy due to drugs, in Dyck PJ, Thomas PK, Lambert EH, et al.: Peripheral Neuropathy, Vol. II, (2nd ed). Philadelphia, W.B. Saunders Co., 1984, pp 2126–2179
31. Molinari R: Therapy of cancer pain in the head and neck, in Bonica JJ, Ventafridda V (Eds): Advances in Pain Research and Therapy, Vol. 2. New York, Raven Press, 1979, pp 131–138
32. Mundy GR, Spiro TP: The mechanisms of bone metastasis and bone destruction by tumor cells, in Weiss L, Gilbert HA (Eds): Bone Metastasis. Boston, G.K. Hall Medical Publishers, 1981, p 65
33. Norton WS, Lack SA: Control of symptoms other than pain, in Twycross RG, Ventafridda V (Eds): The Continuing Care of Patients with Terminal Cancer. Oxford, Pergamon Press, 1980, pp 167–178
34. Olson ME, Chernik NL, Posner JB: Infiltration of the leptomeninges by systemic cancer: a clinical and pathological study. Arch Neurol 30:122–137, 1978
35. Osler MW, Vizel M, Turgeon MS: Pain in terminal cancer patients. Arch Intern Med 138:1801–1802, 1978
36. Palmer JJ: Radiation myelopathy. Brain 95:109–122, 1972
37. Pannuti E, Rossi AP, Marroro D: Natural history of cancer pain, in Continuing Care of Terminal Patients. Proceedings: International Seminars on Continuing Care of Terminal Cancer Patients. New York, Pergamon Press, 1980, pp 75–89
38. Payne R: Anatomy and physiology of cancer pain, in Management of Cancer Pain— Syllabus of the Postgraduate Course, Memorial Sloan-Kettering Cancer Center, November 14–16, 1985, New York City, pp 1–14
39. Payne R: Postchemotherapy and postradiation therapy pain syndromes, in Management of Cancer Pain—Syllabus of the Postgraduate Course, Memorial Sloan-Kettering Cancer Center, November 14–16, 1985, New York City, p 76
40. Payne R: Postchemotherapy and postradiation therapy pain syndromes, in Management of Cancer Pain—Syllabus of the Postgraduate Course, Memorial Sloan-Kettering Cancer Center, November 14–16, 1985, New York City, pp 80–83
41. Portenoy RK, Duma C, Foley KM: Acute herpetic and postherpetic neuralgia: review of clinical features and current therapy. Ann Neurol, 1987 (In press)
42. Posner JB: Back pain and epidural spinal cord compression, in Management of Cancer Pain—Syllabus of the Postgraduate Course, Memorial Sloan-Kettering Cancer Center, November 14–16, 1985, New York City, pp 51–53
43. Price RW: Herpes zoster: an approach to systemic therapy. Med Clin North Am 66:1105–1118, 1982

44. Rotstein J, Good RA: Steroid pseudorheumatism. Arch Int Med 99:545–555, 1957
45. Rubin R, Rogers A, Foley KM: The measurement of pain in children with cancer. (Manuscript in preparation, Memorial Sloan-Kettering Cancer Center)
46. Sherman RA, Sherman CJ, Parker L: Chronic phantom and stump pain among American veterans: results of a survey. Pain 18:83–95, 1984
47. Stoll BA, Andrews JT: Radiation-induced peripheral neuropathy. Br Med J 1:834–837, 1966
48. Taskar R: Deafferentation, in Wall PD, Melzack R (Eds): Textbook of Pain. New York, Churchill Livingstone, 1984, pp 119–132
49. Thomas JE, Cascino TE, Earle JD: Differential diagnosis between radiation and tumor plexopathy of the pelvis. Neurology 35:1–7, 1985
50. Trotter JM, Scott R, MacBeth FR, et al.: Problems of the oncology outpatient: role of the liaison health visitor. Br Med J 282:122–124, 1981
51. Twycross RG: Clinical experience with diamorphine in advanced malignant disease. Int J Clin Pharmacol Ther Toxicol 9:184–198, 1974
52. Twycross RG, Fairfield S: Pain in far-advanced cancer. Pain 14:303–310, 1982
53. Wilkes E: Some problems in cancer management. Proc Roy Soc Med 67:23–27, 1974
54. Young DF, Posner JB: Nervous system toxicity of chemotherapeutic agents, in Vinken PJ, Bruyn GW (Eds): Handbook of Clinical Neurology. Amsterdam, North-Holland Publishing Co., 1980, pp 91–129

C. Richard Chapman, Ph.D.,
Judith Kornell, M.S., R.N., and
Karen L. Syrjala, Ph.D.

3

Painful Complications of Cancer Diagnosis and Therapy

Patients given the diagnosis of cancer dread the treatment as well as the disease. Surgery, chemotherapy, and radiotherapy take a heavy toll: multiple painful conditions, nausea and vomiting, lack of appetite, fatigue, sleeplessness, and disfigurements such as temporary alopecia or permanent dismemberment. These problems contribute heavily to the emotional morbidity of the patient, fostering persistent anxiety, somatic preoccupation, discouragement, and depression. Each encounter with therapy is potentially debilitating and perhaps painful. Accurate information on potential side effects of treatment can prevent patient attribution of toxicity symptoms to the disease, a factor that promotes depression and contributes to a sense of helplessness and hopelessness in cancer patients (Table 3-1).

PATHOPHYSIOLOGY OF PAIN IN CANCER PATIENTS

The incidence and severity of pain associated with cancer have been described by Daut and Cleeland[13] and Foley.[16] Patients with cancer may suffer pain related to early manifestation of a tumor (this is comparatively infrequent); direct or metastatic tumor progression; exacerbation of pre-existing nonmalignant chronic pain problems; and cancer treatment. The focus of this chapter is on cancer treatment, but treatment-induced pain may

Table 3-1
Sources of Pain Associated with Cancer Treatment

I. Diagnostic Procedures
    A. Lumbar punctures
    B. Blood samples
    C. Angiography
    D. Endoscopy
    E. Biopsies
II. Surgery
    A. Acute postoperative pain
    B. Chronic postoperative pain
        1. Mastectomy
        2. Radical neck resection
        3. Lymphedema
        4. Thoracotomy
        5. Phantom-limb
III. Chemotherapy
    A. Acute
        1. Gastrointestinal distress
        2. Mucositis
        3. Myalgia
        4. Joint pain
        5. Cardiomyopathy
        6. Pancreatitis
        7. Extravasation
    B. Chronic
        1. Peripheral neuropathy
        2. Steroid pseudorheumatism
        3. Aseptic osteonecrosis
IV. Radiation
    A. Acute
        1. Skin burn
        2. Gastrointestinal cramping
        3. Proctitis
        4. Mucositis
        5. Itching
    B. Chronic
        1. Osteonecrosis
        2. Fibrosis
        3. Keratitis
        4. Demyelination
        5. Pneumonitis
        6. Bowel ulceration or obstruction
        7. Myelopathy
V. Other Treatments and Treatment Complications

combine additively with the other sources of pain cited to exacerbate the patient's global suffering.

Pain may originate with any of several different pathological conditions or with a combination of such conditions. An understanding of the different mechanisms of pain is valuable. Pain responds selectively to different therapeutic interventions in accordance with its underlying etiological mechanisms. Patients can be prepared in advance to cope with certain predictable pain experiences and the efficacy of coping skills training can be enhanced if the etiological mechanism(s) of the pain are well understood. A clear understanding of the origin(s) of a patient's pain helps ensure that one can avoid procedures or interventions that might inadvertently worsen it. The major causes of pain related to anticancer treatment are primary nociception, pain associated with inflammation, pain related to reflex activity, axonal compression, and deafferentation pain.

Primary Nociception

Pain that results from the direct mechanical, thermal, or chemical stimulation of injury-sensitive free nerve endings, termed *nociceptors*, has been well studied.[49] Cutaneous and deep tissue nociceptors respond to cutting, severe pressure or crushing, and extreme temperature change. Visceral nociceptors are insensitive to cutting or burn but are activated by stretch, distension, or chemical irritation. Two subjectively different types of pain are associated with the two classes of nociceptors. The thinly myelinated A-delta sensory nerve fibers produce a bright, well localized, and distinct pain that is immediately associated with tissue insult. The more slowly conducting unmyelinated C fiber activation results in a poorly localized, particularly aversive, and persistent pain typically described as burning or aching. Roughly 10 to 25 percent of the A-delta sensory nerve fibers respond to tissue injury or stress, as do about one-half of the C fibers. These two types of fibers are found throughout the body, including vascular beds and muscle tissue.

Clinical events that directly stimulate nociceptors include those associated with immediate mechanical injury such as needle penetrations, endoscopies, surgeries and other treatment-related traumatic procedures, and chemical stimulation such as the injection of radiologic contrast agents.

Pain Associated With Inflammation

After injury has occurred, inflammation alters the function of the nociceptors through the release of chemical substances such as the plasmakinins, which may directly excite nerve endings. Endogenously produced chemical stimuli that result in pain are known as *algogenic substances*. Other chemical products released during inflammation, particularly the prostaglandins of the E group, sensitize the nociceptors, lowering their thresholds for excitation. As an example, pain associated with a resting surgical wound is minimally dependent upon mechanical stimulation, except when the injured tissue is moved or stretched; such pain is mediated by algogenic substances.

Pain Related to Reflex Activity

Another cause of pain, which is often a complicating factor in discomfort related to surgical wounds, is extreme or abnormal reflex response to nociception. Both motor and sympathetic reflex responses may occur when nociceptors are activated. Reflex mediated spasm of the skeletal muscles in the vicinity of an injury can produce a condition that, in itself, gives rise to nociception. In acute postoperative pain the painful splinting of chest and abdominal muscles may impair breathing and become a greater source of distress to the patient than the wound itself. Such reflexes may form "vicious circle" mechanisms in which nociception begets further nociception.

Sympathetic reflexes may occur in the acute response to nociception, decreasing the microcirculation in the vicinity of the injury, altering the chemical environment of the nociceptors, and producing painful smooth muscle spasm such as vasospasm. These reflexes are also implicated in certain chronic pain syndromes. *Reflex sympathetic dystrophies* are remarkably painful chronic conditions characterized by persistent, burning pain and a delayed, excruciating over-reaction to noninjurious stimuli, termed *hyperpathia*. The release of norepinephrine in the periphery following traumatic injury may be a mediating factor in this type of pain. Such problems are rarely related to cancer, but less severe forms of this disorder are commonly seen as long range complications of trauma including surgery and are associated with trigger point phenomena in musculoskeletal pain. Inappropriate sweating, either vasodilation or vasoconstriction, and sometimes abnormal growth or lack of body hair, are indications of sympathetic involvement in a chronic pain problem.

Axonal Compression

In addition to the above pain problems, which depend to some extent upon nociception, there are pain syndromes in which nociception plays no role; instead, there is direct stimulation of an axon or neural structure. Acute mechanical stimulation of a nerve trunk may cause ectopic firing with abnormal discharge patterns and produce pain. This can occur in cancer patients, for example, who have spinal nerve root compression from metastatic tumor.[2] Fracture of a vertebra or other bone that lies adjacent to a nerve or nerve root can cause sudden compression, characterized by sharp neuralgic pain that projects to the neurologic segments supplied by the involved nerves.

Chronic compression lesion problems can also occur. Sometimes problems of this sort may elude accurate diagnosis because they are characterized by slow onset. Cancer patients who have received high-dose irradiation treatments may develop fibrosis of the brachial or lumbrosacral plexi six months or more following treatment. Such pain is severe, intractable, and sometimes associated with numbness or paresthesias.

Deafferentation Pain

In some patients with cancer, amputation of a limb or other body part such as a breast is indicated; this may produce both a phantom body sensation and a deafferentation pain syndrome.[39] Such unlikely pain problems as a phantom uterus have been observed in postsurgical patients in addition to the more common phantom limb pain. The patient typically experiences a persistent sense of presence for the lost body part, which is often twisted or contorted in a bizarre way, and the phantom image hurts. For example, upper extremity amputees sometimes report that the fingernails of the phantom hand seem to be digging painfully and unnaturally into the phantom palm. Similar problems are seen in patients who suffer avulsion of the brachial plexus or other denervations. The exact central mechanisms of these pain syndromes are not yet understood.

PAIN RELATED TO DIAGNOSTIC PROCEDURES

Patients with cancer are often subjected to painful diagnostic procedures that are performed not only to detect cancer but also to evaluate its progression. Consequently, patients experience invasive diagnostic procedures initially to assess disease stage, as well as repeatedly in the course of follow-up.

Invasive diagnostic procedures are too numerous and varied to catalog here. However, it is worthwhile to consider a sampling of painful events that cancer patients frequently encounter. Blood samples are taken with such frequency that some patients become sensitized to venous puncture. Lumbar puncture is typically performed when neurological symptomatology is present. In addition to the pain of the procedure, severe headache can ensue for hours or days due to spinal fluid loss or leakage.

Angiography is always distressing, in part because of the mechanical irritation but also because of the chemical irritation of the contrast material. Nociceptors in blood vessels respond to both types of stimuli; discomfort appears to be proportional to the concentration of the contrast agent. Lymphangiograms, which are routine in the work-up for Hodgkins and non-Hodgkins lymphomas, can be extremely painful and exhausting. Dye is injected intradermally into the interdigital webbing of the foot. When it has migrated to the lymphatic channel, a cut-down is performed and the lymphatic channel is cannulated. Contrast material is then injected; the procedure takes about four hours and leaves the patient with a discolored foot that persists for weeks or months.

Cardioangiography also hurts because of the arterial puncture and placement of a catheter in the femoral artery; nociceptors are stimulated by the threading of the catheter through the arterial bed. During inspection of the left ventricle, patients experience "ventricular flush," often characterized by a visual disturbance and bright pain. This experience is coincident with a large bolus of contrast medium required for imaging of the ventricle.

Gastroenterologists are often called upon to perform time-consuming and uncomfortable procedures. Endoscopic retrograde choledochopancreatography is used to evaluate the patency of the common duct and the extent of the disease in patients in whom pancreatic cancer exists or is suspected. Patients can develop a painful pancreatitis secondary to the contrast material that is employed. Percutaneous transhepatic cholangiography is performed by inserting a 23 gauge needle through the skin, between the ribs, and into the liver.[47] By injecting contrast material while withdrawing the needle, the radiologist can visualize the hepatic bile ducts via fluoroscopy. Sites of obstruction within the biliary system can then be determined. Though this procedure can be completed in 30 minutes or less, when complete obstruction is present, the potential for infection and bile stasis dictate that surgery must be performed immediately.

Some diagnostic procedures are surgical in nature. Biopsies are performed on most body tissues; procedures vary from needle punctures to major surgeries that require general anesthesia. In addition to the frank discomfort of most of these procedures, there is also post-procedure pain. Bone marrow aspirations are commonly performed in patients with hematologic malignancies and are invariably painful and distressing.

Repetition of biopsies or other painful procedures may be accompanied by growing fear and aversion, which tends to exacerbate the pain and suffering associated with the procedure. Moreover, the findings may signal either the defeat or the progression of the disease and determine the patient's prognosis. The fear of the procedure can combine additively with apprehension about the results of the laboratory evaluation, and the resultant anxiety state can make the patient hyper-reactive to even minor aversive stimuli.

PAIN RELATED TO CANCER TREATMENT

Among the numerous treatments for cancer, three principal types warrant extended consideration: surgery, chemotherapy, and radiotherapy. Other treatments that may cause pain include hyperthermia and tumor embolization. In addition to these therapeutic interventions, pain may be caused by viral, bacterial, or fungal infection consequent to the suppressing effect of chemotherapy or radiotherapy on the immune system. Many other less common painful effects of cancer treatment and palliation occur, but are beyond the scope of this chapter.

Surgery

Patients who undergo surgery for cancer typically suffer acute pain during their postoperative course. In addition, some develop chronic conditions that result directly from the surgery and are painful.

Acute Postoperative Pain

Recent studies indicate that approximately 30 percent of surgical patients experience little or mild postoperative pain that does not require opioid therapy, 30 percent have moderate pain, and 40 percent have severe or very severe pain.[6] Such pain occurs most frequently and is most intense with intrathoracic and intra-abdominal surgery, extensive surgery of the spine, and major joint operations. Segmental reflexes often play a contributory role in the severity of postoperative pain through increases in skeletal muscle tension, and they may alter gastrointestinal and/or urinary function, ventilation, and circulation as well. Most pain will persist three days to one week following surgery; a few operations may cause pain that persists much longer. Acute postoperative pain may continue beyond its normal duration for a given procedure in some patients because of infection at the site of the incision, muscle tension at the surgical site, formation of neuroma, or contact irritation related to the patient's unique dressing and personal habits.

The management of postoperative pain has always been suboptimal, and this problem continues.[4] In general, physicians tend to under prescribe opioid medications for postoperative pain and nurses typically administer amounts that are notably lower than the physicians' orders. In a classic study, Marks and Sachar[26] determined that house officers at Montefiore Hospital ordered only 50 to 65 percent of the effective dose of opioid analgesic medication for severe pain; the nursing staff then administered only 40 to 50 percent of the inadequate amounts prescribed. Cohen[12] studied 109 patients after surgery and found that 75 percent of those who had been given opioid therapy for postoperative pain continued to experience moderate or marked pain and distress. Of these, 45 percent stated that the pain caused them to "cry out."

There are no statistics defining the incidence and severity of postoperative pain related to cancer. However, cancer surgeries are often more invasive and aggressive than normal surgical procedures, may be mutilating, may be more debilitating than ordinary surgery, are often performed on very sick patients, are often entered into with uncertain outcome, and are sometimes occasioned by oncologic emergencies such as bowel obstruction. Compared to ordinary surgeries, cancer operations are more likely to produce chronically painful conditions.

Chronic Postoperative Pain

There are many examples of conditions that give rise to pain after cancer surgery. Among the best known is the painful arm and shoulder syndrome in women who have undergone radical mastectomy. Pain is experienced in the anterior chest wall, axilla, and posterior arm consequent to surgical damage of the intercostobrachial nerve and other thoracic nerves.[5,17] This pain typically emerges one to two months (sometimes as late as six months) after surgery and is characterized by a burning, constricting quality. It is relieved by immobilization of the limb. Kanner[22] has estimated the incidence of this syndrome to be approximately 5 percent in radical mastectomy patients. He attributes the pain to the formation of a neuroma at the site of surgical section of the intercostal brachial nerve. The persistent discomfort of this pain problem retards the rehabilitation of the patient, limits the type of clothing that she can tolerate, and inhibits the activities that she can perform. Some patients guard movements of the affected limb so fastidiously that a frozen shoulder develops.

Extensive axillary lymph node dissection, which is performed both therapeutically and diagnostically, contributes to the eventual development of lymphedema ipsilateral to the surgical site, typically a mastectomy. Future minor injury such as a pinprick or cat scratch months or years after surgery can lead to this compromising condition. Although the limb is not intensely painful, the entire arm can become swollen, unsightly, and abnormally heavy. Often this is associated with a persisting dull ache. Once the condition has developed, it is relatively intractable. The confinement that this condition can cause detracts substantially from the quality of life, even in a patient who is considered cured of her disease.

Both of the above conditions compromise normal social life, in addition to causing severe discomfort. Such patients are prone to social withdrawal, hypochondriasis, and depression. These psychologic conditions can further complicate and exacerbate the pain problem.

Surgery performed at the base of the skull to treat neoplastic disease can result in chronic pain.[36] This problem may take many forms. Temporomandibular joint pain is among the most common, because paralysis or excision of muscles in the head or neck alter stress on the temporomandibular joint, producing functional asymmetry. The ear, pharynx, jaw, cervical spine, and associated muscle structures may all be foci of pain complaint. Surgery in the posterior fossa is likely to result in musculoskeletal pain because the sectioning of posterior neck muscles can result in asymmetries; sometimes torsion of the neck during surgery can cause muscle injury or damage nerves innervating muscle. Arthritis or other pre-existing conditions can complicate iatrogenic injury.

Patients who undergo radical neck dissection sometimes experience sensory loss with an associated tight burning sensation, dysesthesias, or intermittent lancinating neck pains. These problems may be complicated by musculoskeletal debilitation and pain that mimics a stooped shoulder syndrome.[22]

Patients operated on for carcinoma of the lung or other cancers sometimes develop pain in the distribution of the intercostal nerves that have been severed.[3] Kanner[22] and colleagues at Memorial Sloan-Kettering Cancer Center followed 126 thoracotomy patients in order to better define this syndrome. In 66 of the patients the postoperative pain was reduced substantially at two months, but in 13 others it recurred after a period of similar relief, due to recurrence of tumor. In 20 patients the pain persisted after the operation and increased during follow-up. This was largely due to local recurrence of the disease or to infection. In only 18 of the patients did the pain decrease or remain stable over time without presenting a management problem. These results indicate that the persistence or recurrence of pain in postthoracotomy patients is often associated with recurrent tumor. However, Kanner found that a small proportion of patients experienced persisting postoperative pain due to formation of neuromas.

Cancer patients who have limbs or other body parts surgically removed may experience prolonged stump pain, which is often caused by the formation of neuromas or painful phantom body parts, e.g., phantom limb pain.[39] This can also occur when a body part is surgically denervated. The phantom is perceived as a startling realization rather than as a dim or distant sensation.[27] In some cases the phantom becomes distorted or grotesque and is associated with an abnormal sense of tension or unnatural position. Pain in the phantom may be severe and burning in nature; in other cases it is reported as throbbing. It is not notably different in cancer patients than in noncancer amputees.[48]

Generally, phantom limbs fade with time, disappearing over several weeks in a manner that patients often describe as telescoping or contracting into the stump. In some patients, the phantom persists or only partly contracts with pain, reaching a plateau or steady state in painful intensity. The percentage of patients in whom this is reported varies substantially with the patient population studied and the time window for data collection. Shukla et al.[39] studied 72 amputees during postoperative recovery and found that 86 percent experienced phantom limb pain that was distinctly different from the pain at the surgical site. Sherman, Sherman, and Parker[38] sent questionnaires to 5000 patients with service-related amputations and 55 percent responded. About 78 percent indicated that they still experienced phantom limb pain, even though the average time since amputation was 26 years.

Roth and Sugarbaker[34] found the incidence of painful phantoms to be 97 percent in a sample of 63 cancer patients during the first four weeks following surgery, while in a follow-up period of several years the pain had resolved in 20 percent of the patients. In two of the patients studied, the pain began to increase over time; this was a function of the local recurrence of sarcoma.[45]

The higher the amputation of a limb, the greater the frequency of occurrence of a painful phantom. Roth and Sugarbaker[34] reported the incidence of a painful phantom to be 0 percent in patients with below-the-knee amputations, but 68 percent in hemipelvectomy patients. Although data are not available on the incidence, severity, or time course of these phenomena, painful phantoms have been reported following mastectomy, facial surgeries, and even hysterectomy. Considered together, various clinical reports and the studies cited above indicate that surgical denervation is a major cause of chronic postoperative pain.

Chronic pain of surgical origin may mask the recurrence of disease in cancer patients. In follow-up care of patients who have pain consequent to surgical therapy for neoplasia, it is important to monitor the patients' chronic pain. Exacerbations in otherwise stable patterns of persistent pain may be indicative of tumor recurrence.

Chemotherapy

As chemotherapeutics become more aggressive, the success rates for rescue from cancer increase; however, there is a concomitant increase in toxicity, including treatment-induced pain. Pain is only one problem in a complex spectrum of neurotoxicity and organ toxicity that occurs following chemotherapy. Both transient and permanent neurologic problems are seen. The constellation of problems varies with the chemotherapeutic agents used, as described by Kaplan and Wiernik.[23] Table 3-2 specifies pain-related complaints associated with the most common chemotherapeutic agents.

The vinca alkaloids, particularly vincristine and vinblastine, sometimes produce a toxic peripheral neuropathy characterized by painful paresthesias and dysesthesias, loss of deep tendon reflexes, muscle pain, a colicky abdominal pain, painful myalgia, and a peculiar severe jaw pain that may appear within hours of the first treatment.[9,31] Up to 100 percent of patients treated with the vinca alkaloids may experience dysesthesias and paresthesias; these are usually localized in the extremities, burning in quality, and the pain is typically exacerbated by stimulation of the hand or foot. Peripheral neuropathy can also occur with cisplatin or procarbazine, and in rare cases with misoniadazole and hexamethylmelamine.[31] These problems are not well understood; they may be due to chemical injury of the nociceptors, inflammation or edema within the nerve trunk, or to frank axonal injury that results in ectopic firing or abnormal firing patterns in the affected nerve.

Intrathecal methotrexate can induce immediate or early-onset headache, lethargy, nausea and vomiting, leg pains, paraplegia, and stiff neck. Long-term problems include neurologic damage and associated impairment; in some patients a disseminated necrotizing leucoencephalopathy is seen with associated psychologic abnormalities such as spasticity, somnolence, dementia, and ataxia. Mineralizing microangiography, a disease of the small blood vessels, is observed in some patients, primarily in the gray matter of the brain. Platinum and other heavy metal therapies such as diamminedichloroplatinum may produce a tinnitus secondary to ototoxicity, ophthalmologic symptoms, and peripheral sensory neuropathies including dysesthesias and paresthesias like those described above. Platinum therapy is often associated with renal toxicity. Permanent damage is not uncommon with multiple courses, and patients may require dialysis. While renal function may return, it often fails to return to normal. L-asparaginase does not produce peripheral nerve damage, but infrequently (15 percent or fewer of patients) acute pancreatitis occurs.

Cyclophosphamide and several other chemotherapeutic drugs produce toxic degradation of mucosal tissue, which results in painful oral mucositis and xerostomia developing about one week after treatment.[7,14,19,33,44] The division and maturation of oral epithelial cells are compromised by the chemotherapeutic drugs, with resultant thinning and ulceration of the mucosa. Oral trauma interacts with these processes to produce severe degradation of tissue. Oral mucositis occurs in more than 40 percent of all chemotherapy patients as a direct consequence of treatment.[43] Hemorrhage and infections can complicate the problem. Related problems can occur in other mucosal tissues. Cyclophosphamide, for example, may lead to painful hemorrhagic cystitis.

Oral hemorrhage following chemotherapy can sometimes lead to major coagulopathy, which is caused by combination of low platelets, compromised mucosa, and trauma from normal oral function. Xerostomia, although not painful, commonly accompanies mucositis and coagulopathy, as does transient loss of taste. When mucositis or coagulopathy are severe, patients may inadvertently swallow substantial amounts of mucosal slough and blood, and this can cause or exacerbate existing nausea and vomiting.

Corticosteroids can also produce painful toxic sequelae. The best known is steroid pseudorheumatism, which sometimes appears during the withdrawal of steroid medications. Muscle and joint tenderness or frank pain are the primary manifestations of this condition, together with malaise and fatigue.[1,35] The pain is relieved with reinstitution of steroid treatment; patients may respond favorably with slower withdrawal after return to steroid medications. Steroid treatments for months or years can result in aseptic necrosis of bone, in some patients, particularly the femoral head.[20,41]

Table 3-2
Pain Associated with Chemotherapy

Discomfort-Related Complaints with Most Chemotherapeutic Agents:

Nausea and vomiting
Diarrhea/constipation
Extravasation
Pain at site of injection
Phlebitis
Fever, chills, or sore throat
Swelling of feet or lower legs
Unusual bleeding or bruising

Additional Pain Complaints Possible with Specific Chemotherapeutic Agents:

Agent	Possible Complaints
ALKYLATING AGENTS	
Busulfan	Stomach pain, joint pain
Chlorambucil	Stomatitis, stomach pain, joint pain, skin rash
Cyclophosphamide	Hemorrhagic cystitis, stomatitis, cardiomyopathy, flank and stomach pain, joint pain
Melphalan	Skin rash, stomach pain, joint pain, stomatitis
Mechlorethamine (nitrogen mustard)	Skin rash, flank and stomach pain, joint pain, peripheral neuropathy
ANTIBIOTICS	
Bleomycin	Stomatitis, skin rash or tenderness, chest pain
Dactinomycin	Stomach pain, joint pain, skin rash, cardiomyopathy
Doxorubicin	Cardiomyopathy, stomach pain, joint pain, stomatitis, skin rash
Mitomycin C	Stomatitis
Plicamycin	Headache, myalgia, skin rash, stomatitis
ANTIMETABOLITES	
Cytarabine (cytosine arabinoside)	Stomatitis, stomach pain, heartburn, bone, joint or muscle pain

58

gelfoam, steel coils, or other materials.[8] The procedure may be performed either for cure or for palliative purposes. Since it requires an arterial access, tumor embolism is immediately painful and residual pain ensues that may last up to a week. Renal embolizations are inevitably characterized by severe flank pain, and patients typically develop a temperature of up to 40°C due to foreign object reaction.

Hyperthermia

Palliation of advanced disease in localized areas through the delivery of heat to the tumor has been undertaken experimentally via microwave, ultrasound, and radiofrequency technology.[25,42] Often catheters, such as angiocatheters, are placed within the tumor itself and sutured in place. A heat monitoring probe is placed within each catheter to monitor internal tumor temperature during treatment. These procedures are still developmental; they are often undertaken in combination with irradiation.[32]

Patients are required to hold a fixed position for treatments, which often last about one and one-half hours. In addition to the stress of confinement in the therapy chamber, the sensations of heat and nerve compression are often extremely uncomfortable and unsettling. Patients also complain about the pain resulting from the placement of the catheters into the tumor. Breaks in the skin occur regularly and dry or wet desquamation results in painful, hot, and itchy sensations.

The results of hyperthermia treatment are often impressive in the resolution of massive surface lesions and in the shrinkage of enlarged lymph nodes. However, the local effects of heat for prolonged periods of time may produce painful edema in the tumor as well as in the surrounding tissue. In addition, the edema may constrict local passages such as arteries and airways and cause cardiopulmonary failure in elderly or debilitated patients.

Microbial Infection

Chemotherapy and irradiation weaken the immune system and the patient is vulnerable to viral, bacterial, or fungal infections that can produce pain. In the case of the bone marrow transplant patient, the aggressive chemoradiotherapy regimen completely destroys the immune system. Staphylococcal infections, candidiasis, and other bacterial or fungal infections can usually be managed effectively by medications. Viral infections present significant problems and often are life threatening. Pain is a major symptom of herpetic infections, which involve sensory nerves, and chronic postherpetic neuralgias may ensue in some cases.

Herpes simplex viruses can cause both oral and genital lesions that are markedly painful. Such infections can often be prevented or effectively treated with systematically administered acyclovir.

Varicella infections are frequently seen among cancer patients, particularly those who have had chemotherapy or irradiation. The infection follows a dermatomal distribution, and the associated acute zoster pain is typically described as a continuous aching or burning upon which lancinating pains are superimposed. The latter may be paroxysmal when the skin is stretched or moved. Itch and secondary muscle pain complicate the discomfort of the patient.

A small proportion of patients who have had acute zoster develop chronic postherpetic neuralgia (shingles); the incidence appears to increase with advancing age. The pain of the acute episode persists, often increasing in intensity and changing somewhat in character so that the burning and aching accompany a sense of tightness and perhaps crawling. The affected skin areas are extremely hyperesthetic, and patients may even avoid the light contact of clothing on these areas. This syndrome is generally considered to be a deafferentation pain that involves both peripheral and central pathologies. It is very difficult to manage; in some patients the syndrome spontaneously resolves after many years.

Finally, staphylococcal infection may result in a painful condition termed *scalded skin syndrome*.[11] There is cleavage of the superficial epidermis with erythema and blistering. Presenting symptoms include pain, fever, and widespread erythema, which progresses to raw, red, oozing tissues. Patients at risk include those who are immune-suppressed. This condition responds to antibiotics.

CONCLUSIONS

The extent and severity of pain experienced by patients during diagnosis, treatment, and follow-up related to cancer has not been studied comprehensively. Nonetheless, the literature indicates that both acute and chronic pain related to medical procedures and treatments can be major sources of discomfort and personal misery for many patients. That cancer victims must undergo relentless sequences of aversive events is appalling. This oversight has continued unchecked for decades and must be addressed.

Apart from the pressing humanitarian concern, there are three reasons why good medical and nursing care requires careful attention to the details of treatment-induced pain and toxicity. First, some patients who experience extreme, repeated pain and/or discomfort with diagnostic and therapeutic procedures become sensitized, fearful, and profoundly discouraged so that they reject further, potentially life-saving, therapy. For such patients the cost of treatment in personal misery exceeds the meager hope of cure with additional intervention. Patient judgment in such circumstances often reflects depression and phobia rather than objective appraisal. Improved palliative prophylaxis or care for treatment-induced pain is urgently needed.

Second, iatrogenic chronic pain can mask the recurrence of tumor and delay timely intervention. The presence of chronic pain debilitates the patient and results in depression, fatigue, and hypochondriacal preoccupation. Even symptoms unrelated to pain may be harder to identify in a pain patient when the disease recurs years after an apparently successful course of therapy. Cancer patients with iatrogenically-induced chronic pain require a more thorough and circumspect follow-up examination than do their pain-free counterparts.

Finally, when cancer patients with persisting pain of iatrogenic origin are managed on analgesic medications, problems of tolerance and polypharmacy may develop. This leads to medication toxicity, which produces its own unique pattern of symptoms. Well-intentioned care givers who do not recognize the problem may prescribe medications to control symptoms of medication toxicity, thus complicating the problem. Should the tumor recur or some other life-threatening problem develop (e.g., microbial infection), prompt diagnosis may be confounded or delayed by the confusing symptomatology of medication overuse and polypharmacy.

What can be done to address these problems? There are no simple answers. However, there are four steps that can be achieved in most settings. All clinicians, including nurses, can play a major role in this effort.

First, the pain and toxicity problems unique to each diagnostic or therapeutic setting in which cancer patients are seen must be identified. Where possible, research should be conducted to define the extent and severity of these problems. Second, pharmacologic and psychologic prophylaxis for painful events must be employed so that patients are well-prepared in advance for what they will encounter. Fear of the unknown is often a part of the dread that grips patients as they approach invasive procedures. Psychologic prophylaxis for acute pain has recently been described by Chapman and Turner.[10] Third, efforts should be made to insure that the terminal patient does not feel abandoned. Care and concern about proper medication regimens, psychologic support, and the timely use of antidepressant drugs are useful for this purpose. Proper medications for chronic pain should be used when indicated. Methadone, for example, will help stabilize mood swings in patients who suffer from the psychologic changes associated with the administration of short-acting opioids. Finally, the control of pain related to treatment should be a major concern in the care of cancer patients. The possibility or actuality of severe pain related to tumor should not be allowed to overshadow the importance of controlling procedural pain and discomfort.

ACKNOWLEDGMENT

Preparation of this material was supported by National Cancer Institute Program Project #CA 38552.

REFERENCES

1. Amatruda TT, Hollingsworth DR, D'esopo NK, et al.: A study of the mechanism of the steroid withdrawal syndrome. Evidence for integrity of the hypothalamic-pituitary-adrenal system. J Clin Endocrinol Metab 20:339–354, 1960

2. Asbury AK, Fields HF: Pain due to peripheral nerve damage: an hypothesis. Neurology 34:1587–1590

3. Benedetti C, Bonica JJ: Cancer pain: basic considerations, in Benedetti B, Chapman CR, Moricca G (Eds): Advances in Pain Research and Therapy, Vol. 7. New York, Raven Press, 1984, pp 529–555

4. Benedetti C, Bonica JJ, Bellucci G: Pathophysiology and therapy of postoperative pain: a review, in Benedetti B, Chapman CR, Moricca G (Eds): Advances in Pain Research and Therapy, Vol. 7. New York, Raven Press, 1984, pp 373–407

5. Bonica JJ: The Management of Pain. New York, Lea & Febiger, 1953

6. Bonica JJ, Benedetti C: Postoperative pain, in Condon RD, DeCosse JJ (Eds): Surgical Care: A Physiologic Approach to Clinical Management. Philadelphia, Lea & Febiger, 1980, pp 394–415

7. Bottomly WK, Parlin E, Ross GE: Antineoplastic agents and their oral manifestations. Oral Surg 44:527–534, 1977

8. Chabner BA, Myers CE: Clinical pharmacology of cancer chemotherapy, in DeVita Jr VT, Hellman S, Rosenberg SA (Eds): Cancer: Principles and Practice of Oncology, Vol. 1 (2nd ed). Philadelphia, J.B. Lippincott Co, 1985, pp 287–328

9. Chapman CR, Syrjala KS, Sargur M: Pain as a manifestation of cancer treatment. Semin Oncol Nurs 1:100–108, 1985

10. Chapman CR, Turner JA: Psychological control of acute pain in medical settings. J Pain Sympt Mgmt 1:9–20, 1986

11. Chernecky C, Ramsey P: Critical Nursing Care of the Client with Cancer. Norwalk, Appleton-Century-Crofts, 1984

12. Cohen EL: Postsurgical pain relief: patient's status—nurses' medication choices. Pain 9:265–274, 1980

13. Daut RL, Cleeland CS: The prevalence and severity of pain in cancer. Cancer 50:1913–1918, 1982

14. Dreizen S: Stomatotoxic manifestations of cancer chemotherapy. J Prosthet Dent 40:650–655, 1978

15. Ducatman BS, Scheithauer BW: Postirradiation neurofibrosarcoma. Cancer 51:1028–1033, 1983

16. Foley K: Medical progress: the treatment of cancer pain. N Engl J Med 313:84–95, 1985

17. Foley KM: Current controversies in the management of cancer pain. National Institute on Drug Abuse Research Monograph Series 36:169–181, 1981

18. Foley KM, Woodruff JM, Ellis FT, Posner JB: Radiation-induced malignant and atypical peripheral nerve sheath tumors. Ann Neurol 7:311–318, 1980

19. Guggenheimer J. Verbin RS, Appel BN, et al.: Clinico-pathologic effects of cancer chemotherapeutic agents on human buccal mucosa. Oral Surg 44:58–63, 1977

20. Ihde DC, DeVita VT: Osteonecrosis of the femoral head in patients with lymphoma treated with intermittent combination chemotherapy (including corticosteroids). Cancer 36:1585–1588, 1975

21. Jackel KA, Young DF, Foley KM: The natural history of lumbosacral plexopathy in cancer. Neurology 35:8–15, 1985

22. Kanner R: Postsurgical pain syndromes, in Foley K (course director): Management of Cancer Pain, Syllabus of the postgraduate course of Memorial Sloan-Kettering Cancer Center, November 14–16, 1985, New York City. New York, Memorial Sloan-Kettering Cancer Center, 1985, pp 65–72

23. Kaplan RS, Wiernik PH: Neurotoxicity of antineoplastic drugs. Semin Oncol 9:103–130, 1982
24. Kori S, Foley KMF, Posner JB: Brachial plexus lesions in patients with cancer: 100 cases. Neurology 35:8–15, 1981
25. Kretchman D: Hyperthermia review. Reg Oncol Nurs Q 7:2–3, 1985
26. Marks RD, Sachar EJ: Undertreatment of medical inpatients with narcotic analgesics. Ann Intern Med 78:173–181, 1973
27. Melzack R, Wall PD: The Challenge of Pain. New York, Basic Books, 1982
28. Mulkerin LE: Practical Points in Radiation Oncology. Garden City, Medical Examination Publishing Co, 1979
29. Murphy W: Radiation Therapy. Philadelphia, W.B. Saunders, Co, 1967
30. Palmer JJ: Radiation myelopathy. Brain 95:109–122, 1972
31. Payne R: Post-chemotherapy and post-radiation pain syndromes, in Foley K (course director): Management of Cancer Pain, Syllabus of the postgraduate course of Memorial Sloan-Kettering Cancer Center, November 14–16, 1985, New York City. New York, Memorial Sloan-Kettering Cancer Center, 1985, pp 73–93
32. Perez CA, Nussbaum G, Emami B, VonGerichten D: Clinical results of irradiation combined with local hyperthermia. Cancer 52:1597–1603, 1983
33. Peterson DE, Sonis ST: Oral complications of cancer chemotherapy: present status and future studies. Cancer Treat Rep 66:1251–1256, 1982
34. Roth YF, Sugarbaker PH: Pains and sensations after amputation: character and clinical significance. Arch Phys Med Rehabil 61:490–501, 1980
35. Rotstein J, Good RA: Steroid pseudorheumatism. Arch Intern Med 99:545–555, 1957
36. Sataloff RT, Myers DL, Roberts B-R: Pain following surgery of the skull base. Otolaryngol Clin North Am 17:613–625, 1984
37. Shannon IL: Management of head and neck irradiated patients. Adv Physiol Sci 28:313–322, 1981
38. Sherman RA, Sherman CJ, Parker L: Chronic phantom and stump pain among American veterans: results of a survey. Pain 18:83–95, 1984
39. Shukla GD, Sahu SC, Tripathi RP, et al.: Phanton limb: a phenomenological study. Br J Psychiatry 141:54–48, 1982
40. Silverman S: Radiation effects, in Silverman S (Ed): Oral Cancer. New York American Cancer Society, 1981, pp 66–75
41. Solomon L: Drug-induced arthropathy and necrosis of the femoral head. J Bone Joint Surg 55:246–261, 1973
42. Song CW: Physiological factors in hyperthermia. Natl Cancer Inst Monogr 61:169–176, 1982
43. Sonis A, Sonis S: Oral complications of cancer chemotherapy in pediatric patients. J Periodontol 3:122–128, 1979
44. Sonis ST, Sonis AL, Lieberman A: Oral complications in patients receiving treatment for malignancies other than of the head and neck. J Am Dent Assoc 97:468–472, 1978
45. Sugarbaker PH, Weiss CM, Davidson DD, Roth YF: Increasing phantom limb pain as a symptom of cancer recurrence. Cancer 54:373–375, 1984
46. Thomas JE, Piepgras DG, Scheithauer B, et al.: Neurogenic tumors of the sciatic nerve: a clinicopathologic study of 35 cases. Mayo Clin Proc 58:640–647, 1983
47. Troupin R: Diagnostic Radiology in Clinical Medicine (2nd ed). Chicago, Year Book Medical Publishers, Inc, 1978
48. Wall R, Novotny-Joseph P, MacNamara TE: Does preamputation pain influence phantom limb pain in cancer patients? South Med J 78:34–36, 1985
49. Willis WD: The Pain System: The Neural Basis of Nociceptive Transmission in the Mammalian Nervous System. Pain and Headache, Vol. 8. New York, Karger, 1985
50. Yasko JM: Care of the Client Receiving External Radiation Therapy. Reston, VA, Prentice Hall, 1982

Josie Howard-Ruben, M.S., R.N.

4

Issues in Cancer Pain Management

In no area of nursing practice is there more opportunity for independent action based on sound application of knowledge than in discovering the patient's particular needs for pain relief, in revealing the measures that work best for him and in solving the problem of pain. And I submit that in no area have we overlooked our responsibilities more. Recent findings concerning nurses' reaction to patients who complain of pain lend credence to the need for accepting our responsibility. We must investigate the barriers which we have created and we must overcome them if we are to 'comfort those in distress' . . . (p. 69).[48]

These words were written in 1965 and illustrate the fact that nurses and others have had and still have difficulty dealing with patients in pain. Over these two decades, much research has addressed variables that affect nurses' and physicians' assessment and management of the patient in pain. At present, there are many issues that contribute to the challenge of managing cancer pain. Two major problems are the knowledge and attitudes of health care professionals relative to pain and pain management, and issues related to appropriate pharmacologic management.

KNOWLEDGE AND ATTITUDES OF HEALTH PROFESSIONALS

Knowledge

In spite of recent advances in the field of pain management, the clinical care of patients in pain is frequently inadequate. A major reason is a significant lack of knowledge on the part of health professionals about appropriate methods of pain control. Pain is an abstract, complex, and uniquely subjective phenomenon. Unlike many other clinical problems, there are few screening tests to document and quantify its existence. Health care professionals may be more comfortable treating patients on the basis of objective parameters. Perhaps because of this, there has not been adequate attention to pain in educational programs.

Bonica[11] discussed the inadequate attention to pain in educational programs as well as in clinical textbooks. One recent textbook[33] presented pain as a pertinent clinical concern, with knowledgeable clinicians addressing pain management. However, misinformation and gaps in knowledge still exist. Bonica attributed the difficulties physicians have with pain management to a number of factors. These include lack of organized teaching in the management of cancer pain, a progressive trend toward specialization that contributes to specialists viewing pain in a narrow fashion, an inability of some practitioners to devote the necessary time and effort to provide optimal pain relief, and a meager amount of published information on the proper treatment of cancer pain. Bonica concluded that most health care providers approach pain management empirically rather than scientifically, depending on narcotic analgesics as the therapeutic mainstay, but unfortunately using them in a suboptimal fashion.

Review of the Literature

Many studies of knowledge about pain management have been undertaken, with both nurses and physicians serving as subjects. Marks and Sachar[65] published the first study of this sort in 1973. They found several trends relative to inadequate knowledge about pain management. Widespread misinformation among housestaff physicians about the analgesic properties of meperidine prevailed, including the drug's duration of action and its maximal safe dosage. Additionally, a major concern expressed by the housestaff was a fear of iatrogenic addiction, which led to both the prescription and administration of low dosages of drugs at inappropriately long intervals.

Marks and Sachar also found that the nursing staff compounded the inadequacy of patients' analgesia by failing to administer the maximum amount of drug allowable by physicians' orders. Table 4-1 amplifies this finding for the 12 (of 37 total) patients who reported marked distress. As indicated, care givers administered from between 6 percent and 50 percent of the amount of meperidine actually prescribed, despite obvious marked distress from pain as evidenced by patients' responses to inquiries about global pain relief; difficulties with sleep, nutrition, concentration, and conversation; and feelings of anxiety, depression and irritability. Marks and Sachar's findings have clear implications relevant to the knowledge deficits of both physician and nursing staff caring for patients in pain.

Charap[19] expanded upon this work, focusing on the terminally ill patient

Table 4-1
Amount of Drug Prescribed versus Administered for Patients
Reporting Marked Distress (n = 12)

Patient Distress Score* 13–18 = Marked distress	Dosage of Meperidine Ordered[†]	Dosage of Meperidine Administered[†]	Percentage Actually Given
18	600 mg	300 mg	50
17	450 mg	150 mg	33
17	300 mg	100 mg	33
16	450 mg	175 mg	39
15	450 mg	75 mg	17
14	450 mg	85 mg	19
14	300 mg	100 mg	33
14	300 mg	50 mg	17
14	300 mg	25 mg	8
14	400 mg	25 mg	6
13	450 mg	75 mg	17
13	300 mg	75 mg	25

* 13–18 = marked distress (on a 0–18 scale).
† Dosage noted in mg/day on prn schedule.
Adapted from Marks RM, Sacher EJ: Undertreatment of medical inpatients with narcotic analgesics. Ann Intern Med 78:173–181, 1973. With permission.

with pain. Again, physicians and nurses were found to have a generally inaccurate knowledge base about the pharmacologic properties of analgesics, although the findings should be viewed with caution as the sample size was small. Often, care of the terminally ill patient in the acute care setting was described as haphazard, insensitive, and sometimes even cruel and inhuman. It appeared that few attempts to educate professionals about appropriate care of the patient in pain had been initiated. When asked, most respondents said they had accumulated their knowledge from fellow clinicians and their own experience. Charap recommended a renewed emphasis in professional education on pharmacologic properties of drugs and the clarification of the meaning of addiction, tolerance, and physical dependence, as well as on improving the general knowledge of physicians and nurses about pain management.

Weis et al.[99] used a survey methodology to examine house staff physicians' and nurses' beliefs about the goal of postoperative analgesia, the appropriate use of co-analgesics, the prevalence of addiction and respiratory depression, use of placebos, and knowledge of analgesic drug properties. Results of this survey are summarized in Table 4-2. Several important findings emerged from the responses to the questionnaire. Only 22 percent of respondents viewed *complete* relief of pain as the goal of pain management. Questions related to awareness of pertinent pharmacologic properties of the

Table 4-2
Responses of Housestaff and Nurses to Multiple-Choice
Questions

	(%)	
Category	Housestaff	Nurses
Goal of postoperative analgesic treatment:		
Complete pain relief	22.8	21.4
Enough relief that pain is noticed but not distressing	63.1	54.2
Moderate relief with a small degree of distress	12.2	11.2
Pain relief only at peak periods of pain	0.0	8.6
Unanswered	1.7	4.3
Effect of promethazine when added to a narcotic analgesic:		
Markedly increases the analgesic effect	19.3	44.2
Slightly increases the analgesic effect	71.9	48.6
Decreases the analgesic effect	0.0	0.0
Makes no change in the analgesic effect	7.0	5.7
Unanswered	1.7	1.4
Effect of amphetamine when added to a narcotic analgesic:		
Markedly increases the analgesic effect	10.5	18.6
Slightly increases the analgesic effect	21.1	20.0
Decreases the analgesic effect	29.8	24.2
Makes no change	28.1	20.0
Unanswered	10.0	17.1
Chance of addiction when a 70-kg patient received 100 mg of meperidine intramuscularly every 4 h for 10 days:		
Less than 1%	15.8	11.4
1–5%	28.0	15.7
6–15%	17.5	20.0
16–50%	22.8	27.1
>50%	15.8	21.4
Unanswered	0.0	4.3
Chance of developing respiratory depression when a 70-kg patient received a single dose of 16 mg of morphine intramuscularly:		
Less than 1%	33.3	25.7
1–5%	33.3	28.5
5–10%	12.3	12.8
11–15%	8.8	15.7
>15%	12.3	17.0
Unanswered	0.0	0.0

From Weis OF, Sriwatanakul K, Alloza JL, et al.: Attitudes of patients, housestaff, and nurses toward post-operative analgesic care. Anesth Analg 62:70–74, 1983. Reprinted with permission.

co-analgesics promethazine and amphetamine revealed a fair amount of misinformation among physicians and nurses. For instance, an overwhelming majority of both nurses and physicians agreed that promethazine markedly or slightly increased the analgesic effect of narcotics. Factual support for this belief does not exist, as research findings on the analgesic properties of promethazine are divergent. The general consensus is that sedation and not analgesia is enhanced with concomitant use of promethazine and a narcotic.[55,56,79] In contrast, only 31.6 percent of physicians and 38.6 percent of nurses knew that amphetamines *enhanced* analgesic effects of narcotics, a fact that has been substantiated.[34] There were the usual fears of addiction, but little concern about the potential for respiratory depression in the postoperative patients receiving narcotic analgesics. In summary, this survey clearly illustrated the need for more appropriate instruction about analgesics in the basic education of both nurses and physicians.

Nurses' attitudes, knowledge, and clinical behaviors have been specifically addressed by several researchers.[22,35,39,80] Cohen[22] conducted a study in which she replicated the methodology of Marks and Sachar[65] in a nursing population. The study consisted of two parts, one to assess and describe adequacy of pain relief in hospitalized postoperative patients, and the other to describe how nurses selected analgesics. In part one, Cohen learned that many patients who had marked or moderate distress from their pain were not receiving as much analgesic as they could have, a finding very similar to Marks and Sachar.[65] Additionally, she learned from the results of part two that nurses were unduly concerned about addiction, had inadequate knowledge of analgesics, and made somewhat irrational choices of amounts of medications to administer.

Fox[35] studied attitudes, knowledge, and clinical behaviors of nurses in a two-part exploratory study. Through an audit of medical records, she found that inadequate pain assessment was a major problem in the nursing care of patients with pain. Nurses' notes of "c/o pain × 2" or "no complaints" failed to adequately describe the quality of the pain experienced by patients. In addition, the average number of changes in analgesic regimen was four, with a range from 0 to 11, probably reflecting a nonspecific plan for analgesic management. Through administration of a questionnaire to nurses, Fox sought to identify preferences for narcotic analgesics, awareness of common side effects of narcotics, understanding of equianalgesic dosages, knowledge of potential drug interactions, understanding of PRN versus around-the-clock (ATC) schedules, and cognizance of the concepts of equianalgesia and tolerance. She identified many shortcomings in nurses' knowledge and understanding of pain management, including misunderstanding of narcotic side effects and analgesic schedules. An important finding was that 65 percent of the study participants stated they felt less than adequate, or grossly inadequate, in terms of cancer pain management expertise. Again, the findings indicated a clear need for better education. Fox recommended structured educational programs, with an emphasis on optimal patterns of narcotic analgesia.

In another study, Myers[80] examined knowledge and attitudes toward cancer pain in a sample of 65 nurses. Using a pre- and post-test design, she assessed differences in knowledge, attitude, and comfort-orientation before and after subjects participated in a three-hour educational session. Mean overall scores were lower than post-test scores (p = .01), and knowledge scores increased in 39 percent of the participants. Myers concluded that an educational intervention addressing both knowledge and attitude was beneficial to nurses, thus providing support for implementation of improved nursing education programs related to pain management in various settings.

Another researcher recently evaluated the impact of education on both knowledge and attitudes toward cancer pain using separate tools to measure each.[39] Experimental and control groups completed each instrument at pre- and post-test sessions, with the experimental group participating in a two-hour education program on pain management. Pre-test knowledge scores of the two groups revealed no significant differences. Following the education program, the experimental group demonstrated a significant improvement from their pre-test scores on the knowledge measure, again providing support for education programs on pain management.

Recommendations for Professional Education

Misconceptions about pain are difficult to erase, and information once held as unquestionable clinical wisdom may no longer be appropriate (i.e., use of phenergan and meperidine for pain). The notion that clinical specialists (physicians and nurses) in selected areas (i.e., oncology) may be more attuned to pain because of their specialization may be unfounded. A recent telephone survey of oncology nurses with a practice focus in pain management indicated that they had gained most of their knowledge about pain management from clinical practice and self-directed learning.[75] Respondents expressed the sentiment that baccalaureate nursing programs generally provided inadequate instruction on pain. They also reported that they were exposed to more specialized knowledge of pain at the master's and doctoral levels of study. A multitude of misconceptions plague the assessment and management of pain in the pediatric population, many of which are motivated by lack of knowledge. Several pediatric practitioners review and discuss this area in some depth.[6,28,40,67,83]

Education programs for health professionals have clearly been remiss in their treatment of the clinical management of pain. Most health care providers, including nurses, learn to assess and manage pain using the acute pain model. As a result, many clinicians expect to observe the behaviors seen with acute pain in all patients experiencing pain. Objective signs such as pallor, restlessness, grimacing, and tachycardia are believed to be

Table 4-3
Summary of Position Statement on Drug Therapy for Severe
Chronic Pain in Terminal Illness

1. The goal of drug therapy for severe, chronic pain in terminal illness is to make the patient relatively pain-free.

2. Oral administration of narcotics on a regular basis will relieve the pain of most terminally ill patients as well as relieve them from the fear of pain recurring.

3. No clinical evidence exists to indicate that the availability of heroin will improve pain care for patients with severe, chronic pain of terminal illness.

4. Fear of patients becoming dependent on narcotics is unfounded in the context of terminal illness.

5. The American College of Physicians accepts its responsibility to improve the internist's knowledge of drug therapy in such pain.

6. The American College of Physicians supports expanded research in the field of narcotic therapeutics.

Adapted from Health and Public Policy Commitee, American College of Physicians: Drug therapy for severe, chronic pain in terminal illness. Ann Intern Med 99:870–873, 1983. With permission.

consistent with the presence of pain, so the reports of pain by patients not exhibiting such behaviors are subject to skepticism. This traditional approach to pain assessment and management has been passed on via generations of health professionals, and unfortunately is deeply ingrained in the practice of many individuals. In order to address this problem, considerable reform in education curricula is warranted.

Weis et al.[99] made several recommendations as a result of their findings. Education programs for health professionals should include content reflecting pharmacologic properties of various analgesics, co-analgesics, and narcotic antagonists. Factual data about each drug's duration of action, dosage range, and appropriate dosing intervals must be given. Finally, the importance of the goal of complete pain relief and the need for continuous assessment of pain throughout the clinical trajectory of the pain experience should be stressed. Although these recommendations emanated from a study of postoperative patients with acute pain, the principles are applicable to management of chronic pain as well. The American College of Physicians has published a position statement on drug therapy for severe chronic pain.[41] This should be taught at the basic levels of professional education (see Table 4-3).

Although continuing professional education is a well accepted part of the health professions, its role in helping to improve the management of patients with cancer pain still needs clarification. Several investigators have demonstrated the efficacy of education programs relevant to pain management in improving professionals knowledge and/or attitudes,[37,39,80] but further research is needed.

Attitudes

Educational deficiencies have not been the only issue contributing to problems in the management of pain. Often, clinicians maintain attitudes and biases about pain that distort their view of the patient with pain and interfere with appropriate care. Allport[3] defined the term "attitudes" as a cognitive factor, based on experience that influences an individual's responses to relevant events. Attitudes toward pain, therefore, can directly affect the quality of care by exerting significant control over the clinician's behaviors related to care. McCaffery[66] presented a number of health professionals' misconceptions that hamper assessment of the patient in pain (see Table 4-4). These misconceptions vividly demonstrate the power that professionals' attitudes may wield over their behavior.

Many of the same authors who evaluated the knowledge of health professionals also assessed their attitudes about pain in general, patients in pain, and the optimal care of such patients. Many attitudinal biases revolve around the issue of potential for iatrogenic addiction, as revealed by several of the studies discussed above.[22,65,99] Clearly, these biases were a motivating factor in the care behaviors of health professionals.

Clarification of the meaning of addiction and related terms is important. *Drug abuse* is a voluntary behavioral response where a person uses drugs in a culturally unacceptable manner. *Drug addiction* is a voluntary, overwhelming involvement with obtaining and using drugs for psychic effects, rather than for legitimate therapy of medical problems. *Physical dependence* is an involuntary physiologic event that follows repeated administration of a narcotic, where withdrawal symptoms will occur if the drug is not taken.[66] The correct meanings of these terms need to be shared with oncology clinicians and disseminated in the professional, as well as the lay public, literature.

Many factors related to attitudes about pain were obtained from research about nurses' inferences of patients' pain, suffering, and psychological distress. Davitz and Davitz and their colleagues have made extensive contributions to knowledge in this area. In an early study,[5] physicians and nurses were discovered to discern less suffering in patients than did social workers. In a related study,[61] nurses and physicians again inferred a lesser dimension of pain than did nuns and teachers. In addition, a third study[24] revealed that first year nursing students inferred more physical pain than did second year nursing students, but second year students inferred slightly higher psychological distress. The conceptual thread common to these findings is the tendency for groups with a heavier exposure to the clinical setting to infer lesser degrees of physical pain. Particularly salient to oncology clinicians is whether this tendency to infer less pain with increased

Table 4-4
Misconceptions that Hamper Assessment of the Patient with Pain

Misconception	Correction
1. Health team members are the authorities on the existence and nature of the patient's pain.	The patient is the authority on his pain. Pain is whatever the experiencing person says it is, existing whenever he says it does. The patient is believed.
2. The patient who use his pain to obtain benefits or preferential treatment does not hurt as much as he says and may not hurt at all.	The patient who uses his pain to his own advantage may still hurt as much as he says he does.
3. The patient's pain can always be verified by the presence of certain behavior and/or physiological expressions of pain.	Physiological and behavioral adaptation occur, leading to periods of little or no signs of pain. Lack of pain expression does not mean lack of pain.
4. All "real" pain has an identifiable physical cause.	Not all physical causes of pain can be identified. All pain is real, regardless of its cause. Calling pain imaginary does not make it go away.
5. Psychogenic pain does not really hurt and is almost the same as malingering.	A localized sensation does exist in psychogenic pain.
6. The severity and duration of pain can be predicted accurately on the basis of the stimuli for pain.	There is no direct and invariant relationship between any stimulus and the perception of pain.
7. All patients can and should be encouraged to have a high tolerance for pain.	Pain tolerance is the individual's unique response, varying between patients and in the same patient from one situation to another.
8. Health team members tend to make accurate inferences about the severity and existence of the patient's pain.	Health team members tend to infer less pain than the patient experiences.

From McCaffery M: Nursing Management of the Patient with Pain (2nd ed.). Philadelphia, JB Lippincott, 1979. Reprinted with permission.

patient contact exists in cancer care settings. This author suggests that this phenomenon does not occur, but the question has not been systematically evaluated.

Sociocultural variables were also explored by Davitz and Davitz.[24] Both the cultural background of the nurse and the patient seem to influence inferences of pain and suffering. Collectively, all nurses inferred lesser psychological distress due to pain in children than in adults and in men than in women. However, the nurses often disagreed on degrees of pain and suffering when various ethnic groups were assessed. For example, less pain was inferred in Oriental patients by American nurses than any other group. This research on the influences cultural background has on pain has a profound impact on health care settings, since interactions among clinicians and patients of many cultures are a routine event.

Strategies for Improving Knowledge and Attitudes

It is clear that prevailing educational approaches to pain management are inadequate in preparing health care professionals to manage clinical pain. Issues affecting proper use of drugs in managing pain are summarized in Table 4-5. Less clear is how to address this problem. In the studies evaluating the effect of education on posteducational program test scores, short-term positive effects were noted but little or no follow-up was done to ascertain if the changes persisted over time.[39,80] Whether educational interventions aimed at altering knowledge and attitudes have a lasting effect should be assessed by longitudinal studies.

New implications for professional education also emerge in the context of attitudes toward pain and pain management. With more appropriate teaching about pain management incorporated into the basic education of health professionals, will their attitudes be more comfort-oriented than those of clinicians educated earlier? Further, what specific sorts of educational interventions might create an enduring impact on the attitudes of clinicians already in practice? Reed-Ash[85] recently discussed this problematic area and suggested strategies based on principles of adult education with an emphasis on lifelong learning. She urged the use and evaluation of creative approaches in both basic and continuing education. Recommendations for achieving this broad goal are outlined in Table 4-6.

Another area for attention is the absence of a pertinent role model who displays optimal pain management behaviors in many clinical settings. If

Table 4-5
Issues Affecting Proper Use of Drugs for Pain

- Use of PRN as opposed to around-the-clock analgesia.
- Fear of causing addiction.
- Inappropriate pain assessment.
- Faulty knowledge about drug pharmacology.
- Prescription of inadequate dosages.
- Failure to "titrate to effect."
- Withholding narcotics until death is imminent.
- Failure to manage and prevent expected side effects of narcotics.
- Failure to administer prescribed doses of medication without proper cause.

Table 4-6
Recommendations for Improving Health Care Professionals'
Skills in Pain Management

- Increased participation in continuing education programs on pain management.

- Increased educational exposure to pharmacologic principles relevant to pain care, with emphasis on the commonly used non-narcotic, narcotic, and adjuvant analgesics.

- Exposure to pertinent resources on management of pain.

- Discussion of pain articles in journal clubs.

- Awareness of the influence of attitudes, biases, and beliefs about pain and pain management.

- Examination of research related to inferences of pain.

- Discussion of research findings relevant to clinical specialties (i.e., oncology, hospice care, postoperative pain management).

- Orientation to severe pain in the cancer patient as an oncologic emergency.

- Increased emphasis on the assessment and documentation of pain in the clinical setting.

- Socialization into a clinical setting where pain care is a high priority.

- Exposure to role models with expertise in pain management.

- Referral to consultants for difficult pain management problems.

- Exposure to non-invasive pain relief methods, with clinical experience in the use of these methods.

- Peer pressure when pain is inadequately managed and staff are not assertive in pursuing strategies for relief of pain.

---

specific behaviors and attitudes are not observed in the clinical setting in which the clinician is socialized, the likelihood of those behaviors and attitudes being adopted is decreased. As noted by Strauss et al.,[91] the care of patients with pain must be supported as an organizational priority. In settings where accountability for such care is not expected of the staff, those individuals who pursue changes in patient management may be viewed as deviant. On the other hand, it is possible that observation of others exercising specific positive behaviors and attitudes could be considered a challenge by the individual clinician to improve his or her own pain care practices. Oncology clinical nurse specialists are excellent role models, since many of them possess extensive knowledge about pain management. The potential impact of the oncology clinical nurse specialist on pain management needs to be investigated.

Aside from the strategies presented above, it is also important that clinical settings provide good resources and reference materials for clinicians. McCaffery's[66] text is an excellent resource for nurses and others interested in the care of patients with pain, as is a more recent book by Meinhart and McCaffery.[72] Much material is included in these volumes, making them succinct and pertinent references for problems in pain assessment and management. An additional valuable reference is a book on control of cancer pain by Twycross and Lack.[97] Oncology nurses, as well as other groups of nurses specializing in pain, have addressed the high priority of pain relief in their standards for care.[82] The general care setting is the most critical target area for education about pain management. Health care professionals may not be motivated to learn more about pain care, but as Meinhart and McCaffery[72] have asserted, inattention to pain management may be viewed as inhumane, negligent treatment. Increased knowledge and better attitudes about pain management must be a collective priority of all clinicians.

ISSUES IN APPROPRIATE PHARMACOLOGIC MANAGEMENT

Despite significant advancement in techniques for control of pain, the collective behavior of health care providers often prohibits implementation of the most effective strategies. Fears, attitudes, and prejudices that are probably motivated by a lack of knowledge and understanding are still pervasive enough to prevent control of cancer pain. These sentiments most certainly apply to the use of analgesics and other drugs for cancer patients. Jacox and Rogers[47] commented, "the failure of analgesics to control pain has been primarily due to inadequate knowledge of the pharmacology of analgesics and the misconceptions and attitudes of those health care professionals who are involved in the care of people who have pain caused by cancer . . . (p. 394)."

PRN Versus ATC Scheduling

McCaffery[66] stated that prevention of severe pain is easier than to relieve it once it occurs. Narcotics administered on a regular (around-the-clock or ATC) schedule may result in decreased dosages necessary to control chronic pain because the intensity of pain is consistently less using this schedule.[94] Traditionally, narcotics are administered sparingly because of the problems detailed earlier. As greater knowledge about the clinical application of pain strategies is disseminated, the practice of *pro re nata* (PRN) scheduling appears to be slowly changing. The preponderance of literature supporting ATC administration of narcotics comes from hospice data, much of which originated in England. For instance, Twycross[96] declared, "persistent pain requires preventative therapy" (p. 17), and

Saunders[86] suggested that chronic pain requires continuous treatment. These notions have become more accepted in this country, and many settings have completely replaced PRN scheduling. Unfortunately, there is a paucity of research data examining whether ATC scheduling is the best schedule for pain control.

McGuire et al.[70] examined ATC and PRN analgesics in 47 cancer out-patients. Both the efficacy of each regimen and patients' subjective assess-ments of their regimens were evaluated. Of the 47 patients studied, 27 constituted a comparison group while 20 were in the experimental group. Eight were assigned to a PRN and 12 to an ATC schedule. No differences in pain intensity ratings over a five-day period between patients on the two schedules were observed. Several reasons for these findings were offered, including possibly inadequate doses of narcotics, potentially inadequate intervals between doses, the use of various narcotics, unique responses to narcotic analgesics, problems with pain measurement, and small sample size.

Clearly, McGuire et al.'s research examined an issue that is extremely difficult to evaluate in the clinical setting. The findings did not lend support to the contention that PRN is a deficient method of analgesic administration, nor did they support the use of ATC scheduling, but several important methodologic issues and physiologic factors that warrant further attention by researchers were cited.[70]

A database is needed to support or refute administering narcotics on an ATC schedule, including factors that influence efficacy of schedules. There are numerous ways to generate such information, including collaborative research efforts intra- and interinstitutionally, as well as locally, regionally, and nationally, to increase sample size and generalize results. One potential strategy would assess the pain management regimens of a group of patients, focusing on patterns of analgesic self-care, medication preference, and satisfaction with the degree of pain relief achieved. In a variation of this approach, the distribution of pain diaries to patients upon prescription of narcotics would provide information about self-administration practices and self-reported pain relief scores. In both variations, patients could be retro-spectively assigned to groups based on their medication use, and the effects of schedules evaluated through comparisons of pain relief and/or satisfaction with the regimen.

Prospective studies raise some ethical concerns especially with regard to randomization (i.e., if care givers believe a particular method of drug administration is more efficacious, or if patients believe a particular method is better). However, a potential strategy to overcome this problem would be to thoroughly explain the reasons for the study in the informed consent so that patient participation could be maximized. Controlling for intensity of pain, physical performance status, age, and disease site through stratifica-tion might provide additional information on effects of analgesic schedule in relation to these variables. It may be that individuals with different cancer pain syndromes respond differently to pain control regimens. Perhaps PRN analgesia is effective in instances when pain is intermittent. Although many patients find ATC analgesia necessary and effective, there are some who are satisfied with PRN analgesia. Clearly, this area deserves further attention.

Age may be a real factor in pain management and appropriate analgesic scheduling.[10,52] Ettinger et al.[30] commented on adverse sequelae of methadone used in the elderly. Perhaps various schedules of analgesia have some role in the elderly patient, but exact roles are unclear as yet. Finally, the issue of compliance might also be explored in addressing analgesia schedules for pain control. Donabedian and Rosenfeld[27] found a positive relationship between self-medication compliance and the disability associated with the disease under study. Recent investigators[4] reported that patient non-compliance was an important factor among hospice patients with severe pain. Half of the patients with severe pain did not adhere to the prescribed pain management regimen. When queried, patients often stated that they were concerned about addiction and retention of personal control over their situation. Other authors[36,93] described self-imposed resistance to therapeutic regimens as well, so it is clear that the issue of compliance must be examined in the context of the PRN versus ATC question.

In the absence of clinical trials substantiating the positive effects of ATC analgesia, there is clinical anecdotal experience that affirms ATC as the method of choice for controlling cancer pain in most situations.[43] Individual practitioners, however, must be guided by patients' clinical responses to any course of therapy, with trial and error guiding the plan for management.

Twycross[95] stated that PRN medication has no place in the treatment of chronic pain. Prevention of pain by administering subsequent analgesic doses before previous doses become ineffective allows the patient to become more relaxed and to anticipate that pain will not become worse. Several authors[86,97] suggest that pain is a strong antagonist to analgesia, and that preventive pain therapy ameliorates the anxiety associated with "anticipated" pain.

McCaffery[66] discussed several issues germane to PRN analgesia. The first entailed a lack of clarity about what the term PRN implies. Does it signify giving a drug at the first indication of pain or should medication be administered only when pain is severe? A second issue referred to the way orders are written. Is the nurse allowed latitude in the interpretation of a physician's order? A complete discussion of these and other issues may be found in McCaffery.[66]

An extremely important concept relative to the ATC versus PRN question is the notion of titrating the amount of drug to achieve pain relief but without causing undue toxicity. Obviously, analgesics must be administered on a schedule that is consistent with the pharmacologic properties of each drug. Dosage schedules must be individualized according to both patient-related and drug-related criteria. For instance, in some patients, levorphanol may adequately relieve pain when it is administered every six hours. Other patients may have undue sedation with the same amount and schedule, and thus might benefit from smaller doses at more frequent intervals. This variability exists for virtually all narcotic analgesics, and there are no hard and fast rules for all clinical situations.

This author advocates the administration of ATC analgesia based on clinical experience and anecdotal support in the literature. It may be effective for the control and perhaps prevention of cancer pain. In certain circumstances, patients' analgesic requirements may be so low as to require PRN analgesia. However, in moderate to severe cancer pain, ATC analgesia produces a multitude of benefits, not the least of which is the degree of confidence the patient may have in health care personnel when pain is relieved or decreased. Pain that is prevented or only mild in severity creates less anxiety and possibly less pain for the patient. Because of a decrease in overall pain intensity, less medication may be required to control pain. The absence of pain, or a reduction in its intensity, allows the patient to focus on other aspects of life. And finally, minimal pain allows the patient to erase the memory of a severe pain experience, thereby possibly reducing anxiety and worry. In conclusion, however, one must bear in mind that the contention that ATC analgesia is superior to PRN is based on clinical anecdotal evidence. Substantiation through controlled research is necessary to clearly establish ATC analgesia as the method of choice.

Use of Inappropriate Drugs

Drug therapy in the cancer patient should involve careful scrutiny of the appropriateness of a particular agent in a specific clinical situation. Certain drugs are viewed as inappropriate in the cancer pain setting because of attendant problems associated with their use.

Meperidine

The use of meperidine in the patient with cancer pain is a practice that is not recommended. Several reasons exist for this recommendation. One problem is the need for very large oral (PO) doses (200–300 mg) in order to achieve the equianalgesic effect of 75 mg administered intramuscularly (IM). Since it is unusual for such high PO doses to be prescribed, most patients experience significant reductions in their degree of analgesia when meperidine is converted from the IM to PO route of administration. A second problem is that when meperidine is administered over extended periods of time it is associated with severe fibrosis of muscle tissue, a problem only compounded when it is used in the advanced cancer patient. Finally, its short duration of action (2–3 hours) necessitates repeated administration and excessive tissue trauma.[7] These factors alone constitute meperidine being a poor choice for cancer patients,[68] but recent experimental evidence suggests additional central nervous system (CNS) toxicity.

In a study of 67 patients receiving meperidine for postoperative or chronic pain, Kaiko et al.[50] analyzed the relationship between CNS toxicity and plasma levels of meperidine (and its metabolite, normeperidine). Normeperidine is a potent CNS excitatory agent, so its accumulation is cause for concern. Patients who received repeated administration of meperidine over approximately 6–8 days displayed both increased plasma levels of normeperidine and attendant CNS symptoms such as tremor, twitches, myoclonus, and seizures.[50] A previous investigation indicated that higher serum normeperidine/meperidine levels were documented in patients with renal failure than in cancer patients.[92] Kaiko et al.[50] noted that while altered renal function may be a factor in normeperidine accumulation, patients with normal renal function also exhibited elevated normeperidine levels and the previously described neurologic signs. Another portion of Kaiko et al.'s[51] study assessed mood changes from days one to two in postoperative patients receiving meperidine or another narcotic. Those treated with meperidine reported feeling angry, "blue," sad, restless, pessimistic, apprehensive, and shaky at a significantly higher level than those treated with other drugs.

In summary, these studies demonstrate that chronic administration of meperidine may result in toxic accumulations of normeperidine and associated CNS disturbances. In addition, mood changes may result with prolonged use of this drug. Finally, renal function contributes to exacerbation of these problems, a finding that may have application in the setting of cancer pain. These recent findings, in addition to the problems discussed earlier, clearly limit the usefulness of meperidine as an appropriate analgesic for pain associated with cancer.

Mixed Agonist-Antagonist Drugs

Several agents are included in the narcotic antagonist category, many of which are classified as mixed agonist–antagonists. Pentazocine, nalbuphine, and butorphanol are included in this group, but only pentazocine is available for oral administration. Because of their tendency to produce psychotomimetic effects as doses are increased, these drugs have limited usefulness in cancer pain. Further, they contribute to precipitation of withdrawal in patients who have received previous narcotic analgesics and who are physically dependent on such drugs.[9,38] As noted by Beaver et al.,[9] the role of these agents in cancer pain remains to be ascertained, but may be most appropriate early in the onset of pain, prior to the use of narcotics. Catalano discusses the mixed agonist-antagonist drugs in more detail.[17,18]

The Brompton Cocktail

The lay public as well as many clinicians continue to perceive the pain cocktail as a panacea for the control of cancer pain, despite evidence that such cocktails may have little benefit compared to single analgesics. A variety of pain cocktails have been reported, including Brompton's cocktail,[74]

Schlessinger's solution,[97] and Val-Steck elixir.[98] Since the Brompton's cocktail enjoys the greatest popularity, it will be discussed at length.

Snow[89] was the first to record the use of a morphine and cocaine mixture for the relief of cancer pain in 1896, however, the high cost of cocaine contributed to its deletion from this formulation.[90] The Brompton cocktail was eventually reintroduced at the Brompton Chest Hospital for treatment of postthoracotomy pain. Concurrently, many similar pain cocktails were used throughout Britain.[57] As the hospice concept took hold in the United States, interest in the Brompton cocktail grew. Although the exact drugs vary, the usual mixture contains morphine as the analgesic component, cocaine as a stimulant, ethyl alcohol as a preservative, and syrup for flavoring.[63] Because narcotics are often emetogenic, a phenothiazine is usually dispensed along with the pain cocktail to prevent nausea and vomiting.

The value of such pain cocktails probably has little to do with the unique ingredients of any particular formulation. Increasing evidence suggests that regular dosing is the most important "ingredient" of the Brompton cocktail.[77] In fact, several of the drugs in the cocktail have been scrutinized and the findings are relevant to this issue. Twycross and Lack[97] studied a group of patients in a crossover trial comparing opiate cocktails both with and without cocaine. They found that when cocaine was delivered in small regular doses, tolerance developed within several days and the mental alacrity of all patients remained unaffected, implying that they fared equally well with or without cocaine. A separate study[73] compared the Brompton cocktail to morphine and yielded no significant differences with respect to pain, nausea, drowsiness, or confusion.

Catalano[18] stated that morphine is the primary cause of beneficial effects from the Brompton's cocktail. In institutions where pain cocktails continue to enjoy popularity, special attention is warranted when increasing the dose of analgesic. As the analgesic is increased, so is the stimulant, which can result in toxicity due to excessive CNS stimulation. Thus, for patients requiring a higher dose of analgesic, single entity narcotics are preferable. In patients using pain cocktails who have persistent drowsiness from the narcotic that interferes with quality of life, Twycross and Lack[97] proposed occasional use of dextroamphetamine 2.5 to 5.0 mg administered in the early morning and at about 3:00 p.m. Caffeine or caffeine-containing beverages during waking hours may also counteract the sedative effect of narcotics, allowing increased alertness without side effects.[66]

Ethyl alcohol is also a component of pain cocktails. Melzack et al.[73] analyzed morphine solution (without ethyl alcohol) after a shelf-life of one week, discovering contamination with yeasts, fungi, and bacteria. Inclusion of 1.5 ml of 98 percent ethyl alcohol per 20 ml dose prevented such alterations in the solution and extended the shelf-life of the morphine solution. Some patients, particularly those with oral or esophageal ulcerations,may experience local pain because of the effect of the alcohol on such lesions.[97]

According to Wescoe and Salter,[100] the optimal pain cocktail need only contain an opiate (usually morphine), since the Brompton cocktail is no more effective than single agents. Perhaps the most important point relative to pain cocktails is that their use should be within the context of total patient care. In most instances, when sound pharmacologic principles are adhered to, virtually any narcotic can be as effective as the pain cocktail.[100]

Continuous Intravenous Infusion (CII)

Continuous intravenous infusion (CII) of narcotics has recently been described as a therapeutic alternative for patients with severe, intractable pain.[13,71,81] Because the narcotic is administered on a continuous basis, fluctuating blood levels of analgesic are eliminated and the patient receives better pain relief. In addition, peaks and troughs of analgesic effect are equilibrated, affording a more reliable level of analgesia and fewer untoward side effects. Although CII is particularly useful for patients whose pain is severe and unrelieved by conventional measures, it may be a reasonable choice in some specific situations for patients requiring parenteral analgesics. Thus, CII need *not* be limited to terminally ill patients in their last hours of life.

Selection of patients for CII can be facilitated by use of guidelines such as those presented in Table 4-7, although CII need not be restricted to these patients. McGuire and Wright[71] recommend that CII be considered whenever ATC administration of oral, injected, or rectal narcotics no longer controls a patient's pain. Unfortunately, inadequate trials of oral narcotics are often seen. Provided that an exhaustive trial of oral analgesia has occurred, CII may constitute a logical therapeutic alternative.

Some patients may be incapable of taking oral analgesics for a variety of reasons, including nausea and vomiting, gastrointestinal distress, small bowel obstruction, stomatitis, esophageal stricture, dysphagia, and tracheo-bronchial fistula. Other routes of drug administration, such as rectal, sub-cutaneous, and intramuscular, are not always feasible. Rectal suppositories may be contraindicated because of rectal involvement with tumor, proctitis, bone marrow suppression, or other problems with absorption.[15] The patient's analgesic requirement may also limit the usefulness of rectal suppositories, since efficacy requires a maximum of two suppositories per dose.[62]

Administration of parenteral analgesics is problematic as well. Bleeding dyscrasias, thrombocytopenia, and cachexia make administration difficult. Generally, the subcutaneous route is more easily tolerated and more easily used by patients and families than the intramuscular route.[62] Additionally, these methods of intermittent drug administration may not result in optimal analgesic effect with minimal side effects.

In all of the above situations, CII is a viable option. In addition, a

Table 4-7
General Guidelines for the Institution of Continuous Narcotic
Infusion

1. Does the patient experience inadequate analgesia with oral, rectal, or injectable narcotics?

2. Is the patient N.P.O. for any reason?

3. Does the patient experience nausea, vomiting, diarrhea, or other gastrointestinal distress with the oral route?

4. Does the patient have thrombocytopenia or some other bleeding problem?

5. Is the staff uncomfortable with administering narcotics on a regular schedule?

6. Does respiratory distress create difficulties in swallowing?

7. Is there a problem with inadequate muscle mass or with inadequate absorption due to multiple parenteral injections?

8. When appropriate doses of medication are given, is the patient unable to achieve pain relief?

9. Does the patient have a high narcotic requirement?

10. Does the patient have venous access? Is a venous access device advisable?

Adapted from Howard-Ruben J, McGuire L, Groenwald S: Pain, in Groenwald S (Ed): Cancer Nursing: Principles and Practice. Monterey, CA, Jones and Bartlett (in press). With permission.

number of other clinical situations may be amenable to CII, regardless of the patient's status (i.e., imminent death, expected recovery from an acute problem, etc.). Severe acute postoperative pain or pain occurring as a result of a sudden tissue injury (i.e., pathologic fracture) can be treated with CII. Severe chronic pain that has suddenly worsened and warrants rapid control can be managed with CII. Finally, severe chronic pain previously controlled by oral analgesics that can no longer be administered for a variety of reasons and severe pain associated with terminal cancer may also be treated with CII.

CII is only one method for the continuous infusion of narcotics. Several other routes include subcutaneous, epidural, intrathecal, and intraventricular. This chapter addresses only the intravenous route, as the others are covered elsewhere in this volume.[16,17,87] The discussion will focus on the issues of safety and efficacy of CII, since Catalano discusses the specific techniques used.[17]

Safety and Efficacy

Reports of CII of morphine have appeared with greater frequency in both the medical and nursing literature and are summarized in Table 4-8. Unfortunately, CII of morphine has been used hesitantly or not even considered because patients are not yet deemed "terminal" enough. The

Table 4-8
Studies of Continuous Intravenous Infusion of Narcotics

Report	Age	Dose Range/ Hour	Duration of Infusion	Side Effects	Comments	Drug Preparation
Holmes[42]	NR	40–95 mg/hr	30-70 d	NR	Reasonably alert and coherent, good pain control	500 mg Morphine sulfate in sterile water added through 0.22 micron filter 500 ml of D5W resulting in 1 mg/ml. An infusion pump employed.
Entsworth[29]	NR	5–144 mg/hr	1 pt-6 d 1 pt-at least 5 d	• Local phlebitis. • Agitation. • Restlessness. • Nightmares, tremors & diaphoresis in one patient.	Both patients were alert. One patient free of pain.	Initial drug preparation: 240 mg Morphine Sulfate and 50 mg Chlorpromazine added to 482 ml of D5W, resulting in a concentration of 0.48 mg/ml. An infusion pump was not used; 100 cc of solution was administered by volutrol using a microdrip.
Kowolenko[59]	NR	NR	NR	NR	Patients described as more coherent and less lethargic.	Infusion pump essential. Caution about use of narcotic antagonists. Suggests respiratory depression should be treated by mechanical means.

(continued)

Table 4-8 (*continued*)
Studies of Continuous Intravenous Infusion of Narcotics

Report	Age	Dose Range/ Hour	Duration of Infusion	Side Effects	Comments	Drug Preparation
Miser et al.[76]	3–16 yrs	0.8 to 80 mg/ hr	1–16 d	Constipation, mild drowsiness, decrease in respiratory rate to 10 breaths per minute.	Satisfactory pain relief. The physician, nurse, patient and parent(s) determined the rate of infusion based on achievement of maximal pain relief with minimal drowsiness. Side effects easily controlled.	Continuous infusion in a dextrose-saline vehicle via an infusion pump.
O'Donnell & Papciak[81]	Adults (aged 41, 74)	0.4–3.2 mg/ hr	1–2 d	Sedated, respiratory rate of 6–10. One patient described as restless.	One patient was experiencing liver failure and small bowel obstruction prior to initiation of IV morphine infusion. The second patient did not receive an adequate trial because of an administrative decision to stop the infusion.	100 mg morphine in 250 mg D5W via an infusion pump.

(*continued*)

Table 4-8 (*continued*)
Studies of Continuous Intravenous Infusion of Narcotics

Report	Age	Dose Range/ Hour	Duration of Infusion	Side Effects	Comments	Drug Preparation
Boyer[13]	NR	1-20 mg/hr	NR	Less lethargic, more coherent less short of breath, less anxious. Also noted decreased respiratory rate and slightly increased PC02.	One case was fully described. This patient was pain-free, mentally alert with a normal respiratory rate. This patient's pain, probably due to a pulmonary embolus, eventually resolved and she was discharged on oral analgesia.	50 mg morphine added to 500 cc D5W via rate-controlled infusion pump.
DeChristoforo et al.[25]	19 yr	Increased to maximum dose of 275 mg/hr	52 days Highest dose given for 4 days	Somnolence.	Patient received IV push morphine, methadone, radiotherapy, diazepam, and diphenhydramine, and other therapies to help control her symptoms. The effect of the preservative used in the preparation of morphine was explored and considered as a possible etiology for the patient's somnolence.	Continuous infusion of morphine diluted in 150 cc D5W.

(*continued*)

Table 4-8 (*continued*)
Studies of Continuous Intravenous Infusion of Narcotics

Report	Age	Dose Range/ Hour	Duration of Infusion	Side Effects	Comments	Drug Preparation
Citron et al.[20]	32–60 yrs	20–359 mg/ hr	1–80 d	Somnolence reduced respiratory rate.	A majority of the 13 patients studied experienced significant pain relief. Patients were generally able to walk, eat, and talk without difficulty. In some trials, adequate analgesia was not achieved for over 7 days.	Morphine infusion via IVAC pump.
Portenoy et al.[86]	1.5 yrs to 67 yrs	4-480 mg (mean maximum dose) Various narcotics used; see text.	1–45 days	Sedation & confusion, nausea/ vomiting, constipation, myoclonus, dizziness. Respiratory depression in one patient.	Side effects were difficult to assess because the patients in this survey were experiencing advanced cancer and concomitant medical problems. Sedation occurred with greatest frequency; respiratory depression occurred in 1 patient also receiving intrathecal morphine. Analgesia did not occur in one third of patients evaluated.	NR

NR = not reported.

91

purpose of the following discussion is to familiarize the reader with the literature pertaining to CII so that decisions about its use in the clinical setting may be made with greater facility, thus benefiting more patients.

Holmes[42] reported the use of IV morphine infusion in three patients in the final stages of cancer. Infusions were maintained for as long as 30–70 days; patients remained alert and coherent, and few dosage escalations were necessary once a consistent plasma state of morphine was attained. Entsworth[29] reported two patients treated with CII of morphine. One patient was free of pain at a dose of 144 mg/hr, reached after five days of therapy. The other experienced phlebitis at the infusion site, so it was discontinued; this individual also had untoward side effects (nature unclear) that ceased after the withdrawal of CII.

Kowolenko[59] offered technical recommendations related to IV infusion of morphine in a report of experiences with 12 patients. Caution was advised in the use of narcotic antagonists in the event of respiratory depression, with mechanical ventilation assistance available if an antagonist should precipitate a sympathetic crisis. The use of an infusion pump was mandated to prevent "withdrawal" effects should the infusion be interrupted in any fashion. Finally, alterations in dosage should be instituted only at the recommendation of an experienced clinical observer.

Miser et al.[76] reported eight pediatric patients who achieved satisfactory pain relief and experienced mild but easily controlled side effects. Some children became drowsy but not to the extent that their social interaction and play were affected. Continuous intravenous morphine was judged as a safe and effective intervention for children with severe pain due to malignancy.

Data from two reports in the nursing literature were related to CII of morphine in cancer patients. In one paper, two case reports were presented.[81] Many of the biases of nurses and physicians toward pain management were illustrated. The nursing staff interpreted the morphine infusion as the precipitating cause of one patient's death. The medical chief of staff discontinued the infusion in the other case because approved guidelines for infusion of narcotics were not available. As a result, the authors developed such guidelines, although their procedures for decreased respirations may be questioned on the basis of inadequate scientific rationale. In the other paper, Boyer[13] described experiences with seven patients. Pain relief was described as complete in four patients, satisfactory in one, and partial in the remaining two. The minimal hourly doses reported may have been insufficient; further dose escalation may have resulted in improved overall results.

Citron et al.[20] performed a prospective study of the safety and efficacy of CII of morphine in a group of cancer patients with severe pain. Variables that were studied included vital signs (respiratory rate, pulse, blood pressure), arterial blood gas values, mental status, and degree of pain relief. Vital signs and blood gas values did not vary enough to require intervention during the study period. While a decrease in respiratory rate was noted, there was no direct relationship between changes in respiratory rate and blood gas values for the first 96 hours. Slowing respiratory rate alone was not cause for reducing the rate of morphine infusion, and in the absence of mental status deterioration, the decreased respiratory rates demonstrated no clinical significance. Citron et al. also noted that somnolence *without* change in respiratory rate should alert the clinician to search for causes. For example, one patient who had an onset of somnolence and garbled speech in concert with stable blood gas values was discovered to be hypercalcemic.

Other investigators addressed somnolence and sedation as well. DeChristoforo et al.[25] described a single case where possible sedative effects of the chlorbutanol preservative used in the morphine may have contributed to somnolence. Portenoy et al.[84] suggested a trial of preservative-free morphine if excessive sedation was noted.

A variety of other drugs and dosages have been used in CII, as evidenced by a review of Memorial Sloan-Kettering's experience with opioid infusions.[84] Examples included methadone, hydromorphone, oxymorphone, and levorphanol. The mean starting dose for infusion was 17 mg/hr, with a range of 0.7 mg to 100 mg/hr; the maximum dose range from 4–480 mg/hr with an average of 69 mg/hr. Three dosing patterns were described: a relatively stable dosage range, a rapidly incremental pattern, and a rapidly increasing dosage that did not yield good pain relief, despite the addition of alternative pain relief strategies.

Safe use of CII of morphine in the home has also been described in a case report.[26] The patient received between 7–14 mg of morphine per hour over a ten-week period (via an ambulatory infusion pump) while remaining active, alert, and mobile. As expected, no undue toxicity was experienced by the patient and the therapy was managed at home with nurse visits for pump maintenance. Although Dennis[26] used a Cormed pump (Cormed, Inc., Medina, NY), the technique can easily be adapted to other types of ambulatory infusion pumps and venous access devices.

Recommendations

The studies described above indicate collectively that use of CII has established its potential as a safe and effective alternative to pain control in patients experiencing severe pain. Such infusions can be initiated with relative ease in inpatient and outpatient settings. Judicious use of CII is required, however, with acute awareness of pharmacology of narcotics and potential side effects. Unless a specific allergy or other intolerance to morphine exists, morphine is the drug of choice for CII therapy because of its low cost and wide availability.[71] In the event of intolerance, other narcotic analgesics can be substituted.[84]

The current lack of controlled clinical trials using CII is a problem. Safety, efficacy, and guidelines for initiation and use of CII must be further explored by careful research. The plight of the patient in pain, however, contributes to the difficulty of achieving this goal. In the meantime, few definitive conclusions about safety and efficacy can be stated with accuracy and confidence. However, empirical data from the use of CII in divergent settings (Table 4-8) does substantiate its usefulness and feasibility at the present time.

Co-Analgesics

Divergent opinions exist on the use of co-analgesics (also called adjuvant analgesics) in pain management, and their optimum use with cancer pain is discussed by Catalano.[17] When selecting co-analgesics, the most important consideration is that co-analgesics not be used as a substitute for optimal doses of narcotic analgesics. If the patient's major problem is pain, pain is the symptom that mandates aggressive treatment. The use of tranquilizers and hypnotics instead of adequate analgesics should not be tolerated.

Anti-inflammatory Drugs

Perhaps the most commonly used co-analgesics are aspirin or nonsteroidal anti-inflammatory drugs (NSAIDs) administered with a narcotic. The presence of painful osseous metastases frequently warrants use of an NSAID. If a narcotic is the major choice for pain control, but the patient experiences adverse effects, a possible course of action is to reduce the dose of narcotic and begin an anti-inflammatory agent such as aspirin or indomethacin. Often this simple technique helps take the edge off pain while allowing the patient to remain as alert and active as possible. It has been estimated that approximately 50 percent of patients with cancer have pain which might be controlled by NSAIDs alone.[54]

Steroids

Steroids provide relief for a number of pain syndromes attributable to cancer. Increased intracranial pressure, lymphedema, and spinal cord compression are several examples. Unfortunately, oral candidiasis may result as a sequela of long-term steroid therapy. Careful oral assessment and prophylactic antifungal agents should be used in conjunction with steroids. Another possible untoward effect is steroid myopathy, which may be difficult to diagnose in the oncology patient, as many complications of progressive cancer are manifested in sensorimotor changes.

Psychotropic Drugs

A variety of psychotropic agents may be used effectively in the management of cancer pain. The use of tranquilizers remains subject to debate, since they are sometimes used inappropriately to sedate the patient in an attempt to "quiet" complaints of pain.[69] Diazepam and hydroxyzine are supported as co-analgesics by some clinicians.[97] The former may be beneficial for patients with anxiety or insomnia, and can also relieve muscular tension. The latter has been demonstrated to potentiate the analgesic effects of morphine in postoperative patients,[8] and may also offer increased analgesia in cancer pain.

Antidepressants improve mood and relieve depression in selected patients. The analgesic effects of these drugs are believed to be linked to their enhancement of serotoninergic activity in the central nervous system. Neuroleptics may exercise their effect in a manner similar to opiates, as some influence on opiate receptors has been demonstrated.[21,88] In fact, several butyrophenones possess a greater analgesic effect than propoxyphene and meperidine[23] and their chemical structures are somewhat similar.[64] In summary, the advantages of psychotropic therapy in the oncology patient with pain can include augmented analgesic response in patients unresponsive to usual analgesics, enhanced analgesic effect, possible reductions in the dose of analgesia, and positive psychological benefits.[58]

Stimulants

The use of stimulants in cancer pain is discussed in the section on pain cocktails. Additionally, Forrest et al.[34] suggested that dextroamphetamine potentiates the analgesic effect of morphine, although without an apparent increase in mental alertness. This particular study incorporated a double-blind, single-dose methodology in postoperative patients. Findings revealed that dextroamphetamine 10 mg plus morphine afforded twice the analgesic effects as morphine alone. The results cannot be generalized to the patient receiving repeated doses of narcotic for cancer pain, so further research on the potentiating effect of dextroamphetamine in acute episodes of cancer pain may prove worthwhile. Routine use of this agent is not recommended except under unusual circumstances.

Conclusion

When persistent narcotic therapy offers limited analgesia, co-analgesics may be effective in improving pain control. Polypharmacy without thoughtful consideration of a patient's unique pain problems, however, is to be discouraged. When used judiciously, co-analgesia may be an excellent strategy for pain management. The simplest but most effective combination of drugs should be sought. Specific pain-related symptoms, the quality of pain, the patient's pertinent medical history, and potential drug interactions form the basis for decision-making about choices for co-analgesics.[12]

Heroin

The Compassionate Pain Relief Act, recently introduced in the United States legislative system, attracted much media attention to the issue of legalization of heroin for cancer pain. Some call this the "great non-issue of our day."[2] Proponents for legalization of heroin argue that all possible approaches to pain control should be made available to patients experiencing pain. Others have suggested that heroin possesses unique pharmacologic attributes that make it preferable for the treatment of cancer pain.[45,78] The majority of experienced pain researchers and clinicians feel that morphine and heroin are extremely similar in most aspects and not different enough to warrant legalization of heroin.[18,60] Evans[31] provides a comprehensive discussion on the use of heroin for cancer pain.

Kaiko[49] analyzed the effects of morphine and heroin on the basis of available data. The comparison of the two drugs yielded a number of similarities and some minor differences. Heroin was noted to be different from morphine with respect to its analgesic potency. Although reports vary slightly, milligram for milligram, heroin is said to be 1.5 to 2.0 times as potent as morphine,[46,49] suggesting that less heroin is required than morphine to achieve the same degree of analgesia, but this has no real clinical implication since drug effects can be equalized through the use of equianalgesic doses. In substantiation of this method, Twycross,[96] a proponent of heroin narcotic cocktails, found that equianalgesic doses of morphine and heroin were equally effective in relieving cancer pain, again at a 1.5 to 1.0 ratio, respectively.

Another supposed benefit of heroin is its higher dose per volume concentration for parenteral injection. If volume is a problem, hydromorphone is currently available in high potency preparations and is easily employed. Onset of analgesia differs slightly between morphine and heroin. Heroin analgesia occurs more rapidly than morphine but has a shorter duration. While rapid onset of analgesia might prove useful in certain circumstances, other available drugs or routes of administration can be used if fast analgesia is desired.

Heroin is described as a pro-drug, which implies that its major action occurs as a result of metabolic breakdown to its byproducts, monoacetyl morphine and morphine.[46] Pro-drugs tend to result in more unreliable effects both between and within patients, with a possible result of unpredictable analgesic effects. Thus, optimal dosage scheduling may be more difficult to attain in the patient ingesting ATC heroin than ATC morphine.

Heroin and morphine compare favorably along several parameters. For instance, there is no analgesic ceiling effect with either heroin or morphine. There are no major differences between the two drugs in the patterns of side effects and mood changes. Each has similar low oral bioavailabilities, so that oral equivalencies to parenteral dosage forms often must be escalated and may be somewhat variable.[49]

In practical terms, there are very few differences between the two drugs. While heroin has some properties that make it more convenient in specific circumstances, available data describe no particular unique aspects of heroin that make it preferable to any available narcotic analgesic.[32]

Catalano[18] echoed this sentiment, concluding that legalization of heroin for medicinal purposes does not appear to be a socially responsible position at this time. Because of heroin's potential for abuse, its availability in pharmacies could possibly increase crimes associated with its illegal procurement.[32] Brandt[14] cited a Department of Justice estimate of approximately 2600 pharmacists, employees, or customers either injured or killed as a result of robberies of controlled substances. One can imagine the bureaucracy and red tape that might be associated with dispensing heroin if pharmacists were even willing to stock it. As noted elsewhere in this paper, even many standard narcotic analgesics are often unavailable at pharmacies in a number of geographic settings. It is more appropriate that financial and administrative resources be directed at improving the use of current drugs and technologies than at the popular, though misguided, efforts to include heroin in the therapeutic armamentarium for the treatment of cancer pain.[1]

Experienced Drug Users

A special problem in the management of cancer pain involves the appropriate use of analgesics in the patient who is an experienced drug user. Obviously, previous use of unverifiable quantities of narcotic presents a particular dilemma. Initial narcotic requirements for pain control in such patients may seem incredibly large. Two major errors in patient management are that patients' complaints of pain are not taken seriously, with the staff ignoring requests for analgesics; and/or staff fail to recognize that the patient is indeed an addict, thus allowing unlimited amounts of narcotic to be administered.[97] A third potential problem is conflict among staff members as a result of manipulative behavior by such patients.

It must be emphasized that these problems refer specifically to those patients who truly have a drug addiction problem, not those who have taken narcotics solely for the relief of pain. This difficult situation may be outside the range of skills of oncology clinicians, and it may be advisable to include other professionals on the team caring for such patients. Narcotic addicts may require extremely large doses of narcotics to achieve relief of pain, largely due to the development of tolerance. Thus, recognition of a previous drug habit is crucial to the optimum resolution of this situation. Regardless of an existing drug habit, the patient with a narcotic addiction merits relief of pain just as any other patient.

Consultation with experts on substance dependence can serve several useful purposes in such circumstances. Above all, the patient's complaint of pain is seriously heeded, and intelligent management of the problem can ensue. Staff may experience negative feelings because they are providing drugs to an addict; consultation with experts can assuage some of the anger and guilt experienced by staff, and simultaneously affirm that they are helping the patient to achieve relief from pain. Twycross[97] provides succinct

Table 4-9
Guidelines for Helping the Patient Who was Narcotic-
Dependent Before Becoming Ill

1. Patient should be under the care of an experienced doctor, who is able to reasonably estimate narcotic requirements for the pain commonly associated with
   the patient's disease.
2. Patient should be under the care of an experienced oncology nurse, oncology
   clinical specialist, or hospice nurse who can appropriately tailor the patient's
   plan of care as well as consult with the nursing staff.
3. Narcotic prescription should be managed by only one physician.
4. Contingency plans must be made in the event of breakthrough pain.
5. Outside consultation synthesizing methods of cancer pain control and drug de-
   pendency care may be helpful, as most oncology staff will not be familiar with
   the care of narcotic-dependent patients.
6. Use the oral or rectal routes of drug administration as soon as possible. This
   serves two purposes: to break the association between the street ritual of drug
   injection and pain medicines and to create a new link between drugs and pain
   control. The patient should be instructed about the use of oral narcotics and advised that injectables will not be necessary for the purposes of pain control.

Adapted from Twycross R, Lack S: Symptom Control in Far Advanced Cancer: Pain Relief.
London, Pitman Publishing Limited, 1983.

guidelines for the care of the narcotic-dependent patient with cancer pain
(Table 4-9).

Availability of Narcotics

The prime concern in selecting an analgesic should be efficacy and
safety for a particular patient. It is not uncommon, however, for patients to
report difficulty in filling their narcotic prescriptions at local pharmacies.
Many pharmacies fail to stock specific narcotics because of a fear of robbery
or because they are dispensed so infrequently.[44,53] Kanner and Portenoy[53]
surveyed pharmacies in New York City to ascertain which narcotic analgesics were among their routine inventory. Their results are summarized in
Table 4-10. The apparent unavailability of certain drugs requires careful
planning to ensure that patients have adequate access to narcotics.

CONCLUSION

Clinicians, educators, and researchers have much to keep them busy in
the management of cancer pain. The preceding discussion has focused on
several issues, with an emphasis on the application of flawed knowledge in
the clinical setting. While it is clear that there are many explanations for this

Table 4-10
Availability of Narcotic Analgesics for Ambulatory
Cancer Patients

New York City Survey (N = 94)	
Total pharmacies called	112
Total responding	94 (100%)
No Class II narcotic analgesics	27 (29%)
Oxycodone/ASA/APAP only	24 (25%)
Class II Narcotic Analgesics:	
Levorphanol	19 (20%)
Hydromorphone	14 (15%)
Oral morphine	3 (3%)
Methadone	2 (2%)

From Kanner R, Portenoy R: Unavailability of narcotic analgesics for ambulatory cancer patients in New York City. J Pain Symptom Manag 1:87–89, 1986. With permission.

state of affairs, the really important issue is that problem areas need immediate attention and correction as a first step toward solving the problem of cancer pain.

REFERENCES

1. Angell M: Should heroin be legalized for the treatment of pain? N Engl J Med 311:529–530, 1984
2. Anonymous: Heroin for cancer: a great non-issue of our day.(Editorial.) Lancet 1: 1449–1450, 1984
3. Allport GW: Attitudes, in Murchison C (Ed): Handbook of Social Psychology. Worcester, Clark University Press, 1935, pp 798–844
4. Austin C, Cody P, Eyres PJ et al.: Hospice home care pain management: four critical variables. Cancer Nurs 9:58–65, 1986
5. Baer E, Davitz LJ, Lieb R: Inferences of physical pain and psychological distress. I. In relation to verbal and nonverbal patient communication. Nurs Res 19:388–392, 1970
6. Beales G: Suffer the little children. Nurs Mirror 155:58–59, part 2, 1982
7. Beaver WT: Management of cancer pain with parenteral medication. JAMA 244:2653–2657, 1980
8. Beaver WT, Feise G: Comparison of the analgesic effects of morphine, hydroxyzine and their combination in patients with postoperative pain, in Ng L, Bonica JJ (Eds): Advances in Pain Research and Therapy, Vol I. New York, Raven Press, 1976, pp 135–149
9. Beaver WT, Wallenstein SL, Houde RW, et al.: A comparison of the analgesic effects of pentazocine and morphine in patients with cancer. Clin Pharmacol Ther 7:740–751, 1966
10. Belleville J, Forrest W, Miller E, Brown B: Influence of age on pain relief from analgesics. JAMA 217:1835–1841, 1971
11. Bonica JJ: Pain research and therapy: past and current status and future needs, in Ng L, Bonica JJ (Eds): Pain and Discomfort. Amsterdam, Elsevier, 1980

12. Bouckoms AJ: Analgesic adjuvants: the role of psychotropics, anticonvulsants, and prostaglandin inhibitors. Drug Ther 1:179–186, 1982
13. Boyer M: Continuous drip morphine. Am J Nurs 82:502–504, 1982
14. Brandt E: Compassionate pain relief: is heroin the answer? N Engl J Med 311:530–532, 1984
15. Brook-Williams P, Hoover LH: Morphine suppositories for intractable pain. Can Med Assoc J 126:14, 1982
16. Carson BC: Neurologic and neurosurgical approaches to cancer pain, in McGuire DB, Yarbro CH (Eds): Cancer Pain Management. Orlando, FL, Grune & Stratton, Inc. 1987, pp 223–244
17. Catalano RB: Pharmacologic management in the treatment of cancer pain, in McGuire DB, Yarbro CH (Eds): Cancer Pain Management. Orlando, FL, Grune & Stratton, Inc. 1987, pp 151–202
18. Catalano RB: Pharmacology of analgesic agents used to treat cancer pain. Semin Oncol Nur 1:126–140, 1985
19. Charap AD: The knowledge, attitudes, and experience of medical personnel treating pain in the terminally ill. Mt Sinai J Med (NY) 45:561–580, 1978
20. Citron M, Johnston-Early A, Fossieck B, et al.: Safety and efficacy of continuous intravenous morphine for severe cancer pain. Am J Med 77:199–204, 1984
21. Clay GS, Brougham LR: Haloperidol binding to an opiate receptor site. Biochem Pharmacol 42:1363–1367, 1975
22. Cohen FL: Postsurgical pain relief: patients' status and nurses' medication choices. Pain 9:265–274, 1980
23. Creese J, Feinberg AP, Snyder SH: Butyrophenone influences on opiate receptor. Eur J Pharmacol 36:231–35, 1976
24. Davitz J, Davitz L: Inferences of patients' pain and psychological distress: studies of nursing behaviors. New York, Springer, 1981
25. DeChristoforo R, Corden BJ, Hood JC, et al.: High-dose morphine infusion complicated by chlorobutanol-induced somnolence. Ann Intern Med 98:335–336, 1983
26. Dennis EM: An ambulatory infusion pump for pain control: a nursing approach for home care. Cancer Nurs 7:309–313, 1984
27. Donabedian A, Rosenfeld LS: Follow-up study of chronically ill patients discharged from hospital. J Chronic Dis 17:847–862, 1964
28. Eland J: The child who is hurting. Semin Oncol Nurs 1:116–122, 1985
29. Entsworth S: Morphine IV infusion for chronic pain (letter). Drug Intell Clin Pharm 13:297, 1979
30. Ettinger DS, Vitale PJ, Trump DL: Important clinical considerations in the use of methadone in cancer patients. Cancer Treat Rep 63:457–459, 1979
31. Evans WJ: Is heroin needed for cancer pain? Oncol Nurs Forum 13:49–52, 1986
32. Foley K: Commentary. PRN Forum 4:2, 1985
33. Foley K, Sundaresan N: Management of cancer pain, in DeVita V, Hellman S, Rosenberg S (Eds): Cancer: Principles and Practice of Oncology, Vol 2, (2d ed.). Philadelphia, JB Lippincott, 1985, pp 1940–1962
34. Forrest WH, Brown BW, Brown CR, et al.: Dextroamphetamine with morphine for the treatment of postoperative pain. N Engl J Med 246:712–715, 1977
35. Fox LS: Pain management in the terminally ill cancer patient: an investigation of nurses attitudes, knowledge, and clinical practice. Military Medicine 147:455–460, 1982.
36. Given BA, Given CW: Creating a climate for compliance. Cancer Nurs 7:139–47, 1984
37. Grossman SA, Sheidler VR: Skills of medical students and house officers in prescribing narcotic medication. J Med Educ 60:552–557, 1985
38. Halpern LM: Analgesic drugs in the management of pain. Arch Surg 112:861–869, 1977
39. Hauck SL: Pain: Problem for the person with cancer. Cancer Nurs 9:66–76, 1986

40. Hawley DD: Postoperative pain in children: misconceptions, descriptions, and interventions. Pediatr Nurs 10:20–23, 1984
41. Health and Public Policy Committee, American College of Physicians: Drug therapy for severe, chronic pain in terminal illness. Ann Intern Med 99:870–873, 1983
42. Holmes AH: Morphine intravenous infusion for chronic pain (letter). Drug Intell Clin Pharm 12:556–557, 1978
43. Howard-Ruben J: Around the clock medication for pain. Oncol Nurs Forum 10:60, 1983
44. Howard-Ruben J, McGuire L, Groenwald S: Pain, in Groenwald S (Ed): Cancer Nursing: Principles and Practice. Monterey, CA, Jones and Bartlett (in press)
45. Iles J: Heroin and pain (letters). Can Med Assoc J 132:317, 1985
46. Inturrisi C, Max M, Foley K, et al.: The pharmacokinetics of heroin in patients with chronic pain. N Engl J Med 310:1213–1217, 1984
47. Jacox A, Rogers A: The nursing management of pain, in Marino LB (Ed): Cancer Nursing. St. Louis, CV Mosby, 1981, p 394
48. Jarratt V: The keeper of the keys. Am J Nurs 65:68–70, 1965
49. Kaiko RF: Heroin: facts and comparisons. PRN Forum 4:1–2, 1985
50. Kaiko RF, Foley KM, Grabinski PY, et al.: Central nervous system excitatory effects of meperidine in cancer patients. Ann Neurol 13:180–185, 1983
51. Kaiko R, Wallenstein S, Rogers A, et al.: Analgesic and mood effects of heroin and morphine in cancer patients with post-operative pain. N Engl J Med 304:1501–1505, 1984
52. Kaiko R, Wallenstein S, Rogers A, Houde R: Sources of variation in analgesic responses in cancer patients with chronic pain receiving morphine. Pain 15:191–200, 1983
53. Kanner R, Portenoy, R: Unavailability of narcotic analgesics for ambulatory cancer patients in New York City. J Pain Symptom Manag 1:87–89, 1986
54. Kantor TG: Nonsteroidal anti-inflammatory analgesic agents in the management of cancer pain, in Management of Cancer Pain (monograph). Hosp Prac (Summer, 1984)
55. Keats AS, Telford J, Kurosu Y: "Potentiation" of meperidine by promethazine. Anesthesiology 22: 33–41,1961
56. Keeri-Szanto M: The mode of action of promethazine in potentiating narcotic drugs. Br J Anaesth 46:918–924, 1974
57. Kerrane TA: The Brompton cocktail. Nur Mirror 140:59, 1975
58. Kocher R: The use of psychotropic drugs in the treatment of cancer pain. Recent Results Cancer Res 89:118–126, 1984
59. Kowolenko M: An additional comment on IV morphine infusion (letters). Drug Intell Clin Pharm 14:296–297, 1980
60. Lasagna L: Heroin: a medical "me too." N Engl J Med 304:1539–1540, 1981
61. Lenburg C, Glass H, Davitz LJ: Inferences of physical pain and psychological distress. III. In relation to stage of patient's illness and occupation of the perceiver. Nurs Res 19:392–398, 1970
62. Levy M: Pain management in advanced cancer. Semin Oncol 12:394–410, 1985
63. Lipman AG: Drug therapy in cancer pain. Cancer Nurs 3:39–46, 1980
64. Maltbie AA, Cavenar O, Sullivan JL, Hammet EB: Analgesia and haloperidol: a hypothesis. J Clin Psychiatry 40:323–326, 1979
65. Marks R, Sachar E: Undertreatment of medical inpatients with narcotic analgesics. Ann Intern Med 78:173–181, 1973
66. McCaffery M: Nursing Management of the Patient with Pain (2nd ed.). Philadelphia, JB Lippincott, 1979
67. McCaffery M: Pain relief for the child: problem areas and selected non-pharmacologic methods. Pediatr Nurs 3:11–16, 1977
68. McCaffery M: Problems with IM meperidine (Demerol). PRN Forum 3:1–2, 1984
69. McGee JL, Alexander MR: Phenothiazine analgesia — fact or fantasy? Am J Hosp Pharm 36:633–640, 1979

70. McGuire D, Barbour L, Boxler J, et al.: Analgesic scheduling in cancer outpatients (Abstract). Paper presented at the Ninth Annual Conference of the Midwest Nursing Research Society, Chicago, IL, April 25, 1985
71. McGuire L, Wright A: Continuous narcotic infusion: it's not just for cancer patients. Nurs 84 14:50–55, 1984
72. Meinhart NT, McCaffery M: Pain: A Nursing Approach to Assessment and Analysis. Norwalk, CT, Appleton-Century-Crofts, 1983
73. Melzack R, Mount B, Gordon J: The Brompton mixture versus morphine solution given orally: effects on pain. Can Med Assoc J 120:435–439, 1979
74. Miaskowski C: The Brompton cocktail. Cancer Nurs 1:451–455, 1978
75. Mioduszewski J, McCray N: The evolving role of the oncology nurse in managing cancer pain. Semin Oncol Nurs 1:123–125, 1985
76. Miser A, Miser J, Clark B: Continuous infusion of morphine sulfate for control of severe pain in children with terminal malignancy. J Pediatr 96:930–932,1980
77. Moertel C: Treatment of cancer pain with orally administered medications. JAMA 244:2448–2450, 1980
78. Mondzac A: In defense of reintroduction of heroin into American medical practice and H.R. 5290 — the Compassionate Pain Relief Act. N Engl J Med 311: 532–535,1984
79. Moore J, Dundee JW: Alteration in response to somatic pain associated with anesthesia V. The effect of promethazine. Br J Anaesth 33:38, 1961
80. Myers JS: Cancer pain: assessment of nurses' knowledge and attitudes. Oncol Nurs Forum 12:62–66, 1985
81. O'Donnell L, Papciak B: Continuous morphine infusion for control of intractable pain. Nurs 81 11:69–72, 1981
82. Oncology Nursing Society: Outcome standards for cancer nursing practice. Kansas City: American Nurses' Association, 1979
83. Patterson KL, Klopovich P: Pain in the pediatric oncology patient, in McGuire DB, Yarbro CH (Eds): Cancer Pain Management. Orlando, FL, Grune & Stratton, Inc. 1987, pp 259–272
84. Portenoy RK, Moulin DE, Rogers A, et al.: IV infusions of opioids for cancer pain: clinical review and guidelines for use. Cancer Treat Rep 70:575–582, 1986
85. Reed-Ash C: Education approaches for teaching pain management. Integrated Approach to Management of Pain. National Institute of Health Consensus Development Conference, 1986
86. Saunders C: The Management of Terminal Illness. London, Hospital Medicine Publications, 1967
87. Sheidler VR: New methods in analgesic delivery, in McGuire DB, Yarbro CH (eds): Cancer Pain Management. Orlando, FL, Grune & Stratton, Inc. 1987, pp 203–222
88. Simon J: The opiate receptors. Neurochem Res 1:3–28, 1976
89. Snow H: Opium and cocaine in the treatment of cancerous disease. Br Med J 2:718–719, 1896
90. Snow H: The opium-cocaine treatment of malignant disease. Br Med J 1:1019–1020, 1897
91. Strauss A, Fagerhaugh SY, Glaser B: Pain: an organizational-work-interactional perspective. Nurs Outlook 22-560–566, 1974
92. Szeto H, Inturrisi C, Houde R, et al.: Accumulation of normeperidine, an active metabolite of merperidine, in patients with renal failure or cancer. Ann Intern Med 86:738–741, 1977
93. Trotter JM, Scott R, MacBeth FR, et al.: Problems of the oncology outpatient: role of the liaison health visitor. Br Med Jour 282:122–124, 1981
94. Twycross RG: Bone pain in advanced cancer, in Vere DW (Ed): Topics in Therapeutics IV. Tunbridge Wells, Pitman Medical, 1978, pp 94–110

95. Twycross RG: Medical treatment of chronic cancer pain. Bull Cancer (Paris) 67:209–216, 1980
96. Twycross RG, Lack S.A. Therapeutics in Terminal Cancer. London, Pitman Publishing Limited, 1984.
97. Twycross R, Lack S: Symptom Control in Far Advanced Cancer: Pain Relief. London, Pitman Publishing Limited, 1983
98. Valentine AS, Steckel S, Weintraub, M: Pain relief for cancer patients. Am J Nurs 78:2054–2056, 1978
99. Weis, OF, Sriwatanakul K, Alloza JL, et al.: Attitudes of patients, housestaff, and nurses toward post-operative analgesic care. Anesth Analg 62:70–74, 1983
100. Wescoe G, Salter F: The Brompton cocktail no more effective than oral narcotic analgesics in chronic pain. Hosp Form 15:266–268, 1980

Marilee Ivers Donovan, Ph.D., R.N.

5
Clinical Assessment of Cancer Pain

Assessment of the patient experiencing pain is the foundation upon which all interventions are built. In contrast to measurement of pain for the purposes of research, the assessment of the patient with pain is done specifically to aid in choosing among alternative interventions for the relief of pain. Standard IV of the Outcome Standards for Cancer Nursing Practice developed by the Oncology Nursing Society and the Division on Medical-Surgical Nursing Practice of the American Nurses Association states, "The client and family identify and manage factors that influence comfort."[26] Every cancer patient experiencing pain has the right to expect an accurate, timely assessment of that pain experience and a concerted effort on the part of the involved care givers to help the patient find a way to adequately control the pain experience.

Many methods of measuring pain have been developed, and considerable controversy exists regarding the "best" approaches. The spectrum of these ranges from patient self-reports of pain on the "subjective" end to the use of physiologic correlates such as electromyographic readings, autonomic indices (vital signs, galvanic skin response, and thermography), and central nervous system measures (electroencephalogram and evoked potential) on the "objective" end.[4,27,30]

Physiologic measures have been shown to have limited value in assessing clinical pain. They correlate unpredictably with the subject's self-report of pain. Indeed, it has been impossible to document consistent patterns of physiologic arousal in conjunction with pain even in the controlled environment of a research laboratory. Contradictory findings in replication studies are common.[4,30]

On the other hand, self-report measures are challenged because they are subjective, difficult to validate, and sensitive to response bias.[4,16] Most health professionals accept these challenges as fact. However, subjectivity and response bias should not be considered limitations of clinical assessment of pain. It is often believed that only phenomena that can be observed and quantified exist, thus causing doubt about the reality of anything that does not fit the empirical model. Pain, an inherently subjective phenomenon, is challenged on the very basis of its subjectivity. Because self-report measures correlate poorly with the objective physiologic indices, self-report measures are said to be difficult to validate. If validity is the extent to which a technique measures the phenomenon under study, might it not be more appropriate to question the validity of objective measures? Such a possibility is seldom considered. It has been reported that if the assessment process is unidimensional, that is, the patient is only asked about the quantity/intensity of pain, the answer tends to vary little from assessment to assessment, which suggests response bias. However, in the case of clinical pain for which no effective intervention has been implemented, this lack of variability could actually represent high test–retest reliability rather than response bias.

Not all of the methods of *measuring* pain are appropriate for assessing pain. In an attempt to enhance the validity and reliability of pain measurement, the process and the instrumentation have become increasingly more complex, time-consuming, precise, and even invasive. Much of the scientific literature is written by researchers/practitioners whose primary intent is to find a way to quantify the patient's pain without having to rely on the patient—these techniques include magnitude estimation procedures, mathematical modeling, cross-modality matching, and sensory decision theory (SDT).[4,16,30] Although developed for the precision of laboratory research, these methods and their philosophical foundations are finding their way into the clinical arena.

According to advocates of this objective measurement approach, the "ideal" method of pain measurement should be (1) free from bias; (2) able to predict patient performance; (3) useful in practice as well as research; (4) able to distinguish between the sensory and affective aspects of pain; and (5) able to compare clinical and experimental pain.[15] In considering the problem of cancer pain, it is difficult to conceive (1) how clinical pain can ever be bias free; (2) how one could eliminate the effects of personal and situational variables in order to predict performance from some quantification of pain; (3) how one could compare complex clinical pain in which no variables are controlled with the well controlled experimental pain of the research laboratory; or (4) how one could separate the sensory and affective components of a human experience. Thus, even as science is beginning to demonstrate the extent to which the mind is biochemical and the extent to which autonomic processes are controllable by cognitive process, some research/practitioners are trying to separate pain (a truly mind–body experience) into distinct mind and body components.

Pain is a complex multidimensional, neurophysiologic, and psychosocial process fully known only to the person experiencing it. Therefore, a valid measurement of pain must be both subjective and multidimensional. Since part of the complexity of pain is its variability over time, assessment should be longitudinal as well.

This author and colleagues recently studied 465 randomly selected medical-surgical inpatients to determine the incidence and characteristics of pain in hospitalized patients and to explore the type and perceived effectiveness of pharmacologic and nonpharmacologic therapies used by these patients.[11] A structured interview was developed from the McGill Pain Questionnaire (MPQ),[24] with additional questions establishing the history of the pain, its general characteristics, the patient's perception of the cause, nursing activity in relation to pain assessment, and the effects of 21 factors (such as eating, resting, heat, medications, distraction) on the pain. In addition to the already documented reliability and validity of the MPQ, this questionnaire demonstrated good content validity, internal consistency, and interrater reliabilities greater than .90. Ninety-six of the patients who consented to be interviewed had a confirmed diagnosis of a malignancy. Data from these individuals will be used in conjunction with the literature review and personal clinical experience to discuss the assessment of pain.

It appears that care givers often undervalue assessment or assess because they are required to do so without a clear idea of what to ask or what they will do with the information obtained. In the author's study, the lack of systematic or regular assessment was woefully evident. Seventy-five percent of the subjects reported experiencing pain within the past 72 hours. Fifty-three percent were in pain at the time of the interview, yet only 43 percent were able to recall a nurse ever discussing their pain with them. For more than 70 percent there was neither a note in the patient record relative to pain nor an indication in the care plan that pain was a problem to be considered.[11]

MULTIDIMENSIONAL ASSESSMENT

There are eight dimensions considered to be essential to a thorough assessment of pain: (1) location, (2) intensity, (3) factors influencing the occurrence of pain, (4) observed behaviors including vital signs, (5) psychosocial modifiers, (6) effects of pain, (7) effects of therapy, and (8) established patterns of coping.

Location

Logically, the characteristic of pain that is assessed first is the location of the pain. Failure to consistently validate the location of pain can lead to treatment of the wrong pain; for example, continued treatment of a painful fungating local breast metastasis in a patient who has sustained a pathologic fracture. The patient's answers to questions regarding the location of the pain begin to suggest appropriate interventions as outlined in Figure 5-1. Some assessment tools include a graphic representation to elicit and record the patient's response.

To ask a patient "Where is your pain?" is not sufficient if the data are to be useful for determining treatment. There are two effective methods for assessing location. First, if the patient is able, he or she can mark on an outline of the human body exactly where the pain hurts (Fig. 5-2). The McGill Pain Questionnaire[24] and the Brief Pain Inventory[7] also ask that the patient indicate whether the pain is external/superficial or internal/deep. An equally effective alternative method in clinical practice is to ask the patient to point with one finger to the site of the pain. If the patient can precisely indicate the site of the pain, then it is superficial and localized, and interventions that act locally or regionally are appropriate. If the patient cannot localize the pain or has many separate sites, then systemic, cortical, or thalamic methods of relief are needed (Table 5-1). In the study conducted by the author, one of the 96 cancer patients reported pain "everywhere," and nearly one-third reported multiple sites of pain.[11]

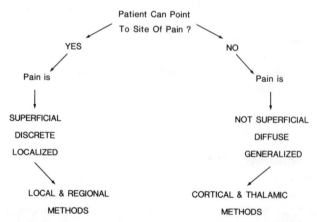

Fig. 5-1. Location as a factor determining the method of intervention.

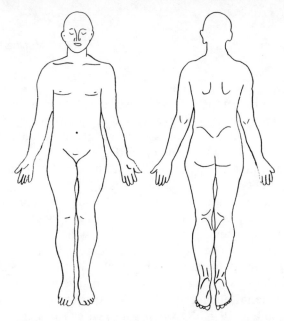

Fig. 5-2. A method for locating the site of pain: The patient is asked to place an X on, circle, or shade the area(s) of pain.

Table 5-1
Classification of Pain Relief Methods

Method	Local	Regional	Thalamic	Cortical
Noninvasive				
Relaxation	X		X	X
Imagery	X		X	
Hypnosis			X	X
Heat	X	X		
Cold	X	X		
Massage	X	X		
Vibration	X	X		
Mentholated rubs	X	X		
Pressure		X		
TENS		X		
Electrical stimulation		X	X	
Systemic				
Anti-inflammatory agents	X			
Nonnarcotic analgesics	X			
Narcotics		X	X	X
Antispasmodics	X	X		
Antidepressants			X	X
Tranquilizers			?	
Anesthetics	X	X	X	
Acupuncture		X	X	X
Neurosurgical procedures	X	X	X	X

TENS, transcutaneous electrical nerve stimulation.

Intensity

The second characteristic to be assessed, and the one most important to the patient, is the intensity (or severity and duration) of the pain. The type, severity, and duration of the pain assist one in choosing the methods of pain relief that are most likely to be effective. The assessment of the quantity of pain is also important as a baseline measure by which to gauge the efficacy of the intervention(s) used to relieve the pain.[12,20]

Visual analogue scales and categorical scales are commonly used to quantify the intensity of pain (Fig. 5-3). Many variations of these scales are in use, but a visual analogue scale (VAS) without intermediate verbal anchors is considered to be the most sensitive, reliable, and valid method of estimating the intensity of pain.[4,30] The simplicity of the VAS allows it to be used with children as young as five years of age.[16] In clinical practice, another technique for quantifying the pain experience is to ask the patient, "If 0 = no pain and 10 = the worst pain you can imagine, what number represents your pain right now?" This method is slightly more difficult for patients to use than a visual analogue scale but is more sensitive than the categorical scale where patients select from words such as No Pain, Mild,

CATEGORICAL SCALE:

0   NO PAIN

1   MILD

2   DISCOMFORTING

3   DISTRESSING

4   HORRIBLE

5   EXCRUTIATING

VISUAL ANALOGUE SCALES:

NO   MOST
PAIN   _____   PAIN

NORMAL 0-1-2-3-4-5-6-7-8-9-10 SEVERE PAIN

Fig. 5-3. Scales for quantifying pain intensity.

Moderate, Severe. Regardless of the method used to estimate the intensity of the pain, it is important to ascertain not only the intensity of the current pain but also the intensity of the pain at its worst, at its best, and the average pain intensity. The answers to these questions can assist the care giver in understanding much about the patient's experience of pain. For instance, if a patient answers, "At its worst the pain is 10,000" when asked to rate the pain from 0 to 10, it may mean that the pain is much worse than anyone could imagine.

A patient whose pain at its worst is reported to be 8 to 10 but which is regularly reduced to 1 to 2 will need a different plan of care from the patient who reports that the pain at its worst is 8 to 10 and pain average is 7. The former pattern suggests that the patient is using an effective intervention for controlling the pain but that the timing of the intervention is suboptimal. The latter pattern indicates that any intervention(s) currently in use are ineffective and a new plan needs to be developed. A decision tree for using the patient's report of pain/pain relief is diagrammed in Figure 5-4.

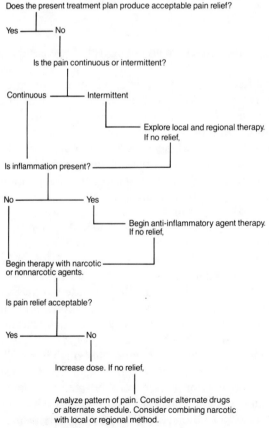

Fig. 5-4. Decision tree for use in planning interventions.

Factors Influencing Pain

Factors that influence the existence of pain are often overlooked. Certain foods, eating or not eating, activity or lack of activity, positions, weather changes, and times of day are all associated with particular painful conditions. Most patients can respond to a direct question, "Have you identified anything that makes your pain worse?" Some need to be asked whether any activities, foods, positions, times of day, or factors in the environment make the pain worse. Not everything that intensifies or causes pain can be eliminated, but it is negligent to ignore those factors that, if identified, could be easily avoided.

Patients with bony metastases may be comfortable with little medication while in bed but may experience severe pain when attempting to move from the bed to a chair. If the patient does not want to get up and go to a chair, the plan of care can easily be adapted to prevent atelectasis and skin breakdown so the patient may remain on bedrest and avoid pain-producing activity.

Observation

From the moment the care giver begins to have contact with the patient, and throughout the period of assessment, it is also important to carefully observe the patient's behavior, ability to interact, and the condition of the environment. The patient lying with his back to the door in a darkened room suggests depression, or a pattern of coping by withdrawal, or somone who has not found distraction and interaction with others to be beneficial in relieving pain. Methods of scoring behavioral observations have been developed by those who believe that behavior analysis is a more valid form of pain assessment than patient's self-report. These include methods of quantifying guarding, rubbing, bracing, and sighing[17] and LeResche's[18] characterization of the prototype of the facial expression of pain. Next it is important to observe how significant individuals, such as family members, nurses, physicians, and friends, interact with the patient. Finally, the environment itself (light, temperature, noise, need to reach for water, telephone, etc.) may affect that patient's pain.

One type of observation that is often misused in the assessment of pain is physiologic measures such as pulse, respirations, and blood pressure. If the patient reports severe pain in the absence of tachycardia, tachypnea, and elevated blood pressure, health care givers commonly question whether the patient is "really having that much pain," although it is well established that chronic pain does not routinely elicit a sympathetic response. Even in response to the application of a controlled painful stimulus in a research laboratory, signs of automatic activation decrease over time and are unpredictably related to the subject's verbal reports of pain.[4]

It is not uncommon that a patient given morphine sulfate 15 mg intramuscularly (IM) who is found asleep 30 minutes later with a respiratory rate of nine would be given naloxone hydrochloride (Narcan, Endo Laboratories, Garden City, NY). This action may occur despite the care giver's awareness that a respiratory rate of 8 to 12 respirations per minute is common during a sound sleep. The relief of pain, especially after many hours of suffering from pain will often result in relaxation and deep sleep. The observation and recording of vital signs is recommended in the assessment of pain primarily for the purpose of serving as a baseline from which to judge the onset of relaxation or the appearance of side effects of certain medications.

Observations are but one dimension of a multidimensional assessment of pain. They are most accurately described as correlates of the pain experience, not measures of pain.[6] They are extremely sensitive to cultural and learning pressures. It is important that the oncology care giver consider these limitations. In a review of the literature on pain assessment, Syrjala and Chapman[30] conclude that nurses respond more to physiologic signs and observed behaviors than to patients' self-reports of pain if the observations and self-reports do not agree. For instance, the patient who is talking on the phone enthusiastically is suspected of not really suffering from pain when, in fact, he may be effectively using distraction. In the study by this author described earlier,[11] 30 percent of the patients in pain identified distraction as an effective method of reducing the pain experienced. The patient who puts his call light on 15 minutes before the next dose of analgesic is due may be labeled a clock watcher, a pest, or an addict, when in fact he may be an expert at analyzing the operations of a busy unit.[20]

Another important observation that the care giver can make involves the patterns of interaction and attitudes within a family, for these may limit the range of interventions that are acceptable and/or feasible for a particular patient. For instance, a wife who is constantly urging her husband to wait a little longer before taking the "shot for pain" will usually have difficulty "remembering" post-discharge to give her husband the analgesic every four hours as scheduled.

Care givers frequently neglect to observe the pattern of use of a pain relief method. For example, one can never assume that the treatment recommended or ordered is used as directed or even used at all. Observation of the use of the method or analysis of the documentation of the *actual* use is necessary (Table 5-2). In the previously described study of 96 cancer inpatients,[11] the average amount of analgesic ordered (converted to milligrams of morphine IM) was 55.7 mg. Observations revealed, however, that the average amount of analgesic given (converted to milligrams of morphine IM) was 13.5 mg, less than a quarter of the amount ordered.

Many pain researchers and practitioners in pain clinics recommend a daily recording of the occurrence and intensity of pain, setting and activities related to the pain, and interventions/medications used and their effect. The most common methods for obtaining such information are pain diaries or pain charts. Underreporting and overreporting are common with this method

Table 5-2
Analysis of Pattern of Use of Pain Relief Method

Ordered: Percodan i–ii q 3–4 hr prn	
Example No. 1	Example No. 2
Pattern	
Mr A. takes:	Mr B. takes:
Percodan i at 1:00 pm, 4:00 pm, 7:00 pm, 10:00 pm	Percodan ii q 3 hr
Percodan ii at 6:00 am, 9:00 am	
Pain varies from 1–9	Pain remains at 7–8
Suggested intervention	
Give Percodan q 4 h on a schedule	Develop a new plan based on a thorough assessment

Ordered: mentholated rub to right trapezius qid	
Example No. 3	Example No. 4
Pattern	
Ms D. has not used mentholated rub because she has no one to apply it	Ms. E. has used the mentholated rub qid for three days with relief for brief periods (<2 hr)
Suggested intervention	
Apply ice pack or heating pad for 20 min qid	Apply transcutaneous electrical nerve stimulation (TENS)

of measurement.[4,16,30] In an attempt to overcome this limitation, some have suggested that a significant other also keep a daily pain diary for the patient as well, and that the two records be compared.[16] It appears that this kind of "checking" on the patient develops from a basic assumption that pain is not inherently subjective and/or that the patient will intentionally deceive the care giver. Although this kind of manipulative behavior is a possiblity in some circumstances, to operate from an assumption that it is a common behavior is counterproductive to therapeutic relationships and contrary to the holistic nature of the human being.

Psychosocial Modifiers

Many variables (psychologic, social, attitudinal, situational, and physiologic) have been implicated in the experience of pain.[23] Clearly, no pain is totally organic. The more that is learned about mood states, the clearer it becomes that moods are not purely psychologic but are mediated by biochemical changes in the central nervous system. All pain has psychologic and physiologic components. It behooves those who are interested in controlling pain to be able to assess and analyze all interacting variables that can intensify the patient's pain and interfere with the effectiveness of the planned interventions. Karoly[16] describes many unidimensional and multi-dimensional methods of assessing chronic pain emphasizing the psychological and social dimensions.

The instrument most commonly employed to assess the qualitative aspects of pain is the Pain Rating Index (PRI) of the McGill Pain Questionnaire.[24] The PRI provides information about three dimensions (subscales) of the pain experience: sensory, affective, and evaluative. Patients are asked to select from 20 sets of descriptors the words that best describe their pain. Each word chosen contributes both to the subscale score and to the total PRI score. Numerous studies have supported the basic structure, reliability, and validity of this tool.[4,30,31] Authors of recent reviews conclude that the PRI is best used as a qualitative tool rather than a quantitative one.[4,31] If the numerical scores are used, the high intercorrelations between subscales make a total score more appropriate than subscale scores.[31]

Fear and anxiety are often identified as increasing the reaction component of pain. The cyclic interaction of pain and anxiety resulting in more pain is well described by Sternbach.[28] Research suggests that depression is even more likely to have an effect on the perception of and the reaction to pain.[32] Derogatis et al.[9] have demonstrated that care givers routinely overestimate the amount of anxiety being experienced by a patient and underestimate the amount of depression being experienced. It is important that a comprehensive assessment of pain include a brief evaluation of the patient's mood state with emphasis on the identification of signs of depression (Table 5-3)[2]. Ahles et al.[1] have demonstrated the validity of a Pain-VAS and a Depression-VAS for use in assessing the sensory and affective components of cancer pain.

Zborowski,[33] among others, has described the reactions of people of various cultural backgrounds to pain. For the clinician, it is most important to understand one's own cultural behaviors surrounding pain and the extent to which these are cultural norms rather than the "right" way to behave. Health care givers from stoic cultures are likely to be judgmental toward patients who are too verbal about their pain. It is equally problematic when care givers who are from expressive cultures *expect* patients to complain in direct proportion to the extent of their pain. The former patients may be stereotyped as "clockwatchers," or anxious, or even "addicts." The latter patients' pain may never be identified as a problem.

The limited research on the factors that impede adequate pain control suggests that the attitudes of patients, families, and care givers are a primary impediment to rational and effective control of pain.[5,14,19,25] Marks and Sachar[19] reported in 1973 that physicians underprescribed analgesics, and nurses repeatedly gave less than was prescribed. The study conducted by this author[11] confirmed that little has changed in the past 13 years. On the

Table 5-3
Assessment of Depression

Sad mood or loss of interest or pleasure in all or almost all of one's usual activities. The mood disturbance must be relatively persistent but need not be the most dominant symptom.

At least four of the following symptoms have each been present nearly every day for at least a two week period:

Poor appetite or significant weight loss or increased appetite or significant weight gain.

Insomnia or hypersomnia (specifically, difficulty falling asleep, awakening 30–90 minutes before it is time to arise, awakening in the middle of the night with difficulty going back to sleep, increased length of sleep, frequent naps).

Psychomotor agitation or retardation (change in activity level is noticed by others—not just a subjective feeling).

Loss of interest or pleasure in usual activities or decrease in sexual drive.

Loss of energy, fatigue.

Feelings of worthlessness, self-reproach, or excessive or inappropriate guilt.

Complaints or evidence of diminished ability to think or concentrate, indecisiveness.

Recurrent thoughts of death, suicidal ideation; wishes to be dead or suicide attempt.

Data from American Psychiatric Association: Diagnostic and Statistical Manual of Mental Disorders (3rd ed.). Washington, DC, American Psychiatric Association, 1981, pp 210–217.

average nurses continue to administer less than a quarter of the amount of analgesic ordered for cancer patients. In fact, this 4:1 ratio prevailed for both cancer patients and non-cancer patients.

Some of the most common misconceptions leading to inadequate use of analgesics have been identified as (1) a patient must be suspected of malingering if there is no proven basis for the pain; (2) health care professionals know more about the existence of pain and the efficacy of treatment than the person experiencing the pain; (3) the changes associated with acute pain are valid indicators of the existence of all pain; (4) autonomic and behavioral cues are more valid indicators of pain than a patient's self-report; (5) addiction and tolerance are major problems and every effort should be made to avoid them; (6) patients who watch the clock are addicted; and (7) waiting as long as possible between doses of an analgesic will prevent addiction.[5,10,19,20]

A plan for managing the patient's pain must consider the attitudes that are operating in the particular patient care setting (hospital, clinic, or home) in order to be successful. The extent to which such attitudes may impede adequate assessment and control of pain must be determined. A method for overcoming the problems imposed by these attitudes must be an integral part of any pain management plan.

The Effects of Pain on the Patient's Life

The uniqueness of the pain experience is most clearly illustrated by the variability in the effects that pain has on the individual patient's life. Though chronic pain is generally accompanied by significant emotional distress (often depression), studies of patients suffering from pain related to cancer fail to confirm that cancer pain causes them extreme emotional distress.[27] Researchers and clinicians who work with patients having chronic benign pain often describe a reaction pattern in which patients with mild pain report extreme emotional distress and significant impairment in their ability to continue to perform the activities of their lives. However, this author has never observed this particular pattern in cancer patients. Rather patients' activities are restricted in proportion to the magnitude of the pain experience and their emotional response is in proportion to the pain, its meaning, and its effect on their lives.

It is valuable in determining the full meaning of the pain to the patient and for the purpose of planning comprehensive care, to obtain information about a number of areas. How much does the pain affect work, mobility, sleep, eating, interpersonal relationships, mood, and goals? Has the patient had to give up or alter normal activities? If so, which ones? What does the patient think is the cause of the pain? What are the patient's goals with respect to the pain? What does the patient think will be effective in attaining these goals? The Wisconsin Brief Pain Questionnare, now called the Brief Pain Inventory (BPI), explores this area exceptionally well.[7] Stromborg[29] and Dean[8] have recently published reviews of the methods available for assessing quality of life. Several of these instruments may be beneficial in assessing the effects of pain on the individual's life.

Previous Therapy and Its Effects

Patients are the best source of information about what is effective for the control of pain. And patients realize that many approaches other than medication are effective for controlling pain. The effectiveness of a variety of methods for controlling pain as reported by 351 medical-surgical inpatients who had experienced pain within the past 72 hours (239 of whom were experiencing pain at the time of the interview) is summarized in Table 5-4.

Table 5-4
Effects of Pain Relief
Measures as Reported by
Patients

Measure	Reduces Pain	No Effect on Pain	Increases Pain
Cold	7%	22%	15%
Distraction	30%	60%	6%
Heat	32%	21%	5%
Massage	23%	18%	6%
Medications	82%	6%	2%
Mild exercise	14%	36%	33%
Pressure	15%	24%	38%
Rest/lying down	56%	33%	10%

Percentages do no equal 100% because some respondents could not evaluate some of the measures. N = 351 patients who had experienced pain within the past 72 hours.
Data from Donovan MI, Dillon P, McGuire L. Incidence and characteristics of pain in a sample of medical-surgical inpatients. *Pain*. Accepted for publication.

Although medications were the most effective of the interventions, it is noteworthy that distraction, rest/lying down, massage, and heat were also effective for more than half of the patients who tried these techniques.[11] The variability among patients is illustrated both by the number of patients who did not benefit from distraction, rest/lying down, heat, or massage and the differences between the findings of this study and the findings of a study by Barbour et al.[3] Although both studies were conducted in the same geographic area at about the same time, there were major differences. In Barbour's sample, decreased pain was reported to result from distraction in 88 percent of the patients, from position change or rest/lying down in 85 percent, from massage in 75 percent, and from heat in 74 percent.

Since patients already know a great deal about what helps control their pain, it is imperative that this area be thoroughly explored if a plan with the greatest chance of success is to be developed. The extent to which a patient's methods of coping with pain can significantly affect the control of the pain is illustrated by the following anecdote.

Mrs. C. was admitted to the hospital for evaluation of her pain. She was known to have advanced carcinomatosis and possible bony metastases. At home Mrs. C. was able to keep her pain below 5 (on a 0 to 10 scale) by the regular use of a parenteral narcotic in conjunction with sitting in a very warm bath for ten minutes immediately after receiving the analgesic. In the hospital, Mrs. C. was not allowed a tub bath without assistance. It was impossible to provide assistance immediately after each dose of narcotic as she had been doing at home. Mrs. C. reported an average pain intensity of 7 to 8 (on a 0 to 10 scale) despite receiving 25 percent more narcotic on a q4h schedule.

The patient must develop trust and respect for the care giver's ability to be of assistance in gaining control of the pain in order for effective pain management to be achieved. It is, therefore, important that the initial approaches be acceptable to the patient and also that they provide a significant amount of relief. Interventions the patient judges to have been unsuccessful in the past should not be instituted again until the credibility and trustworthiness of the initiator of these methods has been established. For example, if the patient reports that adequate relief from oral analgesics has never been achieved, it is possible that this occurred because of inadequate dosage when converting from the parenteral to the oral route. Nonetheless, no attempt should be made to convert the patient to oral analgesics until enough trust has been developed in the care giver to overcome the patient's resistance to the intervention and to minimize the likelihood that high anxiety levels will impede the success of the new plan.

The author is aware of no research in this area, but clinical observations indicate that patients who describe previously effective therapies in graphic detail do not respond well to simple approaches to pain control. In such patients, codeine, a small white tablet, will often be less effective than Darvon Compound (Lilly, Indianapolis), a large colorful capsule. Likewise, morphine in a cherry syrup concoction may seem superior to an equivalent dose of morphine in a plain, small white tablet. (For equivalent doses refer to tables in Donovan and Girton[12] [pp. 234–236] or McCaffery[20] [p. 191]). Patients who describe many interpersonal components of previous encounters with pain and its treatment are better candidates for interventions relying on personal contact (massage, frequent analgesics, coached relaxation techniques, hypnosis) than on interventions with low personal contact (TENS, long-acting analgesics, distraction).

Established Patterns of Coping

Throughout the process of assessment, the care giver needs to be aware of cues the patient is giving about personal ways of perceiving and coping with pain. The patient who answers every question in detail will need a different approach than the patient who gives brief, vague responses. The patient who says that the only effective method of relief is "the pill my doctor ordered" will accept a different choice of approaches to pain control than the person who does not want to take any drugs. Asking the patient to explain how past health problems and crises (illness, pain, smoking cessation, weight loss, loss of a loved one) were handled, will generally aid in identifying acceptable strategies (Table 5-5). For instance, the patient who describes a lifelong pattern of withdrawal from human contact will be

Table 5-5
Use of Assessment Data to Select Alternative Interventions

Behavior		Pain Relief Methods to Consider Based on Observations
Attitude toward noninvasive methods	Accepting	Noninvasive methods
	Skeptical	Start with medications, then sell noninvasive methods
Attitude toward medications	"The Answer"	Start with medications
	Resistant	Noninvasive methods; sell medications
Level of trust in health care system	High	Any intervention may be suggested
	Lacking	Start with what the patient thinks will work best
Perceptions	Detailed	Specify intervention in detail
	Global	Capitalize on trust and previous success
Interactions	Provide relief	Distraction
	No relief	Don't use distraction
Use of medications	Regular and effective	Continue and evaluate for use of noninvasive methods
	Regular/not effective	Titrate dose and add local/regional methods or refer for pain clinical evaluation if pain is severe and not responding to any type of intervention
Depression		Evaluate for use of tricyclic antidepressants
Anxiety	Pain controlled	Listen, psychotherapy, tranquilizers
	Pain not controlled	Control pain
Expectations	Positive	Meet as much as possible, or if not realistic, assist patient to modify
	Negative	Assist patient to modify

unlikely to embrace plans that include massage, coached relaxation, or conversation as a form of distraction.

SYSTEMATIC ASSESSMENT TOOLS

A systematic assessment of the cancer patient's pain is essential in understanding the patient's experience and devising a realistic plan for controlling the pain. Because of the multidimensional and individual nature of the pain experience, assessment of pain can become an unrealistically laborious process for the patient as well as the nurse. Research methods are often complex, time-consuming, require sophisticated technology, and/or may be invasive. Clinical assessment needs to be less complex, more respectful of patient's time and energy, less precise, and as non-burdensome as possible. In pain research, the goal of measurement is often the quantification of the pain experience. The goal of clinical assessment is control of the pain with assessment as the means of accomplishing that goal. An ideal tool for clinical assessment would provide information about the eight dimensions described above to guide the selection of appropriate therapy. Such a tool must also meet the needs of the patient for simplicity, brevity, and relevancy, as well as the constraints the environment places on the time of the care giver. Few of the tools described in this section completely meet all of these criteria, but each has a contribution to make to the process of pain assessment, and each illustrates a different approach to systematic assessment.

McGuire[22] developed a one-page assessment tool to assure the gathering of essential information in a systematic manner. Despite its brevity, this tool closely meets the criteria for a comprehensive yet practical assessment established in this chapter. McGuire developed the tool to formalize this process so that it could be easily taught to staff nurses and students. The McGuire Pain Assessment Tool can be reproduced for use in patient assessment from the March issue of *Nursing* (1981).

The Memorial Pain Assessment Card, developed by the Analgesic Studies Section of Memorial Sloan-Kettering Cancer Center, has been reported to be useful in the assessment of clinical pain in medically ill patients. The MPAC is a short, easy to administer, multidimensional tool consisting of a pain adjective rating scale, a pain intensity VAS, a pain relief VAS, and mood rating scale.[13] The developers report that the MPAC can distinguish pain from psychological distress and that it is nearly as valid as more sophisticated and complex assessment batteries (see Appendix).

The McGill Pain Questionnaire provides information about the sensory, affective, and evaluative dimensions of pain. In addition to these parameters, the MPQ elicits information about the location of the pain; the intensity and periodicity of the pain; accompanying symptoms; effects on sleep, activity, and eating; and the pattern of analgesic use (see Appendix). Construct validity has been repeatedly confirmed by means of factor analysis.[4] Chapman et al.[4] conclude that the MPQ is a powerful tool for obtaining data on both the qualitative and the quantitative aspects of pain. Turk et al.[31] caution that since the three PRI subscale dimensions (discussed earlier in this chapter) are highly intercorrelated, the total PRI score is more appropriate for pain assessment than subscale scores. Syrjala and Chapman[30] stress the importance of using a visual analogue scale in conjunction with the MPQ because of the tendency of some patients to score high on verbal scales such as the PRI while rating the intensity of pain low on a VAS.

The Wisconsin Brief Pain Questionnaire, now called the Brief Pain Inventory, was developed primarily for clinical use with patients in pain who were too ill to be subjected to longer and more exhausting assessment techniques. It assesses the following dimensions: history of pain; site of pain; intensity of pain at its worst, as it usually is, and as it is now; medications and treatments used to relieve the pain; relief obtained; effect of pain on mood, interpersonal relations, walking, sleep, work, and enjoyment of life (see Appendix). Validity is supported by the facts that (1) test–retest reliability was low in a sample of cancer patients (r=.22–.34); (2) pain intensity increased with advancing disease; (3) increased pain scores were related to increased use of analgesics (p<.002); and (4) worst pain was moderately correlated with interference scores (r=.32–.48).[7] Chapman et al.[4] conclude that the multidimensional nature of the BPI frees it from the limitations of the simpler VAS scales and makes it both useful and reliable as a clinical assessment tool (see Appendix).

There are many more comprehensive methods of measuring and assessing pain. Four recent reviews provide excellent up-to-date information on the spectrum of pain measurement.[4,16,21,30] The first and the last two references are scientific review articles that attempt to present unbiased discussions of the various methods of pain measurement. The emphasis is on the validity and reliability of the instruments for both clinical and research purposes. The limitations of each method are clearly outlined as well. Karoly[16] reviews assessment of pain for those involved in the psychological treatment of medically ill patients. The author is clearly biased in the direction of believing that patients have overwhelming psychological components to their pain and displays a lack of concern for the physical-sensory component of pain. Despite this obvious bias, Karoly's chapter is an excellent source of information about a variety of methods for assessing pain.

SUMMARY

Accurate assessment of pain is the first step toward understanding the experience as the patient perceives it, determining the best methods for alleviating the associated physical and psychological distress, structuring the environment to assist the patient in efforts to prevent the pain from controlling him, and knowing whether the efforts have been effective or not. Good baseline assessment promotes the patient–care giver alliance, directs the choice of intervention among an ever increasing armamentarium of pain management techniques, and is the yardstick by which the degree of pain control is measured.

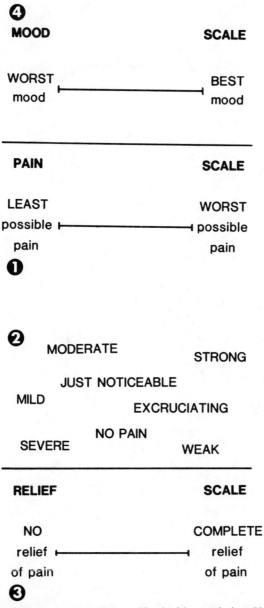

Memorial Pain Assessment Card. Used with permission. Validation and administration information are available in Fishman B, Pasternak S, Wallenstein SL, Houde RW, Holland JC, and Foley KM: The Memorial Pain Assessment Card: A valid instrument for the evaluation of cancer pain. Submitted for publication, 1986. For copies of this paper and the MPAC, please write to K. M. Foley, M.D., Memorial Sloan-Kettering Cancer Center, 1275 York Avenue, New York, NY 10021.

McGILL - MELZACK PAIN QUESTIONNAIRE

Patient's Name_____ Date_____ Time_____am/pm
Analgesic(s)_____ Dosage_____ Time Given_____am/pm
_____ Dosage_____ Time Given_____am/pm

Analgesic Time Difference (hours): +4 +1 +2 +3

PRI: S_____ A_____ E_____ M(S)_____ M(AE)_____ M(T)_____ PRI(T)_____
     (1-10)   (11-15)   (16)   (17-19)   (20)   (17-20)   (1-20)

1 FLICKERING ☐	11 TIRING ☐
QUIVERING ☐	EXHAUSTING ☐
PULSING ☐	
THROBBING ☐	12 SICKENING ☐
BEATING ☐	SUFFOCATING ☐
POUNDING ☐	

PPI_____ COMMENTS:

2 JUMPING ☐
FLASHING ☐
SHOOTING ☐

13 FEARFUL ☐
FRIGHTFUL ☐
TERRIFYING ☐

3 PRICKING ☐
BORING ☐
DRILLING ☐
STABBING ☐
LANCINATING ☐

14 PUNISHING ☐
GRUELLING ☐
CRUEL ☐
VICIOUS ☐
KILLING ☐

4 SHARP ☐
CUTTING ☐
LACERATING ☐

15 WRETCHED ☐
BLINDING ☐

5 PINCHING ☐
PRESSING ☐
GNAWING ☐
CRAMPING ☐
CRUSHING ☐

16 ANNOYING ☐
TROUBLESOME ☐
MISERABLE ☐
INTENSE ☐
UNBEARABLE ☐

6 TUGGING ☐
PULLING ☐
WRENCHING ☐

17 SPREADING ☐
RADIATING ☐
PENETRATING ☐
PIERCING ☐

7 HOT ☐
BURNING ☐
SCALDING ☐
SEARING ☐

18 TIGHT ☐
NUMB ☐
DRAWING ☐
SQUEEZING ☐
TEARING ☐

CONSTANT ☐
PERIODIC ☐
BRIEF ☐

8 TINGLING ☐
ITCHY ☐
SMARTING ☐
STINGING ☐

19 COOL ☐
COLD ☐
FREEZING ☐

20 NAGGING ☐
NAUSEATING ☐
AGONIZING ☐
DREADFUL ☐
TORTURING ☐

9 DULL ☐
SORE ☐
HURTING ☐
ACHING ☐
HEAVY ☐

PPI
0 NO PAIN ☐
1 MILD ☐
2 DISCOMFORTING ☐
3 DISTRESSING ☐
4 HORRIBLE ☐
5 EXCRUCIATING ☐

10 TENDER ☐
TAUT ☐
RASPING ☐
SPLITTING ☐

ACCOMPANYING
SYMPTOMS:
NAUSEA ☐
HEADACHE ☐
DIZZINESS ☐
DROWSINESS ☐
CONSTIPATION ☐
DIARRHEA ☐

COMMENTS:

SLEEP:
GOOD ☐
FITFUL ☐
CAN'T SLEEP ☐

COMMENTS:

ACTIVITY:
GOOD ☐
SOME ☐
LITTLE ☐
NONE ☐

FOOD INTAKE:
GOOD ☐
SOME ☐
LITTLE ☐
NONE ☐

COMMENTS:

COMMENTS:

McGill Pain Questionnaire. Used with permission of Ronald Melzack. For additional information or authorization to use this instrument, please write Ronald Melzack, M.D., Pain Clinic, McGill University, Montreal, Canada.

Brief Pain Questionnaire

Date: _____/_____/_____

Name: _____
      Last   First   Middle

Phone: _____   Sex: Female _____   Male _____

Date of Birth: _____/_____/_____

1) Marital Status (at present)

    1. _____ Single   4. _____ Widowed

    2. _____ Married   5. _____ Separated

    3. _____ Divorced

2) Education (circle only the highest grade or degree completed)

    Grade 0   1   2   3   4   5   6   7   8   9

           10   11   12   13   14   15   16   M.A./M.S.

           Professional degree (please specify) _____

3) Current occupation _____
    (specify titles; if you are not now working, tell us your previous occupation)

4) Spouse's Occupation_____

5) Which of the following best describe your current job status?
    1. Employed outside the home, full-time
    2. Employed outside the home, part-time
    3. Homemaker
    4. Retired
    5. Unemployed
    6. Other _____

6) How long has it been since you first learned your diagnosis? _____ months.

7) Have you ever had pain due to your present disease?

          1. _____ Yes   2. _____ No   3. _____ Uncertain

8) When you first received your diagnosis, was pain one of your symptoms?

      1. _____ Yes   2. _____ No   3. _____ Uncertain

9) Have you had surgery in the past month?   1. _____ Yes   2. _____ No

10) Throughout our lives, most of us have had pain from time to time (such as minor headaches, sprains, and toothaches). Have you had pain other than these everyday kinds of pain during the last week?

      1. _____ Yes   2. _____ No

IF YOU ANSWERED YES TO THE LAST QUESTION, PLEASE GO ON TO QUESTION 11 AND FINISH THIS QUESTIONNAIRE. IF YOU ANSWERED NO, GO ON TO PAGE 7 AND COMPLETE THE REMAINING QUESTIONS.

11) Indicate on this diagram where your pain occurs by shading the affected area. Label the drawings with "S" for pain near the surface of your body, or with "D" for pain that is deeper. Also, label the drawing with "P" for the body site where your *PRIMARY* or *WORST* pain is located.

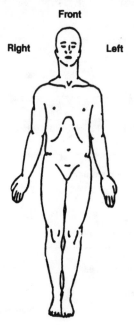
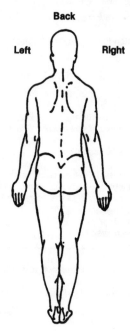

12) Please rate your pain by circling the one number that best describes your pain at its *worst* in the last week.

0	1	2	3	4	5	6	7	8	9	10
No pain										Pain as bad as you can imagine

13) Please rate your pain by circling the one number that best describes your pain at its *least* in the last week.

0	1	2	3	4	5	6	7	8	9	10
No pain										Pain as bad as you can imagine

14) Please rate your pain by circling the one number that best describes your pain on the *average*.

0	1	2	3	4	5	6	7	8	9	10
No pain										Pain as bad as you can imagine

15) Please rate your pain by circling the one number that tells how much pain you have *right now*.

0	1	2	3	4	5	6	7	8	9	10
No pain										Pain as bad as you can imagine

16. What kinds of things make your pain feel better (for example, heat, medicine, rest)?

_____

_____

17) What kinds of things make your pain worse (for example, walking, standing, lifting)?

_____

_____

18) What treatment or medications are you receiving for pain?

_____

_____

19) In the last week, how much relief have pain treatments or medications provided? Please circle the one percentage that most shows how much relief you have received.

0%	10%	20%	30%	40%	50%	60%	70%	80%	90%	100%
No relief										Complete relief

20) If you take pain medication, how many hours does it take before the pain returns?

1. Pain medication doesn't help at all.   5. Four hours.
2. One hour.   6. Five to twelve hours.
3. Two hours.   7. More than twelve hours.
4. Three hours.   8. I do not take pain medication.

21) Circle the appropriate answer for each item.
    I believe my pain is due to:

Yes   No   1. The effects of treatment (for example, medication, surgery, radiation, prosthetic device).
Yes   No   2. My primary disease (meaning the disease currently being treated and evaluated).
Yes   No   3. A medical condition unrelated to primary disease (for example, arthritis).

22) For each of the following words, circle the one number that best corresponds to how well that adjective describes your pain.

	Not at all									Extremely well	
Aching	0	1	2	3	4	5	6	7	8	9	10
Throbbing	0	1	2	3	4	5	6	7	8	9	10
Shooting	0	1	2	3	4	5	6	7	8	9	10
Stabbing	0	1	2	3	4	5	6	7	8	9	10
Gnawing	0	1	2	3	4	5	6	7	8	9	10
Sharp	0	1	2	3	4	5	6	7	8	9	10
Tender	0	1	2	3	4	5	6	7	8	9	10
Burning	0	1	2	3	4	5	6	7	8	9	10
Exhausting	0	1	2	3	4	5	6	7	8	9	10
Tiring	0	1	2	3	4	5	6	7	8	9	10
Penetrating	0	1	2	3	4	5	6	7	8	9	10
Nagging	0	1	2	3	4	5	6	7	8	9	10
Numb	0	1	2	3	4	5	6	7	8	9	10
Miserable	0	1	2	3	4	5	6	7	8	9	10
Unbearable	0	1	2	3	4	5	6	7	8	9	10

23) Circle the one number that describes how, during the past week, pain has interfered with your:

A. General Activity

| 0 | 1 | 2 | 3 | 4 | 5 | 6 | 7 | 8 | 9 | 10 |
Does not interfere / Completely interferes

B. Mood

| 0 | 1 | 2 | 3 | 4 | 5 | 6 | 7 | 8 | 9 | 10 |
Does not interfere / Completely interferes

C. Walking ability

| 0 | 1 | 2 | 3 | 4 | 5 | 6 | 7 | 8 | 9 | 10 |
Does not interfere / Completely interferes

D. Normal work (includes both work outside the home and housework)

| 0 | 1 | 2 | 3 | 4 | 5 | 6 | 7 | 8 | 9 | 10 |
Does not interfere / Completely interferes

E. Relations with other people

| 0 | 1 | 2 | 3 | 4 | 5 | 6 | 7 | 8 | 9 | 10 |
Does not interfere / Completely interferes

F. Sleep

| 0 | 1 | 2 | 3 | 4 | 5 | 6 | 7 | 8 | 9 | 10 |
Does not interfere / Completely interferes

G. Enjoyment of life

| 0 | 1 | 2 | 3 | 4 | 5 | 6 | 7 | 8 | 9 | 10 |
Does not interfere / Completely interferes

Brief Pain Inventory. Used with permission. For additional information or authorization to use this instrument, please write to C. S. Cleeland, Ph.D., Professor, Neurology, University of Wisconsin Medical School, 600 Highland Ave., Madison, WI 53792.

REFERENCES

1. Ahles TA, Ruckdeschel JR, Blanchard EB: Cancer-related pain II. Assessment with visual analogue scales. J Psychosom Res 28:121–124, 1984
2. American Psychiatric Association: Diagnostic and Statistical Manual of Mental Disorders (3rd ed.). Washington, DC, American Psychiatric Association, 1981, pp 210–217.
3. Barbour LA, McGuire DB, Kirchhoff KT: Nonanalgesic methods of pain control used by cancer outpatients. Oncol Nurs Forum 13:(6) 56–60, November/December, 1986
4. Chapman DD, Casey KL, Dubner R, et al.: Pain measurement: an overview. Pain 22:1–31, 1985
5. Charap AD: The knowledge, attitudes and experience of medical personnel treating pain in the terminally ill. Mt Sinai J Med (NY) 45:561–580, 1978
6. Cleeland CS: Measurement and prevalence of pain in cancer. Semin Oncol Nurs 1:87–92, 1985
7. Daut RL, Cleeland CS, Flanery RC: Development of the Wisconsin Brief Pain Questionnaire to assess pain in cancer and other diseases. Pain 17:197–210, 1983
8. Dean H: Selecting a tool for measuring quality of life: multiple tools, in Stromborg M (Ed): Instruments for Use in Clinical Nursing Research. East Norwalk, CT, Appleton-Century-Crofts, 1987
9. Derogatis LR, Abeloff MD, McBeth CD: Cancer patients and their physicians in the perception of psychological symptoms. Psychosomatics 17:197–201, 1976
10. Donovan MI: Cancer pain: you can help! Nurs Clin North Am 17:713–728, 1982
11. Donovan MI, Dillon P, McGuire L: Incidence and characteristics of pain in a sample of medical-surgical inpatients. Pain (Accepted for publication)
12. Donovan MI, Girton SE: Cancer Care Nursing (2nd ed.). Norwalk, CT, Appleton-Century-Crofts, 1984, pp 165–276
13. Fishman B, Pasternak S, Wallenstein RW, et al.: The Memorial pain assessment card: a valid instrument for evaluation of cancer pain. Proc Am Soc Clin Oncol 5:239, March 1986 (abstract)
14. Goodwin JS, Goodwin JM, Vogel AV: Knowledge and use of placebos in house officers and nurses. Ann Intern Med 91:106–110, 1979
15. Gracely RH, Dubner R: Pain assessment in humans—a reply to Hall. Pain 11:109–120, 1981
16. Karoly P: The assessment of pain: concepts and procedures, in Karoly P (Ed): Measurement Strategies in Health Psychology. New York-Wiley Interscience, 1985, pp 461–519
17. Keefe FJ, Block AR: Development of an observation method for assessing pain behavior in chronic low back pain patients. Behav Ther 13:363–375, 1982
18. LeResche L: Facial expression of pain: a study of candid photographs. J Nonverb Behav 7:46–56, 1982
19. Marks RM, Sachar EJ: Undertreatment of medical inpatients with narcotic analgesics. Ann Intern Med 78:172–181, 1973
20. McCaffery M: Nursing Management of the Patient with Pain (2nd ed.). Philadelphia, JB Lippincott, 1979
21. McGuire DB: The measurement of clinical pain. Nurs Res 33:152–156, 1984
22. McGuire L: A short, simple tool for assessing your patient's pain. Nursing 81 11:48–49, 1981
23. Meinhart NT, McCaffery M: Pain: A Nursing Approach to Assessment and Analysis. Norwalk, CT, Appleton-Century-Crofts, 1983
24. Melzack R: The McGill pain questionnaire: major properties and scoring methods. Pain 1:277–299, 1975
25. Myers JS: Cancer pain: assessment of nurses' knowledge and attitudes. Oncol Nurs Forum 12(4):62–66, 1985

26. Outcome Standards for Cancer Nursing Practice. Kansas City, MO, American Nurses' Association, 1979, pp 3–4
27. Shacham S, Reinhardt LC, Raubertas RF, et al.: Emotional states and pain: intraindividual and interindividual measures of association. J Behav Med 6:405–419, 1983
28. Sternbach RA: Pain Patients: Traits and Treatment. Orlando, FL, Academic Press, 1974
29. Stromborg M: Selecting a tool for measuring quality of life: single instruments, in Stromborg M (Ed): Instruments for Use in Clinical Nursing Research. East Norwalk, CT: Appleton-Century-Crofts, 1987.
30. Syrjala KL, Chapman CR: Measurement of clinical pain: a review and integration of research findings. Adv Pain Res Ther 7:71–101, 1984
31. Turk DC, Rudy RE, Salovey P: The McGill Pain Questionnaire reconsidered: confirming the factor structure and examining appropriate uses. Pain 21:385–397, 1985
32. Ward NG, Bloom VL, Friedel RO: The effectiveness of tricyclic antidepressants in the treatment of coexisting pain and depression. Pain 7:331–341, 1979
33. Zborowski M: People in Pain. San Francisco, Jossey-Bass, 1969

Karen L. Syrjala, Ph.D.

6

The Measurement of Pain

Pain is a complex, aversive, and subjective experience that cannot be reduced to a single number or defined purely as a sensation. Despite the complex physical and mental interactions that comprise an experience of pain, evaluation of a clinical problem often requires that pain be quantified. Newer methods for measuring pain are designed to permit this quantification without oversimplification. Measures of pain discussed in this chapter are not intended solely for use in research, although each instrument has met standards of reliability and validity adequate for research purposes. These instruments are also designed to help the clinician in overall assessment of a patient's treatment needs or treatment success.

There are many types of pain associated with cancer. The etiology and nature of pain may be procedure-related and brief, treatment-related and persistent, tumor- or treatment-related and chronic, or a combination of these. The pain exists as a component of a patient's total experience of suffering, including emotional aspects. Therefore, it is difficult to separate discomfort that is specific to pain from general disease-related discomfort. One patient may have severe infiltrates of tumor and rate pain as high, while another may have little physical evidence of injury, but also may report a high level of pain. In fact, both of these patients are processing their experiences of pain, labeling them, having thoughts and feelings about them, changing or not changing their behaviors in an effort to manage them, and reacting to their social environment in relation to whether others recognize their suffering.

CONCEPTS IN MEASURING PAIN

Multiple Dimensions

It is well accepted that pain has sensory, affective, cognitive and behavioral dimensions (see Table 6-1).[46,47] The patient in pain is usually able to describe the qualities of the pain, which are often *sensory* in nature and may include terms such as "burning, stabbing, pressure, or tingling." This sensory dimension appears to be most closely tied to type and extent of tissue injury.

Alternatively, pain may be described in *affective* terms that convey how much the pain bothers the person, e.g., "unpleasant, exhausting, or agonizing." Affect may be measured as it relates specifically to the experience of pain or it may be assessed more globally as depression or anxiety. Ahles et al.[2] found evidence that activity level in cancer patients was not associated with sensory qualities of pain nor with generalized depression or anxiety, but was linked with affective and cognitive responses specific to the experience of pain.

The words people use to describe pain indicate that they think about the intensity and meaning of their pain experience in addition to processing sensory and affective information. This *cognitive* appraisal has direct impact on the affective or emotional dimension of the pain experience since it may include beliefs about the cause of the pain, expected course of pain, and associations of pain with images of decay or loss of control. The pain may be viewed as an indicator that cancer is spreading, pain will worsen, "I don't know what will happen next," and "there is no explanation for why this is happening to me." Cognitive appraisal may be in the form of complete thoughts, a single word, or a visual image of decay that implies many unspoken beliefs. Such thoughts or images may lead to feelings of fear, loss of control, anxiety, helplessness, and perhaps a focus on the pain as a symbol of the disease process. These thoughts, together with a focus on the experience of pain, are likely to have some impact on the level of pain reported by the patient as well as on the words used to describe pain.

Only limited standardized measures of the cognitive dimension of pain exist. These instruments do not measure thoughts about pain, or accuracy of

Table 6-1
Dimensions of the Pain Experience

Dimension	Description
Sensory	Burning, stabbing, pressure, tingling
Affective	Tiring, unpleasant, agonizing
Cognitive	Pain intensity, beliefs about pain
Behavioral	Grimacing, groaning, holding or guarding afflicted area

information about a specific pain problem. Since measurement tools are not available, thoughts about a pain problem must be addressed during the broader assessment process. It is possible, though, to develop an instrument that will define the information that has been provided to a patient and will assess retention of that information. Although research has demonstrated that the provision of information can reduce distress in patients with pain,[27,59,62] one group of investigators found that 74 percent of the cancer patients studied did not recall receiving any information concerning the source or expected course of their pain.[2] It is not known whether these patients were not given information or forgot what they were told. An understanding of the patient's cognitive and affective appraisal of pain may provide as valuable an insight into necessary approaches to treatment as can a number reflecting pain intensity on a tool such as a linear scale.

The *behavioral* dimension of measurement of pain includes both verbal and non-verbal expressions that can be observed by others. The observation of elements such as medication intake, activity level, moaning, and rubbing or guarding of afflicted areas enriches the quantification of pain. However, observation alone is no more valid a measure of pain than is a single report of intensity. Two patients with the same cause of pain may behave very differently. Some patients may cope with pain by conveying their distress to others, while other patients may use activity and ordinary conversation to distract themselves from the perception of pain. Observations, when combined with subjective reports, are helpful in determining appropriate treatment directions for both kinds of patients.

Physiological Correlates of Pain

No direct, reliable physiological measures of pain have been found, although certain physiological responses are clearly associated with acute pain. Autonomic arousal (e.g., increases in heart rate, blood pressure, and respiration) is often seen at the onset of acute pain, but with time this arousal fades. In addition, these physiologic indicators are non-specific responses to stress and may reflect anxiety or fear rather than level of pain. Technological devices for measuring pain, including thermography, evoked potentials, and electromyography, have shown at best an association with pain severity in certain syndromes, but are also vulnerable to contamination by autonomic arousal or tension.

Special Considerations in the Measurement of Cancer Pain

Cancer pain requires particular attention to certain concepts within the realm of pain measurement. Cancer patients differ from patients with benign syndromes, particularly in the affective/emotional dimension.

Research supports the importance of measuring affect specific to cancer pain rather than as general depression or anxiety. In comparing cancer and benign pain patients' responses on the McGill Pain Questionnaire (MPQ), Kremer, Atkinson, and Ignelzi[35] reported similar scores on the affective dimension when intensity of pain was high. However, when intensity was low, cancer patients reported significantly greater affective responses to their pain than did benign patients. The researchers speculated that this difference reflected the differential meaning of the pain. Interestingly, high or low affective responses by cancer patients on the MPQ were not related to their reports of general mood disturbance or functional impairment, contrary to the benign pain patients. In a study assessing the relationship of pain to measures of general distress in cancer patients, Ahles, Blanchard, and Ruckdeschel[2] found that intensity of pain was not related to general distress. The affective dimension of the MPQ, however, was consistently positively correlated with depression, but not related to anxiety. Patients who believed that pain indicated progression of their disease had elevated scores on standard measures of both depression and anxiety, thus supporting the role of cognition in the experience of pain. On the behavioral end, medication intake was associated with intensity, affective, sensory and evaluative dimensions of pain as measured by the MPQ. Activity level was associated with affective and evaluative dimensions but not with intensity.

The results from these studies support three contentions important when measuring cancer pain. The first is that cancer patients are clearly different from patients with benign pain in their emotional reactions to pain. The second is that affective dimensions specific to pain rather than general in nature need to be measured in cancer patients. Finally, the interpretation of personal meaning has a significant impact on reports of pain in the cancer patient.

Cancer pain does not represent a single domain of problems, as other chapters in this monograph attest, but rather encompasses a vast assortment of difficulties that may overlap; the pain problem may be present within a context of multiple symptoms such as nausea, anorexia, or general weakness; and the pain problem may or may not relate to the cancer or its treatment. The duration and source of pain are important considerations when deciding on appropriate measurement tools; however, these factors must be placed within the context of the patient's needs as a whole. For a patient with multiple symptoms it may not be possible to identify how much of the dysfunction is specifically related to pain, mood, or other problems.

Acute versus Chronic Pain

Duration of pain is an important determinant in selecting appropriate measurement tools. A distinction is often made between clinical pain that is acute and chronic. For cancer patients, this traditional dichotomy does not address the broad spectrum of sources or temporal qualities of pain. In the literature, acute pain is generally considered to be associated with an injury or disease process and to be of short duration. Chronic pain is commonly defined as extending for months and having a less clearly defined organic source, or as resulting from long-term illness.[8,16]

The definition of acute pain encompasses both brief and persistent problems. A cancer patient may experience a pain from a procedure that lasts minutes but causes discomfort that requires analgesia. On the other hand, a patient may have treatment-related pain, such as stomatitis, that lasts weeks, or pain from metastases that endures until effective treatment is provided. Both treatment and appropriate measurement will vary depending on the brief or persistent nature of the problem.

Foley[16] has described three types of chronic cancer pain patients. The first is the patient for whom pain is an ongoing part of the disease process, such as with metastatic disease. These patients may have continuous, fairly constant discomfort with intermittent exacerbations of pain. The second type of patient has chronic pain that begins as a definable pain syndrome that gradually becomes a disease unto itself. Chronic cancer pain occurring as a sequela of treatment (e.g., phantom limb pain or post-mastectomy pain) may fit this description. In benign, non-progressive problems, this type of chronic pain usually does not worsen, although tolerance to medications and dimensions of pain other than sensation may change. The third type of patient has chronic pain (e.g., myalgias or arthralgias) that has a less definable cause. These latter two groups of patients are likely to report significant limitations on their activities and impact on their daily lives; additionally, they may be most similar to patients described in the chronic benign pain literature.

Whether pain is brief, persistent, intermittent, or continuous and chronic, each situation is likely to require choices designed to address the individual characteristics of the pain and to meet the goal of measurement. Physiologic responses certainly alter as the body adjusts to pain, but in addition, cognitive appraisal is likely to shift, and affective and behavioral responses to transform with time. Thus, the goal of measurement will differ if pain relief must be maintained for months or years rather than hours or minutes.

INSTRUMENTS FOR MEASURING PAIN

To qualify as a useful tool for measuring pain in the clinical setting an instrument must meet several criteria. First, both staff and patient must be able to understand and complete the tool in a reasonable amount of time. Reasonable time will depend on the duration of pain, the health or illness of the patient, and time constraints of staff. Second, the measure must be able to reflect differences between patients as well as changes within a patient. It also must show clinically useful sensitivity to analgesic effects and, ideally, demonstrate patterns of response that are unique to different syndromes of pain. Finally, a measure must have reliability and validity documented through such techniques as internal consistency, repeated testing, agreement between independent judges, relationship to other measures of pain, and ability to predict or reflect differing treatment outcomes.

Simple Self-Report Measures of Pain Severity

A number of scales are available that allow patients to report their subjective perception of pain severity. These scales measure single dimensions, but have also been used to measure multiple dimensions by repeating the scale format with varied instructions.

The most commonly used and simplest self-report measures of pain are the numerical rating scale (NRS) or the visual analogue scale (VAS). A third alternative is the verbal descriptor scale (VDS) (Table 6-2). Each of these scales has had reliability and validity demonstrated in previous research, although whether they reliably or validly reflect the pain experience is questionable.[7,47] The NRS may be given in oral or written form simply by asking the patient to rate pain on a 0 to 10 or 0 to 100 scale with 0 being "no pain at all" and 10 or 100 being "worst pain imaginable." The VAS is presented as a 10-centimeter line with verbal anchors similar to those on the NRS. Patients mark the line at a point representing the severity of their pain. Theoretically there are an infinite number of points possible on the VAS, but in practice 100 points (corresponding to millimeters) are usually scored. VDS employ rank-ordered words such as "none, mild, moderate, and severe" from which patients choose words that best represent their levels of pain.

A great deal of research has focused on comparing these scales. Each

Table 6-2
Simple Self-Report Measures of Pain Severity

Visual Analogue Scale
Instruction: Mark on the line below how strong your pain is
   No   pain / _____ 10 cm _____ / The   worst
                                                                         pain possible

Numerical Rating Scale
Instruction: On a scale from 0 to 10, how strong is your pain?
   0 = No pain 1   2   3   4   5   6   7   8   9   10 = The worst pain possible

Verbal Descriptor Scale
Instruction: Which word best describes how your pain feels?
   None   Mild   Moderate   Severe   Excruciating

has advantages, disadvantages, and situations in which it is the preferable instrument for measurement of pain. Verbal descriptors, as they are used in unidimensional scaling, have the primary advantage of being easy to understand. In one study,[34] 100 percent of patients were able to complete a VDS, whereas 2 percent were unable to complete the NRS and 11 percent failed to complete the VAS. Failures on the VAS were most common in older patients (mean = 75.3 years) as compared to those who completed the VAS (mean = 54.4 years). All three scales were significantly positively correlated although the NRS (using a 100-point scale), and the VAS were most highly correlated at r = .86. Conflict exists in the literature as to whether patients prefer the VDS or VAS. Although Kremer et al.[34] reported a preference for the VDS, others[24,28,47,52] have found that the VAS was preferred, more often completed, and closer to the patient's actual experience as long as clear explanation and opportunity for practice were given.

In the clinical setting, children and young to middle-aged adults usually have no difficulty comprehending instructions on the VAS. With very sick patients, oral versions of the NRS are easily administered, or patients can hold up fingers from none to ten. Alternatively, if a VAS is used, a staff person can run a pencil along the line and ask the patient to nod or raise a finger at the point that corresponds to the current level of pain. The scales have face validity with both patients and staff; however, any changes in administration may change the reliability of scores when compared between or within patients. Age and ability, as demonstrated in practice sessions, are factors that should be considered in choosing the best instrument in a given circumstance. For patients who have difficulty with the VAS, the NRS is a reasonable alternative.

Beyond patient preference and ease of understanding, the NRS and VAS appear to have certain advantages for the scaling of intensity of pain, while the VDS is useful for ratings on multiple dimensions of pain as described further below. By virtue of their greater number of points for rating, the VAS and NRS provide greater sensitivity and freedom to vary. The VAS most closely approximates an interval scale from which parametric statistics may be used in data analyses.[57] The VDS has the fewest number of points, the least freedom to vary, and is not as sensitive as the VAS. In addition, the VDS is an ordinal scale without proven equal distances between points and as such does not legitimately meet criteria for the use of parametric statistics.

A plethora of alternative forms have been explored to make the VAS or NRS optimally useful. These have included using an unmarked line for the VAS, putting numbers or words under the VAS, horizontal versus vertical placement of the VAS line, the use of faces as an alternative to words, the use of thermometers or chromatics to indicate growing intensity, and a variety of words as anchors.[20,22,54,60] A VAS or NRS format with a horizontal line and no intermediate anchors appears to be easiest to use and to have greatest reliability and validity.

The question of what can be measured with a VAS or NRS has not been fully answered. Current pain intensity appears to be the most frequently and reliably measured dimension. It is also possible to ask patients to rate their worst, least, and average pain. Research on memory for pain suggests that a pain that has ceased may be measured up to a week afterward. However, memory for continuous pain is apparently not reliable for time periods further than 24 hours into the past.[13,23,37]

In measuring affective dimensions such as anxiety or depression with the VAS or NRS, a number of issues merit attention. Affective experience specific to pain may be measured by having patients rate how much their pain "bothers" them. Additionally, VAS and NRS scales can be used as a general "mood" rating or as multiple ratings of specific affects such as anxiety and depression. Depression rated on a VAS has been shown to correlate with other more extensive measures of depression such as the Beck Depression Inventory and SCL-90. Anxiety measured on a VAS did not similarly correlate with standardized measures of anxiety, and therefore may not be a valid use of the scale.[3] There are no data on how many times a VAS may be reliably administered as a measure of pain and/or affect. If ratings are repeated, a halo effect is possible in which the patient's report of affect is influenced by the report of pain intensity. To reduce this possible contamination, scales should be presented in different formats or on separate pages so that comparison with previous scores is less likely. Multidimensional measurements have been designed in an attempt to eliminate these difficulties and should be considered in all but the extremely sick patient or time-limited situation.

Multidimensional Self-Report Measures

Multidimensional self-report measures provide for reporting of multiple dimensions of pain without the vulnerability to halo effects found by repeating the VAS or NRS. This is accomplished by measuring each dimension with a different set of words or scaling format. Each of the measures includes an intensity and affective dimension; most also have subscales for measuring sensory and behavioral components of pain. The duration and type of pain requiring measurement will help to determine the most appropriate instrument in a given situation.

The McGill Pain Questionnaire (MPQ) is the most widely studied multidimensional measure of pain available. It uses the verbal descriptor technique to measure sensory, affective, and evaluative dimensions of pain. In addition, the MPQ provides information on location of pain, changes over time, and compares current pain to other types of pain such as toothaches and headaches.[45] Consistent patterns of word use have been demonstrated in cancer patients given the MPQ.[21,41,42,45]

The verbal descriptor sections of the MPQ are most well-tested and the only subscales that can be reliably and validly used in research comparisons. The verbal descriptors consist of 20 sets of words that are rank-ordered for severity. The subsets can be summed to obtain scores on sensory, affective, and evaluative dimensions as well as a total pain rating index and total number of words chosen. A "present pain intensity" scale (0 = none to 5 = excruciating) provides an intensity rating that has validity, but does not have the range of responses available in a VAS or NRS. Disadvantages of the MPQ reside with several words that may be unfamiliar to some people (e.g., "lancinating") and the burden placed on the responder, since completion time can range from 5 to 15 minutes. It is advisable to review the words with a patient and to define any that are unfamiliar. Both oral and written forms of the MPQ are reliable and valid but not necessarily equivalent.[33] With very sick patients, Walsh and Bowman[61] recommended a combined oral and written format to assist with comprehension.

The *Dartmouth Pain Questionnaire* (DPQ) has been developed as an adjunct to the MPQ.[10] The tool includes measurement of general affect, time course of pain, and behaviors affected by pain. The DPQ may be self-administered in 5 to 20 minutes after a 20 to 40 minute training session and may be repeated for daily monitoring of pain. The authors of the tool[10] have done some standardization with cancer patients, but more work is needed.

The *West Haven-Yale Multidimensional Pain Inventory* (WHYMPI) was developed specifically for patients with chronic pain and has been tested for general reliability and validity.[32] The WHYMPI is derived from cognitive-behavioral theory, and includes measures of subjective pain, impact of pain on daily living, responses of others to patients' pain behaviors, and involvement in activities. The tool has 52 items, each measured on a six- or seven-point scale, and is divided into three parts, each with several subscales. The WHYMPI will likely be of greatest value in measuring pain-related problems in patients with chronic pain who are well enough to spend 15 to 30 minutes completing the form. The initial reliability and validity testing did not include cancer patients, but the instrument is potentially useful for this group. Further work needs to be done on the applicability of the WHYMPI to cancer populations.

The *Brief Pain Inventory* (BPI) was developed to measure pain in cancer patients and can be completed in 5 to 15 minutes.[9,11] With minimal demand on the patient, the BPI has been reported to reliably and validly assess worst, average, and current pain; use of and relief from medication; cognitive dimensions of cause and evaluation of pain; and interference of pain with mood and functioning. A major advantage of the BPI is that it is brief and focused.

The *Memorial Pain Assessment Card* (MPAC) is an even shorter measure of pain or analgesic effectiveness. It consists of three VAS scales for pain intensity, pain relief, and mood; and one VDS for evaluation of pain.[15] The advantages of the scale are its attention to multiple (though very simplified) dimensions, and to the possibility of halo effects. The MPAC is on a card divided in halves with scales on front and back so that a patient sees only one scale at a time. Initial reliability and validity testing indicate that the pain scale correlates with the MPQ and the mood scale correlates with the Profile of Mood States. Although further testing is needed, the MPAC appears to be a 20-second method of validly measuring cancer pain when more extensive measurement is not possible.[15]

MEASURES OF BEHAVIOR

Self-Report Measures of Behavior

In an extension of the self-report approach to measurement, patients, families, or clinicians can complete diaries of daily activities, report on use of medication, or indicate other aspects of behavior that provide information about the impact of pain on functioning. These methods are incorporated into some of the instruments described above and have also been used independently as indicators of pain behavior. A common format is the *Pain Diary*, used to record a patient's standing, walking, and reclining activities in conjunction with hourly recordings of level of pain and medication use. No standardized scoring methods have been developed for the diary, and its reliability and validity are unclear.[17,19] Nonetheless, it may be useful in determining the relationship between pain and activity and in assessing a patient's physical function and participation in activities.

One specific pain behavior, the use of medication, is important in pain measurement, but medication use alone is not an accurate representation of pain severity. Rather it is only one variable within the overall dimension of pain behavior. Patients with the same pattern of medication use may report very different levels of unrelieved pain and activity. Fordyce et al.[19] found no significant correlations between self-reported intensity of pain and use of analgesic medication or time spent sitting, standing, and reclining.

The reliability of self-report measures of pain behavior is an issue of concern. Errors in self-report are common and not predictable. Ready, Sarkis, and Turner[50] found, when comparing reported and observed rates of drug use, that chronic pain patients significantly underestimated their drug use. Kremer, Block, and Gaylor[36] found substantial discrepancies between staff observation and patient reports of activity and social behavior, with some patients reporting significantly lower levels of activity than were observed. Sanders[51] found that chronic back pain patients, normal controls, and psychiatric patients all reported less uptime than was obtained by automated recording devices despite a positive correlation between the two forms of measurement. In contrast, other researchers have found highly significant relationships between observed and self-reported behaviors.[17]

Possible reasons for the greater accuracy reported in some studies may include patients' awareness that other observational measures are being completed and the use of precise operational definitions for recording data. However, it is not yet clear how to achieve accurate self-reports of behavior. Thus, even when patients have no covert or overt reasons to distort information, the reliability of self-reported behaviors is questionable.

Observation of Behavior

The rating of presence or absence of specific behaviors by observers represents an attempt to record more reliable overt indicators of pain, thus providing a closer approximation to objective measurement. The primary limitation of these measures is the need to tailor each one to type or location of pain. The behavior one expects to see, and would use as an indicator of pain, is quite different in a terminal, bedridden cancer patient with metastatic pain than in an active, postmastectomy patient with chronic pain but no evidence of progressive disease. In addition, both patients would exhibit different behaviors than those seen in acute procedural or postsurgical pain.

An observational measure of low back pain has been developed by Keefe and Block[30] and is being extended into the area of cancer pain.[31,40] In studying head and neck cancer patients, Keefe et al.[31] have devised the *Behavioral Dysfunction Index* (BDI), which includes direct observation of pain behavior during activity as well as self-report of specific activities that are painful, general level of activity, pain relief methods, intake of pain medication, and weight loss. The system used by the BDI for scoring guarded movement, grimacing, rubbing, and sighing may be applicable to other types of pain and may provide a model for development of similar systems.

In the development of observational methods for measuring chronic or persisting acute pain, it is important to include actions that are relevant to daily activities, possible for the patient to do, not likely to induce increased pain, but likely to evoke pain behavior if present. For example, talking may be a relevant and painful activity for a patient with severe stomatitis, but neither relevant or painful for a patient with bone pain. The recording method for behaviors is usually the frequency of occurrence in a specific time period or simply occurrence/non-occurrence. Reliability can be evaluated by having more than one observer perform ratings and checking agreement. Validity is often assessed by the relationship of behavior scores to other measures of pain, functioning, and by predicted pre- to post-treatment behavior changes. Additionally, differences in scores between patients with and without the pain problem can be compared.

The approach to behavior measurement described above relates largely to persistent pain where adjustment to the pain has often been made. In situations of brief acute pain there may be more vocalization of pain, autonomic arousal, crying, and abrupt movement. The primary difficulty in measuring acute pain behaviors is the task of distinguishing anxiety from pain, which may even be impossible.[56] Observational checklists for measuring behaviors associated with acute pain have focused on children having bone marrow aspirations. Behaviors that have been scored include crying, screaming, need for physical restraint, verbal resistance, requests for emotional support, muscular rigidity, verbal fear, verbal pain, flailing, nervous behavior, and information seeking.[25,29,38]

MEASURING PAIN LOCATION

In addition to measuring subjective qualities of pain and observed behaviors, it is often helpful to document the location of pain. This is best accomplished with *Pain Drawings*, which require a patient to indicate the pain location on a drawing of a human figure.[39,49] The drawings can also identify the extent of the painful area and provide potentially useful diagnostic information based on the anatomical distribution of the pain. A number of the instruments described above (e.g., MPQ) include drawings that provide clinically relevant information but do not have a standard scoring system. Margolis, Tait, and Krause[39] developed a reliable and valid system that involves scoring the presence or absence of pain in each of 45 possible body areas. Efforts have been made to use pain drawings in determining the relative contributions of psychological and physiological factors to a pain problem, but the usefulness of this approach is not consistently supported in the literature.

IMPACT OF PAIN ON FUNCTIONING

Pain can be the most feared element of cancer and with good reason, as severe pain influences all areas of functioning. In addition, the side effects of medication used to treat pain can impair cognition and capacity to continue with normal activities. Measurements of quality of life can provide valuable information to clinicians about the impact of pain on a patient's physical function and emotions. It is particularly important with chronic pain to assess not only pain but also "wellness," that is, the extent to which the patient is able to balance pain with more positive experiences and activities. Many of the scales described above for evaluating chronic pain include some measurement of emotion and functioning. Many well-standardized measures of emotional and functional status may be used to assess quality of life, including the Beck Depression Inventory, the Profile of Mood States, the Symptom Checklist 90 (SCL-90), or the shorter version of the SCL-90, the Brief Symptom Inventory.[4,12,44,55] Broader measures of quality of life are receiving increasing attention, but a complete review is beyond the scope of this chapter.

The *Sickness Impact Profile* (SIP)[5] is a 136-item instrument that measures functioning. It has had extensive validation, can be completed fairly quickly by patients, and appears both relevant to and easy for most patients. The exception is patients with far-advanced disease who may find it too fatiguing. The SIP provides summary scores for psychosocial, physical, and overall impairment, as well as scores on 12 specific dimensions including ambulation, body care, mobility, emotional behavior, social interaction, alertness, communication, work, sleep and rest, eating, home management, and recreational activities. In a study of chronic pain patients, Follick, Smith and Ahern[18] found that the psychosocial dimension was significantly related to other measures of emotional distress, and the physical dimension correlated with activity level as measured by the pain diary. For some patients, completing the SIP may increase reflection on their changes in function and, as a result, create emotional reactions requiring clinical attention. However, many patients appreciate an opportunity to report on their feelings and functioning.

MEASUREMENT OF PAIN IN CHILDREN

Adequate measurement of pain in children requires a sensitivity to issues of development, as discussed by Patterson and Klopovich in this monograph.[48] Infants cannot report pain verbally, so gross motor indicators of pain such as reflex withdrawal, crying, and other generalized body reaction are used as measures. Pain behavior in toddlers as described by Jeans[26] is likely to include rocking, mouth clenching, rubbing, kicking, hitting, biting, attempting to run away, or opening the eyes wide.

From age three on, a greater variety of tools are available for both self-report and behavioral observation of childhood pain. Although a number of instruments have been developed to make the self-report task more interesting and understandable to children, research indicates that children five years or older can reliably complete a VAS.[1,53] With young children, it is helpful to practice using the VAS with ordinary pain such as from a skinned knee before having them rate their current pain. For children who have difficulty with the VAS, a number of alternatives have been developed including the use of a thermometer, a color-matching technique in which children choose a color that best represents their pain and the "Oucher," a picture scale of happy and sad "painful" faces that has been validated with children as young as three.[6,14,58] The MPQ has been validated with children as young as 12.[26]

Behavioral observation measures are required for infants and toddlers, as discussed above. It has been reported that younger children display a greater variety of anxiety behaviors over a longer time than older children.[29] Older children tend to exhibit more withdrawal and muscle tensing behaviors in response to acute pain. Thus, consideration of the age of the child being evaluated is essential in choosing or designing a behavioral observation measure.

As with adults, it is difficult to distinguish pain from distress in children. Multidimensional measurement can enhance the determination of appropriate interventions and the assessment of treatment outcomes. As noted by Patterson and Klopovich,[48] the traditional tendency to ignore child issues in pain measurement, or to ascribe to children a reduced level of pain experience not requiring the same attention as adults, will no longer be accepted by thoughtful algologists. In all probability, distress and pain in children will need to be treated simultaneously and should both decrease with adequate intervention.

CONCLUSIONS

Several factors need to be considered in choosing which instruments to use (see Table 6-3). Duration of the pain being addressed is important. A shorter, less comprehensive scale would be required to measure a brief, procedural pain than an enduring chronic pain such as phantom limb pain. Likewise, the goal of measurement must be considered. If the goal is to measure analgesic effectiveness, most clinicians are unlikely to complete a comprehensive assessment of functioning. On the other hand, if behavioral measures are not included, critical information may be missed because patients may produce biased self-reports in an effort to please staff or may be influenced by placebo effects. It is necessary to consider patient variables such as age and capacity to respond to the questions included in the measure chosen. Third, reliability is important, and validity is a particularly problematic issue in pain measurement.[43] Many tools have been developed that

Table 6-3
Factors Determining Instrument Choice

External factors	Duration, goal of assessment
Patient variables	Age, patient health
Psychometric properties	Validity, reliability
Setting	Time availability, staff availability, ability to score and use results

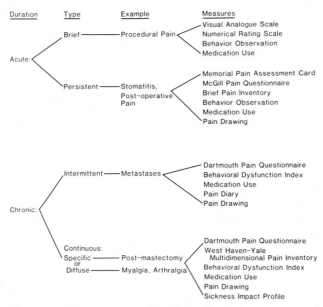

Fig. 6-1. Measures available for scaling different types of pain.

have not had adequate reliability and validity testing and therefore were not reviewed in this chapter.

Finally, although it is always advisable to consider measuring each dimension of pain, the realities of the clinical setting, the availability of staff to administer the instruments, and the likelihood that instruments will be scored and used will play a large role in selecting which measure is best for a particular setting. Not only must instructions to patients be clear and consistent with what is known about memory and validity of responses, but they must also be presented in a way that conveys the importance of the information. Measures can be interpreted by patients as an intrusive, distressing burden or as an indication that staff truly care about and want to understand the patient's experience. Figure 6-1 suggests measures that can be used depending on the duration of pain, although certainly the other factors described above will influence the final choice of instruments.

ACKNOWLEDGMENT

Preparation of this material was supported in part by the National Cancer Institute Program Project #CA 38552.

REFERENCES

1. Abu-Saad H., Holzemer WL: Measuring children's self-assessment of pain. Iss Compr Ped Nurs 5:337–349, 1981
2. Ahles TA, Blanchard EB, Ruckdeschel JC: The multidimensional nature of cancer related pain. Pain 17:277–288, 1983
3. Ahles TA, Ruckdeschel JC, Blanchard EB: Cancer-related pain. II. Assessment with visual analogue scales. J Psychosom Res 28:121–124, 1984
4. Beck AT, Ward CH, Mendelson M, et al.: An inventory for measuring depression. Arch Gen Psychiat 4:53–63, 1961
5. Bergner M, Bobbitt RA, Carter WB, et al.: The Sickness Impact Profile: development and final revision of health status meaure. Med Care 19:787–805, 1981
6. Beyer JE: Development of a new instrument for measuring intensity of childrens' pain. Pain 2:S421, 1984
7. Carlsson AM: Assessment of chronic pain. I. Aspects of the reliability and validity of the visual analogue scale. Pain 16:87–101, 1983
8. Chapman CR, Syrjala KL: Pain measurement in Bonica JJ, Chapman CR, Fordyce WE, Loeser JD (Eds): Management of Pain in Clinical Practice. Philadelphia, Lea & Febiger (in press)
9. Cleeland CS: Measurement and prevalence of pain in cancer. Semin Oncol Nurs 1:87–92, 1985
10. Corson JA, Schneider MJ: The Dartmouth Pain Questionnaire: an adjunct to the McGill Pain Questionnaire. Pain 19:59–69, 1984
11. Daut RW, Cleeland CS, Flannery RC: Development of the Wisconsin Brief Pain Questionnaire to assess pain in cancer and other diseases. Pain 17:197–210, 1983
12. Derogatis LR: Administration, Scoring and Procedures Manual for the SCL-90-R. Baltimore, Clinical Psychometrics Research, 1977
13. Eich E, Reeves JL, Jaegar B, et al.: Memory for pain: relation between past and present pain intensity. Pain 23:375–379, 1985
14. Eland JM: Minimizing pain associated with prekindergarten intramuscular injections. Iss Compr Ped Nurs 5:362–372, 1981
15. Fishman B, Pasternak S, Wallenstein S, et al.: The Memorial Pain Assessment Card: a valid instrument for evaluation of cancer pain. Proc Am Soc Clin Oncol 5:239, 1986 (abstract)
16. Foley KM: Clinical assessment of cancer pain. Acta Anaesthesiol Scand 74:91–96, 1982 (suppl)
17. Follick MJ, Ahern DK, Lawer-Wolston N: Evaluation of a daily activities diary for chronic pain patients. Pain 19:373–382, 1984
18. Folick MJ, Smith TW, Ahern DK: The Sickness Impact Profile: a global measure of disability in chronic low back pain. Pain 21:67–76, 1985
19. Fordyce WE, Lansky D, Calsyn DA, et al.: Pain measurement and pain behavior. Pain 18:52–69, 1984
20. Frank AJM, Moll JMH, Hort JF: A comparison of three ways of measuring pain. Rheumatol Rehab 21:211–217, 1982
21. Graham C, Bond SS, Gerkovich MM, et al.: Use of the McGill Pain Questionnaire in the assessment of cancer pain: replicability and consistency. Pain 8:377–387, 1980
22. Grossi E, Borghi C, Cerchiari EL, et al.: Analogue chromatic continuous scale (ACCS): a new method for pain assessment. Clin Exp Rheumatol 1:337–340, 1983
23. Hunter M, Phillips C, Rachman S: Memory for pain. Pain 6:35–46, 1979
24. Huskisson EC, Jones J, Scott PJ: Application of visual analogue scales to the measurement of functional capacity. Rheumatol Rehabil 15:185–187, 1976
25. Jay S, Ozolins M, Elliot CH, et al.: Assessment of children's distress during painful medical procedures. Health Psychol 2:133–147, 1983

26. Jeans ME: The measurement of pain in children, in Melzack R (Ed): Pain Measurement and Assessment. New York, Raven Press, 1983, pp 183–189
27. Johnson JE, Rice VH, Fuller SS, et al.: Sensory information, instruction in a coping strategy, and recovery from surgery. Res Nurs Health 1:4–17, 1978
28. Joyce CRB, Zutish DW, Hrubes V, et al.: Comparison of fixed interval and visual analogue scales for rating chronic pain. Eur J Clin Pharmacol 18:415–420, 1975
29. Katz ER, Kelleran J, Siegel SE: Behavioral distress in children with cancer undergoing medical procedures: developmental considerations. J Consult Clin Psychol 48:356–365, 1980
30. Keefe FJ, Block AR: Development of an observation method for assessing pain behavior in chronic low back pain patients. Behav Ther 13:363–375, 1982
31. Keefe FJ, Brantley A, Manuel G, et al.: Behavioral assessment of head and neck cancer pain. Pain 23:327–336, 1985
32. Kerns RD, Turk DC, Rudy TE: The West Haven-Yale Multidimensional Pain Inventory (WHYMPI). Pain 23:345–356, 1985
33. Klepac RK, Dowling J, Rokke P, et al.: Interview vs paper and pencil administration of the McGill Pain Questionnaire. Pain 11:241–246, 1981
34. Kremer E, Atkinson JH, Ignelzi RJ: Measurement of pain: patient preference does not confound pain measurement. Pain 10:241–248, 1981
35. Kremer E, Atkinson JH, Ignelzi RJ: Pain measurement: the affective dimensional measure of the McGill Pain Questionnaire with a cancer pain population. Pain 12:153–163, 1982
36. Kremer EF, Block A, Gaylor MS: Behavioral approaches to treatment of chronic pain: the inaccuracy of patient self-report measures. Arch Phys Med Rehab 62:188–191, 1981
37. Kwilosz DM, Gracely RH, Torgerson WS: Memory for postsurgical dental pain. Pain 2:426, 1984 (suppl)
38. LeBaron S, Zeltzer L: Assessment of acute pain and anxiety in children and adolescents by self-reports, observer-reports, and a behavior checklist. J Consult Clin Psychol 52:729–738, 1984
39. Margolis RB, Tait RC, Krause SJ: A rating system for use with patient pain drawings. Pain 24:57–65, 1986
40. McDaniel LK, Anderson KO, Bradley LA, et al.: Development of an observation method for assessing pain behavior in rheumatoid arthritis patients. Pain 24:1165–1184, 1986
41. McGuire DB: Assessment of chronic pain in cancer inpatients using the McGill Pain Questionnaire. Oncol Nurs Forum 11:32–37, 1984
42. McGuire DB: Selecting an instrument to measure cancer-related pain. Oncol Nurs Forum 11:85–87, 1984
43. McGuire DB: The measurement of clinical pain. Nurs Res 33:152–156, 1984
44. McNair DM, Lorr M, Droppleman LF: Profile of mood states. Educational and Industrial Testing Service, San Diego, 1971
45. Melzack R: The McGill Pain Questionnaire: major properties and scoring methods. Pain 1:277–299, 1975
46. Melzack R, Wall PD: Pain mechanisms: a new theory. Science 150:971–979, 1965
47. Ohnhaus EE, Adler R: Methodological problems in the measurement of pain: a comparison between the verbal rating scale and the visual analogue scale. Pain 1:379–384, 1975
48. Patterson K, Klopovich P: Pain in the pediatric oncology patient, in McGuire DB, Yarbro CH (Eds): Cancer Pain Management, Orlando, FL, Grune & Stratton, 1987, pp 259–272
49. Ransford AO, Cairns D, Mooney V: The pain drawing as an aid to the psychologic evaluation of patients with low-back pain. Spine 1:127–134, 1976
50. Ready LB, Sarkis E, Turner J: Self-reported vs actual use of medications in chronic pain patients. Pain 12:285–294, 1982
51. Sanders SH: Automated vs self-help monitoring of 'up-time' in chronic low back pain patients: a comparative study. Pain 15:399–405, 1983

52. Scott J, Huskisson ED: Graphic representation of pain. Pain 2:175–184, 1976
53. Scott PJ, Ansell BM, Huskisson EC: Measurement of pain in juvenile chronic polyarthritis. Ann Rheum Dis 36:186–187, 1977
54. Seymour RA, Simpson JM, Charlton JE, et al.: An evaluation of length and end-phrase of visual analogue scales in dental pain. Pain 21:177–185, 1985
55. Shacham S: A shortened version of the profile of mood states. J Pers Assess 47:305–306, 1983
56. Shacham S, Daut R: Anxiety or pain: what does the scale measure? J Consult Clin Psychol 49:468–469, 1981
57. Syrjala KL, Chapman CR: Measurement of clinical pain: a review and integration of research findings, in Benedetti C, Chapman CR, Moricca G (Eds): Advances in Pain Research and Therapy, Vol. 7. New York, Raven Press, 1984, pp 71–97
58. Szyfelbein SK, Osgood PF, Carr D: The assessment of pain and plasma β-endorphin immunoactivity in burn children. Pain 22:173–182, 1985
59. Thompson SC: Will it hurt less if I can control it? A complex answer to a simple question. Psychol Bull 90:89–101, 1981
60. Wallenstein SL: Measurement of pain and analgesia in cancer patients. Cancer 53:2260–2266, 1984 (suppl)
61. Walsh TD, Bowman K: Letter to the editor. Pain 14:75, 1982
62. Wilson JF, Moore RW, Randolph S, et al.: Behavioral preparation of patients for gastrointestinal endoscopy: Information, relaxation, and coping style. J Human Stress 8:13–23, 1982

Robert B. Catalano, Pharm. D.

7

Pharmacologic Management in the Treatment of Cancer Pain

The patient with cancer may experience a number of distressing symptoms, the most common one being pain. Most people strongly associate pain with cancer and regard it as an inevitable and feared aspect of the terminal phases of this disease. This unfortunate generalization usually stems from an experience of having known, or known of, someone who has suffered excruciating pain due to terminal cancer. In truth, there is no need for most patients to suffer from pain. If properly applied, the current state of knowledge of the causes of pain and methods of controlling it allow successful palliation in 95 to 99 percent of the patients with pain related to cancer.[13,47,93] Nevertheless, for many terminal cancer patients in this country, pain relief will be far from optimal because of inadequate knowledge and improper application of current knowledge on the part of primary health care professionals.

Marks and Sachar[59] found that medical inpatients were almost universally undertreated with narcotic analgesics, according to standard pharmacologic guidelines. Even experienced clinicians hesitate to prescribe adequate doses or administration schedules of narcotic analgesics for cancer patients despite the terminal aspects of many patients, often because of a nonverbalized fear of "addiction." Nevertheless, the findings of Saunders[91] and others[48,94] indicate significant tolerance develops infrequently in patients with terminal cancer.

A failure to achieve adequate palliation in potentially manageable

CANCER PAIN MANAGEMENT
ISBN 0-8089-1868-0

situations supports the conclusion that counterproductive attitudes in the approach to cancer patients with pain stem primarily from a failure of the primary providers of medical education to stray from the goals of the traditional "rescue-mode" model of medical care. This model is based on "cure," or at least prolongation of life, with symptom control being an expected consequence. The better approach would be to allow sufficient priority to the principles of supportive care, which are primarily an attempt to palliate symptoms and optimize the quality of remaining life for each patient. This needed transition from "rescue-mode" to "palliative-mode" therapy should best be looked at as an overlapping approach.

In discussing the management of pain, recognizing these concepts is extremely important. In understanding the basis of appropriate pharmacologic intervention to control pain, one must focus on the most important of the supportive care principles—the evaluation and control of a symptom. Cancer pain is hard to quantify or study, surrounded by folklore, emotionally charged, and potentially difficult to resolve. Yet, as a patient-oriented system would demonstrate, it goes to the heart of what physicians and other health care personnel are supposed to provide, "to heal sometimes, to relieve often, to comfort always" (Edward Trudeau).

GENERAL CONSIDERATIONS

For the purposes of our discussions, pain will be considered to present clinically as two distinct types: acute and chronic. This classification provides the best example of differing pharmacologic approaches, depending on the type of pain being treated (Table 7-1).

Acute pain is probably the most common complaint of patients seeking medical care. It is the kind of pain that most physicians are used to treating and the type most often studied in laboratories with nerve potentials and monitoring of biochemical substances. It should be considered linear (begins and ends), usually reversible, with the meaningful purpose of being a warning sign of underlying pathology. Acute pain serves this useful function only for as long as it is evaluated and treated for what it represents, a symptom and not a primary disease process. Primary efforts to control pain symptomatology should then be directed toward the elimination of the cause of the noxious stimuli rather than suppression of symptomatology. This general concept also applies to some extent to the management of pain associated with malignant disease. Unfortunately, the pain that complicates cancer is often a difficult, frustrating clinical problem. The complexity of pain problems in patients with cancer is of particular importance, since available treatment to control the primary malignant process is often palliative or non-curative in nature. While the incidence of severe, intractable pain in advanced cancer is relatively low, there are many instances when

Table 7-1.
Analgesic Therapy of Acute versus Chronic Pain

	Acute	Chronic
Pain Character	Meaningful, linear, reversible.	Meaningless, cyclical, irreversible.
Therapeutic goal	Pain relief	Pain prevention
Sedation	Often desirable	Usually undesirable
Rapid onset of effect	Important	Unnecessary
Desired duration of effect	2–4 hours	As long as possible
Timing	As needed (on demand)	Regularly (in anticipation)
Dose	Usually standard	Individually titrated
Route	Parenteral	Oral
Adjuvant medication	Uncommon	Common

Adapted from Twycross RG: Relief of pain, in Saunders L M (ed): The Management of Terminal Disease. London, Edward Arnold, 1978, p 65

pain becomes the major problem due to the tumor's refractoriness to specific antineoplastic therapy.

Chronic pain differs from acute pain in that it no longer serves a protective or warning function, but has become an end unto itself, leading to the so-called "agony" of cancer. The chronic pain of cancer is something few clinicians have personally experienced, and this makes understanding the differing nature of chronic pain so difficult for most medical personnel to comprehend. An adequate definition of the "pain syndrome" accepts that pain is whatever the experiencing person says it is and exists whenever he says it does and to the severity he has determined.

The therapeutic goal one strives for in treating chronic pain is pain prevention, not simply pain relief as in acute pain.[70] This goal is achieved by giving an individually titrated dose of analgesia sufficient to relieve the pain and then determining an appropriate schedule for repeating this dose in a time frame that administers it before the pain actually recurs. In such a model, the administration of the analgesia is no longer dependent on the pain being present to initiate each dose, but rather its intent is to maintain a pain-free state and, therefore, erase the pain memory.

Evaluating Pain

Despite the poor prognosis associated with recurrent or advanced malignancies, evaluation and successful control of pain is an important and complex clinical problem that deserves an intelligent appraisal of the patient's physical, mental, and moral resources. Selection of appropriate therapy can be accomplished only after thorough consideration and evaluation of several parameters, all of which contribute to the patient's total pain.[71,88]

A physician, unfamiliar with the complexities of the problems seen in cancer patients, may be prone to attribute all subsequent complaints of pain to the patient's primary disease. It is important to evaluate each new complaint of pain by performing an adequate evaluation to determine the true etiology. Because of the connotation assigned to cancer in our society as always fatal, always painful, and usually prolonged, the nonmalignant causes of pain are often overlooked. In many cases, pain symptomatology is debilitating, and since definitive therapy is dependent on correct diagnosis, the need for detailed history and a complete diagnostic workup should seem obvious.

One particularly important aspect of any pain management program is the realization that diagnosis of cancer does not necessarily mean the malignant process is responsible for a particular episode of pain. As described by Foley, [30] the etiology of pain may be classified into three major categories: (1) pain associated with direct tumor involvement; (2) pain associated with cancer therapy; and (3) pain unrelated to the cancer or cancer therapy. In evaluating all complaints of pain in a general cancer patient population, one will find that pain is caused by direct tumor involvement in approximately 75 percent of the complaints. Twenty percent may be directly attributed to the cancer therapy, and about 5 percent will be unrelated to the patient's malignant disease.

Psychologic Aspects of Pain

Psychological variables as well as sensory input play an important role in the perception of chronic pain and have been well addressed in other areas of this monograph. These variables may be the underlying explanation of the success or failure of any given management program for pain and, therefore, worth mentioning once again. Depending on the emotional state of the patient, the perception of pain may vary considerably. Most patients who know or suspect their pain may be due to cancer manifest emotional factors such as fear, apprehension, anxiety, and depression, which accentuate painful stimuli. Long-standing or chronic pain may eventually affect every aspect of the patient's life, with a gradual but complete alteration in his attitude towards his environment. If allowed to continue, the pain becomes an overwhelming problem that completely dominates his life. Patients with chronic pain often do not become tolerant or accustomed to it, but rather seem to become increasingly more sensitive, and to suffer more as their disease progresses.

Table 7-2
Existing Methods of Alleviating Cancer-Related Pain

I. Primary Control Methods
  A. Therapy directed toward control of the disease process itself.
    1. Surgery.
    2. Radiation therapy.
    3. Chemotherapy (cytotoxic & hormonal agents).
  B. Therapy directed toward a specific disease related (reversible pathophysiologic event).
    1. Infection with antibiotics.
    2. Inflammation with anti-inflammatory drugs.
    3. Gout with antihyperuricemic agents.
II. Symptomatic Control Methods
  A. Systemic analgesics.
    1. Interference with specific chemical substances involved in pain perception peripherally (Anti-inflammatory/antipyretic agents).
    2. Interference with conduction of pain away from affected site (local anesthetics).
    3. Interference with central nervous system perception of pain and the development of affective responses (narcotic analgesics).
    4. Interference with anxiety, tension, or depression (sedative/hypnotics, phenothiazines, tricyclic antidepressants).
    5. Interference with consciousness (general anesthetics).
  B. Surgical procedures on the spinal cord and brain.

PRINCIPLES OF PAIN CONTROL

The management of cancer-related pain may be divided into two distinct approaches. These are attempts at primary control by reversal of the specific pathophysiologic events ultimately producing the pain, and symptomatic control by alteration of the perception of pain (Table 7-2).

Primary Control

The best treatment for any symptom is the treatment of the disease itself. In dealing with malignant disease, primary efforts to control pain involve, when feasible, surgical, radiotherapeutic, or chemical removal of the tumor, with ultimate control of the pain being an expected consequence. Even in pain known to be a direct cause of an incurable primary disease process, or resulting from a potentially treatable problem that is coincidental with an incurable cancer, specific disease-oriented or problem-oriented therapy may provide the best long-term relief of pain and should always be considered before resorting solely to symptomatic attempts at pain control.

In general, primary methods for pain control (e.g., palliative antitumor therapy) should only be attempted at an intensity that is proportional to the expected benefit. In most situations, disease or problem-oriented therapy for primary pain control must be delivered along with analgesia, at least until the maximum tumor response has been achieved. If indicated, efforts may then be directed toward determining the need, if any, for further symptomatic control of residual pain.

An in-depth review of the current state of the art of successful primary methods of cancer control as they relate to the overall planning for pain management is beyond the scope of this chapter. However, several general concepts of primary therapy for cancer that can result in control of the related pain are reviewed.

Surgery

Certain types of cancer-related pain may be controlled with surgical intervention, which should be considered part of the overall pain management program independent of their potential for cure of cancer. Operative procedures considered palliative in nature are commonly performed for known incurable cases. Examples of such procedures are bypass operations of tumors causing obstruction of a hollow viscus or large blood vessel (vein or artery). Pain due to this process is often severe, persistent, and not adequately relieved by systemic analgesics or neurosurgical interruption of the ascending pathways.

Surgical ablation of endocrine glands (e.g. castration) not only has caused regression of advanced carcinoma of the breast and of the prostate gland, but also has produced dramatic relief of pain and generalized improvement in the patients' performance status.[31,92] Adrenalectomy and hypophysectomy, once performed as secondary endocrine manipulative procedures, have similar effects, particularly in tumors suspected of being hormone-dependent, such as breast carcinoma.[72,76] Hormone antagonists are more commonly used today.

Neurosurgical interventions are another group of surgical procedures appropriately used to control pain in the cancer patient. These techniques are addressed in detail in Chapter 9 of this monograph.

Radiation

Although radiation therapy, as a primary treatment modality, is considered as potentially curative in certain malignant diseases, a large segment of the practice of radiotherapy is palliative care of incurable patients. When the problem of pain is secondary to a primary incurable disease, but potentially amenable to focal disease-oriented therapy, the relief produced by palliative radiation therapy, while being sometimes unpredictable, is sufficiently striking in many situations to warrant its consideration. When used in the treatment of metastatic disease, radiation therapy can produce a somewhat rapid relief of pain as a consequence of local cytotoxic effect and retardation of neoplastic spread in the area of the treatment.

The types of patients most likely to benefit from radiation therapy are those with metastatic bone metastases.[89] Osseous metastases often represent the first findings of metastatic disease in many cancer patients. Depending upon the site of origin of the primary tumor and means of detection, the overall incidence of bony involvement ranges from 23 to 84 percent.[100] The major symptom of bone metastases is pain, which can be either a chronic or acute process. Recent studies reported by the Radiation Therapy Oncology Group (RTOG)[46] to determine the palliative effectiveness of radiation in patients with osseous metastases demonstrate that 90 percent of patients experiencing pain secondary to bone metastases experienced some relief as a consequence of local radiation therapy. More important, 54 percent can achieve complete pain relief using radiation therapy as the primary pain control vehicle. Recognizing that palliation is the primary concern, the same study compared different dose fractionation schedules in an attempt to provide the simplest schedule giving maximum relief with minimum morbidity. Interestingly, the low dose, short course schedules of radiation fractionation were as effective as the high dose protracted programs. The most important predictors of the ultimate success of the pain control program were the site of the primary disease, as patients with prostate and breast cancer received more frequent complete relief than those with lung and other primary lesions; and initial pain evaluation scores, as patients with lower scores did better than those with high scores at the start of treatment. Of special interest was the method of scoring pain, which allowed it to be quantitated in such a way as to permit evaluation of the palliation achieved based on relative changes in scores.

Other confirmative studies evaluating subjective pain relief with the use of radiation therapy confirm its use in primary diseases of thyroid and kidney.[89] In the management of severe headaches associated with metastatic cancer to the brain, concomitant use of relatively high doses of corticosteroids for acute relief of symptoms, coupled with palliative radiotherapy to the contents of the calvaria, can improve or completely control the pain in greater than 85 percent of the patients.[12,15,105]

Chemotherapy

Control of pain with the use of systemic cytotoxic chemotherapy is usually a consequence of objective response with shrinkage of the tumor mass. As a result, this method of control is often slow and unpredictable. Therefore, concurrent therapy with some form of systemic analgesia usually must be administered with the chemotherapy. Success or failure of the primary control methods in alleviating chronic pain can be evaluated on the basis of the subsequent need for this concurrently administered analgesia. An example is control of liver pain caused by hepatic metastases with the use of regional intrahepatic arterial infusion of chemotherapy.[25,60] Administration of antineoplastic agents via the hepatic artery permits a higher tissue-dose concentration while minimizing the potential systemic toxicity. This method of chemotherapy has been reported to produce symptomatic relief in up to 70 percent of those patients treated.[25] However, despite the overall objective response rate of 70 percent, the effect on patient survival is questionable.

Symptomatic Control

To achieve symptomatic control of chronic pain, one must either modify the pain threshold within the central nervous system or block the pain pathways leading to the central perception of pain.[30] Attempts to achieve this pharmacologically involve the use of analgesics which, by definition, are drugs that decrease pain without causing a loss of consciousness. Individualization of dosing and constant monitoring and titration for effect are extremely important.

Physicians treating pain must recognize there will be considerable variation among patients in their individual responses to systemic analgesics. Based on this observation, it is unreasonable to assume that one drug, at one fixed dosage schedule will suffice in all patients. Those that advocate the empiric use of one agent (i.e., heroin) or a fixed combination of several agents (i.e., Brompton's Cocktail) are demonstrating their lack of insight into the overall complexity of chronic cancer pain. In truth, the analgesic regimen of choice is the one that achieves a pain-free state at a tolerable dose for an adequate duration of time. This can only be determined by constant monitoring and reassessment of the individual patient response to the administered agent.

For purposes of discussion, analgesics will be divided into classes based on their clinical use relative to the severity of pain (Table 7-3). These include agents suitable for mild pain, generally non-narcotic agents; those suitable for moderate pain, usually narcotic agonists or mixed agonist-antagonists with low addiction potential; and those suitable for severe pain, generally narcotic agonists.[48,49,101]

The basic strategy in treating chronic pain is to begin with the mildest agents that demonstrate effective pain control and add stronger agents or analgesic adjuvants only when the mild agents fail to work. Each drug selected should always be given to its therapeutic/toxic limit before going to a stronger agent or adding a coanalgesic. Initial doses and escalation should be individualized to each patient, paying special attention to liver and kidney function, as these may alter normal pharmacokinetics.[101]

Table 7-3
Recommended Analgesic Therapy Based on the
Severity of Pain

Degree of Pain Symptom	Suggested Agent for Control
Mild Pain	Aspirin or acetaminophen
Moderate pain	Add codeine or oxycodone to above Rx
Severe pain	Morphine, hydromorphone, levorphanol, methadone
Very severe pain	As above in appropriate doses
Overwhelming pain	As above *plus* adjunctive pharmachologic agents and non-pharmacologic maneuvers

GENERAL PRINCIPLES OF ANALGESIC USE

Successful pain management using systemic analgesics requires a drug appropriate for the pain. One needs a basic understanding of the pathophysiology of the perception of pain, the basic principles of drug mechanisms of action, and a thorough knowledge of the pharmacologic actions contributing to analgesic activity. One needs a working knowledge of the terminology used in the selection process for these agents, including efficacy, dose-response, relative analgesic potency, and relative analgesic potential.

Efficacy and effectiveness are synonymous and refer to the degree of analgesia provided by a given dose of an analgesic administered under a particular set of conditions. Efficacy depends on many variables and is not an absolute; neither is the relative efficacy of two analgesic drugs. Aspirin may be more effective than morphine. Maximal efficacy is the degree to which a drug is capable of relieving pain with increasing dose.

There is a dose below which only placebo analgesia occurs. Above this minimum effective dose, increases in doses are accompanied by increases in effectiveness. The relationship between increasing dose and increasing effectiveness is logarithmic, with every doubling of the dose there is an equivalent incremental increase in effectiveness. There is a point, however, where progressive doubling of doses produces smaller increments in effectiveness. This plateau in the dose-response curve is called the "ceiling effect," and defines maximal efficacy.

Relative analgesic potency refers to the ratio of doses of two drugs, or of the same drug administered by different routes, that provides equivalent analgesic effectiveness. Relative analgesic potencies tell us how many milligrams of one drug are therapeutically equivalent to given doses of other drugs. Table 7-4 provides a quick reference to accepted equivalent doses of the commonly employed analgesics.

Table 7-4
An Equianalgesic Comparison of the Most Common Analgesics

Generic and (Trade) Name	Dose	Equivalent to*	Peak Effect	Duration	Plasma Half-Life	Comments	Precautions
NON-NARCOTICS							
Acetaminophen (Tylenol, Tempra, etc)	600 mg po 600 mg rectal suppos.	Aspirin 600 mg po	2 hrs Slower than oral	3–4 hrs	1–4 hrs	Antipyretic and anti-inflammatory action is weak	In large doses, may cause liver toxicity
Acetylsalicylic acid (aspirin)	600 mg po 600 mg rectal suppos.	Morphine 2 mg IM	2 hrs Slower than oral	3–4 hrs	15 min	Has antipyretic and anti-inflammatory activity	Used with steroids, it may increase gastric bleeding
Methotrimeprazine (Levoprome)	20 mg IM	Morphine 10 mg IM	1 hr	4–6 hrs	Unknown	A phenothiazine; recommend starting with 5 mg dose	May cause over-sedation, orthostatic hypotension, liver toxicity
Zomepirac (Zomax)	100 mg po	Morphine 16 mg IM	1–2 hrs	4–6 hrs	1–4 hrs	Has anti-inflammatory and antipyretic activity	Use with caution in patients with urinary tract infection, elevated BUN, creatinine, and in patients with aspirin

160

Generic and (Trade) Name	Dose	Equivalent to*	Peak Effect	Duration	Plasma Half-Life	Comments	Precautions
NARCOTIC ANTAGONISTS							
Butorphanol tartrate (Stadol)	2 mg IM	Morphine 10 mg IM	1 hr	3–4 hrs	2.7 hrs	Mixed agonist-antagonist; may produce psychotomimetic effect	May cause abstinence reaction in patients physically dependent on narcotics
	2 mg IV		30 min	3–4 hrs			
Nalbuphine HCl (Nubain)	10 mg IM	Morphine 10 mg IM	1 hr	4–5 hrs	5 hrs	Mixed agonist-antagonist, but less psychotomimetic effect than pentazocine	Same precautions as with butorphanol
	10 mg IV	Pentazocine 60 mg IM	30 min	3–4 hrs			
Pentazocine HCl (Talwin)	60 mg IM	Morphine 10 mg IM	1 hr	3–4 hrs	2–3 hrs	Mixed agonist-antagonist, may cause psychotomimetic side effects	Same precautions as with butorphanol; use with caution in patients with cardiac abnormalities
	30 mg po	Aspirin 600 mg	2 hrs	3–4 hrs	2–3 hrs		
	180 mg po	Morphine 10 mg IM					
		Pentazocine 60 mg IM					

(continued)

Table 7-4 (continued)

Generic and (Trade) Name	Dose	Equivalent to*	Peak Effect	Duration	Plasma Half-Life	Comments	Precautions
NARCOTICS							
Codeine sulfate	30–60 mg po	Aspirin 600 mg	2 hrs	3–4 hrs	2½–3 hrs	Same as morphine, but weaker	Not for IV use
	200 mg po	Morphine 10 mg IM					
		Codeine 120 mg IM					
Hydromorphone HCl (Dilaudid)	7.5 mg po	Morphine 10 mg IM	1 hr	3–4 hrs	2–3 hrs	Quick onset of action	Same precautions as with morphine
	3 mg rectal suppos.	Hydromorphone 1.5 mg IM					
	1.5 mg IM	Morphine 10 mg IM	30 min	3 hrs	2–3 hrs	Has similar time effect as heroin; highly soluble	Same precautions as with morphine
	1 mg IV		15 min	2–3 hrs			

(continued)

Table 7-4 (continued)

Generic and (Trade) Name	Dose	Equivalent to*	Peak Effect	Duration	Plasma Half-Life	Comments	Precautions
Levorphanol tartrate (LevoDromoran)	4 mg po	Morphine 10 mg IM	2 hrs	4–5 hrs	15 hrs	Same as morphine	Same precautions as with morphine
		Levorphanol 2 mg IM					
	2 mg IM	Morphine 10 mg IM	1 hr	4–5 hrs			
	1 mg IV		15–30 min	3–4 hrs			
Meperidine HCl (Demerol, Pethadol)	50 mg po	Aspirin 600 mg	2 hrs	3–4 hrs	3 hrs	Causes CNS excitation ranging from irritability to seizures	Not for chronic administration in patients with renal dysfunction
	300 mg po	Morphine 10 mg IM					
		Meperidine 75 mg IM					
	75 mg IM	Morphine 10 mg IM	1hr	2–4 hrs			
	50 mg IV		5–15 min	2–3 hrs			

(continued)

Table 7-4 (continued)

Generic and (Trade) Name	Dose	Equivalent to*	Peak Effect	Duration	Plasma Half-Life	Comments	Precautions
Methadone HCl	20 mg po	Morphine 10 mg IM / Methadone 10 mg IM	2 hrs	4–5 hrs	15–22 hrs	Same as morphine	Same precautions as with morphine
	10 mg IM	Morphine 10 mg IM	1 hr	4–5 hrs			
	5 mg IV		15–30 min	3–4 hrs			
Morphine sulfate	60 mg po	Morphine 10 mg IM	2 hrs	4–5 hrs	2½–3 hrs	May cause oversedation, confusion, visual disturbances, urinary retention	Contraindicated in patients with: impaired ventilation, asthma, elevated intracranial pressure, liver failure
	10 mg IM		1 hr	4–5 hrs			
	5 mg IV		15–30 min	2–4 hrs			
Oxycodone (with aspirin-Percodan; with acetaminophen-Percocet)	5 mg po	Codeine 60 mg po	1 hr	3–4 hrs	2–3 hrs	Not available in IM or IV form	
	30 mg po	Morphine 10 mg IM					

(continued)

Table 7-4 (continued)

Generic and (Trade) Name	Dose	Equivalent to*	Peak Effect	Duration	Plasma Half-Life	Comments	Precautions
Oxymorphone HCl (Numorphan)	1 mg IM	Morphine 10 mg IM	1 hr	4–5 hrs	Unknown	Highly soluble; not available orally	Same precautions as with morphine
	.5 mg IV		15–30 min	3–4 hrs			
	10 mg rectal suppos.	Morphine 10 mg IM	2 hrs	6 hrs			
		Oxymorphone 1 mg IM					
Propoxyphene HCl (Darvon, Dolene)	65 mg po	Aspirin 600 mg	2 hrs	3–4 hrs	12 hrs	A "weak" narcotic; structurally related to methadone	Overdose can be complicated by convulsions
Propoxyphene napsylate (Darvon N) (with acetaminophen-Darvocet N)	100 mg po	Aspirin 600 mg	2 hrs	3–4 hrs	12 hrs		

* The oral/parenteral efficacy ratio refers to the ratio of doses given by the two routes of administration necessary to produce equivalent "total" analgesic effect when both intensity and duration of effect are taken into account. If only maximal intensity or "peak" effect is considered, however, oral administration yields even less effective analgesia than parenteral administration. These studies were done on cancer patients. In other types of pain, equivalencies may not be the same.

165

While the maximal efficacy of agonists is represented by complete pain relief, the development of adverse effects limits this potential in many patients. A clinically useful concept is that of analgesic potential, which refers to the relationship between efficacy and adverse effects. If a drug produces fewer adverse effects than another drug having the same degree of efficacy, the former drug is said to possess a greater analgesic potential than the latter. Drugs that are generally considered to possess comparable relative analgesic potential may differ significantly in this regard in an individual patient, many times necessitating a "trial and error" situation until the most appropriate agent is found. The availability of a wide variety of analgesic preparations allows the clinician the opportunity to achieve the maximal benefit of pain relief with minimal undesirable effects in each patient when this rational matching of drug to pain etiology is achieved.

The clinician who is treating pain symptomatically has quite a large number of available analgesics from which to select. Since there are redundant aspects of many agents within the same therapeutic class of drugs, it is reasonable to select a few agents, learn their characteristics in regard to site, mechanism of action, pharmacokinetics, potency, formulation, onset, duration of effect, and adverse reactions. As the clinician learns the best methods for using these agents, increased confidence in the degree of dosage and administration flexibility allows better use of these agents to reach their therapeutic maximal potential.[23]

The events leading to the perception of pain are transmitted on several levels.[78] A peripheral (afferent) mechanism involves receptors in the skin and body tissue that are activated by injurious stimuli. Peripheral receptors stimulate the central nervous system via pathways in the spinal cord and higher brain centers. Central acknowledgement of what is considered pain allows appreciation and avoidance of the pain stimuli by means of the activation of a descending (efferent) mechanism that transmits information from the central nervous system back to the periphery.

The complex interactions of these various systems and the electrical and neurochemical substances involved have been studied extensively. Of particular importance was the discovery and isolation of an opiate receptor in the mid-1970s, which eventually led to the discovery of naturally occurring opiate-like substances in the body called endorphins and enkephalins located in the synapses between nerve fibers.[3,38,43,58,97,98,107] The "three-receptor model" of opiate receptors suggests the probable function of both transmitters and blockers to modify and possibly inhibit noxious stimuli. Their inhibitory role probably is derived from their ability to inhibit release of another peptide, substance P, which transmits noxious stimuli. The current state of knowledge suggests that these agents serve as endogenous opiates and act not only in the brain, but in many parts of the body, especially within the spinal cord. Endorphins allay pain centrally and may block its afferent transmission of efferent impulse conductance in the spinal cord and periphery. These substances have a short half-life and their serum and tissue levels are increased in both acute and chronic pain.

Noxious stimuli received by the skin and body tissue can initiate events that result in inflammation and pain. A complete biochemical enzyme system is involved that exists in all cells of the human body that contain microsomes.[103] Arachidonic acid, an essential fatty acid, exists as an inactive precursor of prostaglandin in the cell wall until molecular oxygen is incorporated into it by microcosmal enzymes called cyclo-oxygenases.[82,83]

The incorporation of oxygen into arachidonic acid produces highly potent unstable peroxides (cyclic endoperoxides) that in turn form many biologically active prostaglandin products. These prostaglandins are believed to play an important role in cell homeostasis, both in health and disease. Their status as true primary mediators of inflammation has not been proven, but blocking their production has been shown to help alleviate inflammation and its attendant symptoms,[83] such as pain.

NON-NARCOTIC ANALGESICS

The non-narcotic analgesics are non-addictive agents and include the general classes of agents known as salicylates, acetaminophen, and the ever enlarging class of agents grouped under the name of non-steroidal anti-inflammatory drugs (NSAIDs). Generally speaking, the clinically useful doses of these agents are without psychotropic activity except for changes in affective behavior concomitant with the relief of fever, inflammation, and pain.

Aspirin

Within the complexities of chronic pain management, there is one observation that has been, and remains, almost universally accepted: in the field of non-narcotic analgesia, none of the newer agents demonstrate superiority over plain aspirin as the agent of choice.[7,65,66,86] As a drug, aspirin calls for superlatives. It is probably the most widely used of all medications; thousands of tons are consumed annually in the United States.[1] It is one of the oldest and least expensive of all drugs, and most certainly the most underestimated by the people who use it. If aspirin were to be introduced in 1986 as a new agent, it would be heralded as a wonder drug because of its effectiveness over a variety of different maladies. It would most certainly be available only by prescription, if it were able to receive approval for generalized marketing by the Food and Drug Administration (FDA), because of the dangers associated with its use, and it would no doubt be extremely expensive to the patient.

Studies done by Moertel et al.[65,66] comparing the relative effectiveness

Table 7-5
Relative Therapeutic Effect of Oral Analgesics According to
Mean Percentage of Relief of Pain Achieved in 57 Patients

Analgesic Agent	Dose (mg)	Relief of Pain (%)	
Aspirin	650	62	
Pentazocine	50	54	Significantly
Acetaminophan	650	50	superior
Phenacetin	650	48	to placebo
Mefenamic acid	250	47	($p < 0.05$)
Codeine	65	46	
Propoxyphene	65	43	Significantly
Ethoheptazine	75	38	inferior
Promazine	25	37	to aspirin
Placebo	—	32	($p < 0.05$)

Adapted from Moertel CG, Ohmann DL, Taylor WF, et al.: A comparative evaluation of
marketed analgesic drugs. N Engl J Med 286:813–815, 1972. Reprinted with permission.

of nine analgesics given by the oral route to relieve cancer pain reaffirm
aspirin's place in the overall management of pain. The first study,[65] utilizing
57 ambulatory patients who had definite pain resulting from nonresectable
cancer, compared analgesic effect in a double-blind crossover study (see
Table 7-5). Of the nine agents studied, aspirin 650 mg was superior to all
agents tested. Mefenamic acid 250 mg, pentazocine 50 mg, acetaminophen
650 mg, phenacetin 650 mg, and codeine 65 mg, also showed significant
advantage over placebo. Propoxyphene 65 mg, ethoheptazine 75 mg, and
promazine 25 mg, gave no significant evidence of therapeutic activity, and
each of these agents was significantly inferior to aspirin in analgesic effects.

In a follow-up comparison of analgesics given in combination to 100
patients with pain due to cancer, the results were similar (see Figure 7-1).[66]
The combination of aspirin 650 mg, plus the addition of either codeine 65 mg,
oxycodone 9.76 mg, or pentazocine 25 mg, produced significantly greater
pain relief than aspirin alone. The combination of aspirin 650 mg, plus either
caffeine 65 mg, pentobarbital 32 mg, promazine 25 mg, ethoheptazine 75 mg,
or propoxyphene napsylate 100 mg, did not show significant advantage in
analgesic efficacy over aspirin alone. The side effects for a single dose of the
effective combinations were essentially equal and clinically tolerable.

When evaluating these studies, it must be stressed that they were simply
single-dose comparisons and did not address the more important issue of the
clinical comparison of these dosage forms under steady-state conditions of
chronic use. The studies did, however, provide scientific evidence in a
controlled way of the clinical efficacy of comparative administration of these
analgesics.

It has never been demonstrated that aspirin, phenacetin, and caffeine

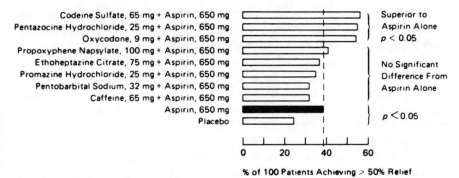

Fig. 7-1. Comparative therapeutic effect of placebo, aspirin alone, and aspirin combinations according to the percentage of patients achieving significant (i.e., more that 50 percent) relief of pain. From Moertel CG, Ohmann DL, Taylor WF, et al.: Relief of pain by oral medications. JAMA 229:55–59, 1974. Reprinted with permission.

(APC) are superior to aspirin alone in providing relief from pain of any etiology.[1,33,61,77] There is much evidence that persons who overuse this type of combination are at risk of developing what is now called "analgesic nephropathy," characterized by papillary necrosis and interstitial nephritis.[33,61,77]

There are, of course, conditions that preclude the use of aspirin despite its superiority to other agents. Among these are pre-existing histories of gastrointestinal ulceration or hemorrhage, hypersensitivity reactions, and certain asthmatic conditions. Increasing emphasis is being given to aspirin as a major cause of hospital admissions due to gastrointestinal bleeding. Most reports on the incidence of aspirin-induced gastrointestinal hemorrhage conclude that at least 50 percent and up to 94 percent of patients admitted with the diagnosis have a positive history of recent salicylate ingestion. Perry and Wood[77] stated that almost 100 percent of patients admitted to hospitals bleeding from acute gastric erosions and with no radiologically demonstrable lesion have given a history of prior consumption of aspirin.

Intolerance to aspirin can also manifest itself in the form of an allergic response.[18] This is particularly important in evaluating a patient with a history of asthma. Signs and symptoms of allergic response observed when patients allergic to aspirin were challenged with other commonly used analgesics make clear the need for caution in prescribing analgesic agents to patients sensitive to aspirin.[95]

The clinical signs of aspirin allergy are usually first seen in the third or fourth decade of life. Watery nasal discharge and nasal polypi are generally the first signs. Bronchial asthma develops after a variable interval of weeks to years; it is often precipitated by nasal polypectomy or by ingestion of aspirin. Thereafter, persistent wheezing occurs with severe life-threatening attacks of asthma after aspirin is taken. The asthma is not abolished by avoiding aspirin, but it is usually well controlled by small regular doses of corticosteroids. Alcohol, indomethacin, antipyrine, and other drugs and chemicals may precipitate asthmatic attacks in patients with this condition.

In one study,[95] five patients who had a clear history of asthmatic attacks after taking aspirin were challenged with the following drugs: acetaminophen, 500 mg; mefenamic acid, 250 mg; indomethacin, 25 mg; dextropropoxyphene, 65 mg; phenylbutazone, 100 mg; and inert white lactose tablets. Aspirin itself was not used, for fear of producing a dangerous attack. The forced expiratory volume (in 1 second) was measured every 30 minutes on a spirometer. Marked decreases in forced expiratory volume, accompanied in some cases by asthma and rhinitis, were observed after administration of most of these analgesics. Acetaminophen, indomethacin, and mefenamic acid caused the most severe and frequent rhinitis reactions. Dextropropoxyphene caused a severe reaction in one case. Phenylbutazone did not have any untoward effects in any of the patients tested.[95]

The results of the study underline the need for great caution when prescribing analgesic drugs to patients sensitive to aspirin. Exacerbations of asthma or increases in steroid requirements in patients with conditions requiring analgesics should be evaluated in light of the evidence that analgesics may cause severe bronchoconstriction. This sensitivity will most likely manifest itself after ingestion of any agent of the NSAID class. Care should be taken to make known the existence of this cross-sensitivity.

Aspirin has also demonstrated an ability to inhibit collagen-induced release of adenine diphosphate (ADP) from platelets resulting in impaired aggregation of platelets.[40,41,106] This effect may prove to be therapeutically beneficial in patients with ischemic heart disease[4,41]; however, it may be detrimental if used concomitantly with other agents known to affect the clotting mechanisms. Clinicians desiring to avoid prescribing aspirin or to warn patients to avoid aspirin-containing products will find over 500 products available on the market with at least one of many salicylate derivatives as their active ingredient.[99]

The analgesic activity attributed to aspirin is primarily due to its interruption of prostaglandin synthesis via the blockade of prostaglandin synthetase enzyme.[29] The subsequent analgesic and anti-inflammatory effect from aspirin is thought to be due to this inhibition of formation of prostaglandin E2 at the chemoreceptor sites, which may sensitize these receptors to stimulation. The major site of action of aspirin should, therefore, be considered peripheral, in contrast to the central action of the narcotic analgesics. Aspirin, therefore, does not change the perception of sensory modalities other than pain. Most data are consistent with the hypothesis that aspirin-like drugs are effective as analgesics primarily in conditions where prostaglandins are synthesized locally and constitute a major contributing factor in the ultimate pain syndrome.[28] The type of characteristics usually associated with this are the dull, "throbbing" pain of inflammation where prostaglandins are apparently sensitizing the nerve endings. In contrast, the sharp, "stabbing" pain caused by direct stimulation of the nerves is usually less responsive to aspirin analgesia.

Acetaminophen

Acetaminophen, while being devoid of any substantial anti-inflammatory action at normal doses, provides a suitable therapeutic alternative to aspirin as an effective non-narcotic analgesic/anti-pyretic agent.[2,22,54,63] Like aspirin, it is effective in control of mild to moderate chronic pain associated with cancer.[22] It possesses the advantage of not causing the gastritis associated with aspirin ingestion.[63] Chronic high dose abuse of acetaminophen has been associated with production of the hepatotoxicity and also the analgesic nephropathy described previously.[110]

NSAIDs

The release of ibuprofen in 1974 marked the first of what has become an increasing number of agents generally classified as non-steroidal, anti-inflammatory agents.[5] These agents share a common mechanism of analgesic, anti-inflammatory and anti-pyretic activity with aspirin; an inhibition of prostaglandin at the cyclo-oxygenase level with subsequent blockage of the formation of prostaglandin E2.[52]

Making a rational decision as to which non-steroidal anti-inflammatory agent should be used as a first choice for a specific patient is difficult. Although the half-life, chemistry, and other individual characteristics of non-steroidal anti-inflammatory drugs may vary (see Tables 7-6 and 7-7), their profiles are similar and the prescriber's choice is reduced to trial and error to arrive at an agent that is effective. One agent may work very well in one patient and may not work in another patient with the same disease.

Several non-steroidal agents cause acute renal failure with oliguria, proteinuria, and increased blood urea nitrogen and creatinine levels.[53,79,87,96] Patients with congestive heart failure, systemic lupus, cirrhosis, or chronic renal failure seem to be more at risk to develop this syndrome. It is thought that these patients have increased renal prostaglandin production as a compensatory mechanism for their disease; blocking prostaglandin production removes this compensatory mechanism and may induce acute renal failure. Because all non-steriodal, anti-inflammatory agents are excreted through the kidney and prostaglandins play an important physiologic role in renal homeostasis, patients on long-term non-steriodal, anti-inflammatory therapy should have their renal functions monitored periodically.[79]

Table 7-6
Differential Profile of the Nonnarcotic Analgesics

Generic (Trade)	Starting Dose	Maximum Received Daily Dose	Milligram/Tablet: Price per 100*	Comments
Acetaminophen	650 mg q 4 h	4,000 mg	325 mg: 1.65/100	Therapeutically equivalent to aspirin except where anti-inflammatory action needed
Aspirin	650 mg q 4 h	3,900 mg	325 mg: 0.87/100	Agent of choice if not contraindicated
Fenoprofen (Nalfon)	600 mg qid	3,200 mg	300 mg: 29.79/100	$t\frac{1}{2}$ = 2–3 h If gastrointestinal complaints occur, administer with meals or milk
Ibuprofen (Motrin, Rufen)	400 mg qid	2,400 mg	400 mg: 11.48/100	$t\frac{1}{2}$ = 3–4 h FDA-authorized as analgesic and anti-inflammatory
Indomethacin (Indocin)	25 mg bid or tid	200 mg	25 mg: 26.50/100	$t\frac{1}{2}$ = 4–5 h FDA-approved for rheumatoid arthritis, degenerative joint disease, acute gout, acute painful shoulder Not indicated for simple analgesia Most adverse effects are dose dependent, so use the lowest effective dose possible

(continued)

Generic (Trade)	Starting Dose	Maximum Received Daily Dose	Milligram/Tablet: Price per 100*	Comments
Mefenamic acid (Ponstel)	500 mg initially	250 mg Q 6 h	250 mg: 32.07/100	$t\frac{1}{2}$ = 4–6 h Not recommended for use longer than one week due to possible serious side effects
Naproxen (Naprosyn)	250 mg bid	750 mg	250 mg: 47.00/100	$t\frac{1}{2}$ = 13 h Urinary clearance increases with increasing doses
Phenylbutazone (Butazolidin, Azolid)	300–600 mg daily	600 mg	100 mg: 34.13/100	$t\frac{1}{2}$ of phenylbutazone = 84 h, oxyphenbutazone = 72 h Indicated for short-term acute use Not indicated as simple analgesics
Oxyphenbutazone (Tandearil, Oxalid)	300–600 mg daily	600 mg	100 mg: 36.50/100	Serious side effects preclude chronic use in patients over 60 Careful patient selection and close supervision are essential Serious blood dyscrasias are possible
Sulindac (Clinoril)	150 mg bid	400 mg	150 mg: 44.87/100	a. $t\frac{1}{2}$ of sulfide metabolite = 18 h b. Parent drug is inactive; activity is due to active sulfide metabolite
Tolmetin (Tolectin)	400 mg tid	2,000 mg	200 mg: 27.68/100	a. $t\frac{1}{2}$ = about 1 h b. Chemically related to indomethacin, but action and toxicity are similar to propionic acid derivatives

* Average wholesale price, Jan, 1987

Table 7-7
General Characteristics of Non-steroidal Anti-inflammatory
Agents

All non-steroidal anti-inflammatory agents:

- are as effective as aspirin as analgesic, anti-inflammatory and antipyretic agents
- act by inhibiting prostaglandin biosynthesis
- can cause gastrointestinal toxicity (irritation, nausea, vomiting, bleeding), although usually less than does aspirin
- are more expensive than aspirin
- share many of the side effects of aspirin
- inhibit collagen-induced platelet aggregation; platelet effects are less significant clinically than aspirin's effects on platelets (more bleeding with aspirin)
- can cause significant sodium retention
- have the propensity for cross-sensitization in patients with aspirin tolerance
- are excreted via the kidney
- can cause central nervous system side effects
- can cause rashes

Propoxyphene

Until recently, the propoxyphene series of prescription drugs remained one of the most frequently prescribed agents of any class in the United States despite eight known controlled prospective studies disputing their effectiveness.[11,16,19,35,45,65,66,81] Much of the popularity is based on claims of less adverse effects when compared to equal doses of codeine, but this may not be true for equinanalgesic doses.

Usual adverse effects noted with the use of therapeutic doses of propoxyphene include nausea, vomiting, constipation, dizziness, and drowsiness. While the addiction potential of propoxyphene is low as compared to the opioids, it is important to note the increasing incidence of over-dosage and subsequent deaths due to propoxyphene abuse. Young[109] reported nine deaths due to propoxyphene over-dosage; the probable cause for death being apnea followed by convulsions. Due to the structural similarity between propoxyphene and methadone, the prompt use of the narcotic antagonist naloxone can effectively reverse the respiratory depression and avoid most deaths.

In summary, aspirin and acetaminophen remain the agents of choice when mild to moderate pain associated with cancer is being treated. If patients obtain satisfactory relief with aspirin or acetaminophen, substitution is certainly not needed. However, if the pain is not controlled with these older agents, or if they are not tolerated, use of a non-steroidal anti-inflammatory agent such as ibuprofen or equivalent seems to be an appropriate alternative and should be tried. It may also be the next logical agent to be used for moderate to severe pain in place of the combination containing narcotics for the patients who can take oral medications. Alternatively, because of NSAIDs' action on peripheral sites it is rational to give one in conjunction with a carefully titrated dose of an orally effective narcotic. The combination of an opiate and non-opiate has been shown to provide a greater degree of pain relief than either agent used alone. Narcotic preparations should not be abruptly discontinued; instead, the NSAID may be added to the regimen and the narcotic gradually withdrawn if possible, depending on the overall pain control achieved.

NARCOTIC ANALGESICS

Narcotic analgesics (opioids) are a group of naturally occurring, semi-synthetic, and synthetic drugs that effectively relieve pain without producing loss of consciousness and have the potential to produce physical dependence. Although the different narcotic analgesics may vary in quantitative and qualitative effects, the similarity of the pharmacologic and therapeutic properties of these drugs permits their discussion as a class. The relative differences of the available agents are summarized in Table 7-8.[17]

Opioids and their effects have recently been classified according to a model proposing three types of opiate receptors: mu, kappa, and sigma.[51] The mu receptor is associated with analgesia and respiratory depression; the kappa receptor with sedative effects; and the sigma receptor with psychotomimetic effects. The differences in affinity and intrinsic activity have been postulated to account for the differing profiles of opioid classes. Those agents with the highest receptor affinity have been labeled as "narcotic agonists."

Agonists

Agonists produce their effects via activity at the mu receptor and, in part, the kappa receptor. Interaction with the mu receptor is associated with supraspinally mediated analgesia, respiratory depression, euphoria, and physical dependence. Interaction with the kappa receptor is associated with spinally mediated analgesia, miosis, and sedation. Agonists do not interact with the sigma receptor and do not, therefore, produce psychotomimetic effects. Examples of pure agonists are codeine, levorphanol, meperidine, methadone, morphine, oxycodone, oxymorphine, hydromorphone, and propoxyphene.

Mixed Agonist-Antagonists

Mixed agonist-antagonist activity within the same moiety is possible and can produce psychotomimetic effects. In addition, they are capable of precipitating abstinence in agonist-dependent persons and do not suppress it

Table 7-8
Pharmacologic Activity of Analgesics

Drugs	Analgesic[a]	Anti-tussive	Sedation	Emesis	Respiratory depressant	Constipation	Addictive	Equi-analgesic mg dose[b]	Average adult mg dose[c]
Morphine	V++	++	++	++	++	++	++	10	10–15
Diecetylmorphine (Heroin)	V++	++	++	+	++	+	+++	4	illegal
Ethylmorphine (Dionin)	V+	+++			++		?		15–60
Nalorphine (Nalline)	V++	+	+ or 0	+	++	+		8	15–10[d]
Codeine	V+	+++	+	+	+	++	+	120	15–60 (8–20)
Hydromorphone (Dilaudid)	V++	++	+	+	++	+	++	1	1–2
Methyldihydromorphinone (Metopon)	V+++	++	++	++	+++	+	+	3	3–9
Hydrocodone (Dicodid, etc.)	V++	+++				?	++		(5–10)
Dihydrocodeine (Paracodin, etc.)	V++	+++		+	+		+	60	30–60
Dihydrodesoxymorphine-D (Desomorphine)	V+++					+	+++	1	
Oxymorphone (Numorphan)	V++	+	++	+++	+++	+++	+++	1	½–1
Oxycodone (Percodan)	V++	+++	++	++	++	++	++	10	10–15 (3–5)
Nalmexone (EN-1620A)	V++	++	++	+	++		?	70–90	
Levorphanol (Levo-Dromoran)	V++	++	++	+	++	?	++	2	2–4
Racemorphan (Dromoran)	V++	++	+	+	++	+	++	2½	1–5
Dextromethorphan (Romilar)	V+++	+++	?	?					(10–20)

Drugs	Analgesic[a]	Anti-tussive	Sedation	Emesis	Respira-tory de-pressant	Constipa-tion	Addictive	Equi-anal-gesic mg dose[b]	Average adult mg dose[c]
Levallorphan (Lorfan)	V++	+	+	+	++			2	1[d]
Pentazocine (Talwin)	V++		++ or 0	++	++	+	+	30	20–30
Naloxone (Narcan)									½–1[d]
Naltrexone (EN-1639A)									½[d]
Methadone (Dolophine, etc.)	V++	++	+	+	++	+	+	8	5–15
Propoxyphene (Darvon)	V+		+	+	+	?	+	130	32–65
Levopropoxyphene (Novrad)		+++	+	+					(50–100)
Noracymethadol	V++	++	++	++	++	+	+	10	8–30
Dextromoramide (Palfium, etc.)	V++	++	+	++	++	+	++	5	5–10
Meperidine (Demerol, etc.)	V++		+	?	++	+	++	100	30–75
Alphaprodine (Nisentil)	V++		++	+	++	+	++	40	25–60
Anileridine (Leritine)	V++	+	++	?	++	+	++	30	25–50
Piminodine (Alvodine)	V++		+	+	++	+	++	7½	10–20
Ethoheptazine (Zectane)	V+				++		+	200	100

From Catalano RB: Supportive care of the seriously ill cancer patient: Control of pain, in Yarbro JW, Bornstein RS (Eds): Oncologic Emergencies. New York, Grune & Stratton, 1981, pp 365–393. Reprinted with permission.

[a] V = visceral and deep traumatic pain in contrast to somatic and joint pains.
+ = degree of activity from the least (+) to the greatest (+++) activity.
0 = produces the opposite effect.
? = questionable activity.
Blank space indicates that no such activity has been reported for this compound.
[b] Equianalgesic to morphine sulfate, 10 mg SC.
[c] Oral antitussive dose in parentheses.
[d] Used solely as narcotic antagonist and not as analgesic.

in high-dose agonist-dependent persons. While analgesic "ceiling effects" have not been established for the mixed agonist-antagonists, there is some question as to their maximal analgesic efficacy. Mixed agonist-antagonists have limited abuse-liability. Examples of mixed agonist-antagonist include butorphanol, nalbuphine, and pentazocine.

Pentazocine is a benzomorphan derivative of this mixed agonist-antagonist class. In early clinical studies, 30 mg of pentazocine was found to have an analgesic activity equivalent to 75–100 mg of meperidine or 10 mg of morphine. After intramuscular administration of pentazocine the onset of analgesia is noticeable after 20 minutes. The duration of analgesic effect is only about three hours.

The disadvantages of pentazocine as an analgesic are its irritative effect at the site of injection and its relatively short duration of action. The analgesia produced by oral administration of pentazocine is not dependable, possibly because of the poor absorption of the drug in the gastrointestinal tract and its extensive metabolism when given orally.

Beaver et al.[8,9] showed that it required 90 mg of oral pentazocine to produce analgesia equivalent to that produced with 30 mg of parenteral pentazocine for cancer patients with chronic pain. The same investigators had previously shown it required 30 mg of pentazocine, intramuscularly, to produce an equianalgesic effect of 5 mg of morphine in the same type of patients.

The most common side effects of pentazocine consist of sedation, drowsiness, nausea, vomiting, and blurring of vision. Side effects that have also occurred include hallucinations, fever, urinary retention, euphoria, changes in mood, constipation, dry mouth, and respiratory depression. The propensity for producing central nervous system side effects, particularly vertigo, reduces substantially the value of this drug in ambulatory patients.[10]

The original claims that pentazocine was non-addicting have proved incorrect. Its dependence potential is substantially less than that of morphine or meperidine. However, at this point no conclusion may be drawn as to whether pentazocine has less addiction potential than codeine, the drug to which it is frequently compared in the commercial literature. Dependence on parenteral pentazocine has been reported by several investigators.[57] Doses exceeding 180 mg daily for at least one month predispose susceptible individuals to morphine-like dependence. To date, there are no reports of dependence with the oral form of the drug.

The final limiting factor in the use of pentazocine is in respect to its respiratory depressant effects.[84] Bellville and Green,[10] in reporting a case of pentazocine-induced respiratory depression, suggested that the problems seen with morphine in patients with limited respiratory function are also seen with pentazocine.

PHARMACOLOGIC ACTIONS
OF NARCOTIC ANALGESICS

Central Nervous System Effects

Narcotic analgesics exert their primary effect on the central nervous system. The precise biochemical mechanism by which they produce their effects is presumed to be a direct interaction with the opiate receptors identified both centrally and in the spinal cord. It has been suggested that opiates may also act on the diencephalon and frontal lobes of the brain to cause modification of the central nervous system response to pain[75] or affect the patient's emotional response (perception) to pain.

In addition to analgesia, the central nervous system response to the administration of an opiate may produce a broad spectrum of effects. The type and degree of response seems to be attributed largely to the conditions under which an opiate is administered.[75,103] In the presence of significant pain, the narcotic-induced analgesia is accompanied by sedation and alteration of mood characterized by euphoria. In this case, the sedative action and sleep may be an incidental occurrence resulting from the relief of pain and accompanying mental and physical exhaustion. When a narcotic is given in the absence of pain, the resultant effect may be one of dysphoria, apprehension, apathy, or mental confusion, and rarely hallucinations and delirium. In certain patients, especially those with a history of seizure disorders, administration of a narcotic analgesic produces a stimulating effect in the motor sphere causing a lowering of the seizure threshold that may precipitate convulsions in a previously controlled patient.

Other centrally mediated effects of narcotic analgesics are discussed in relation to their importance on end-organ function (Table 7-9).[49]

Respiratory Effects

Opiates produce respiratory depression by a direct effect on the chemoreceptors of the respiratory centers in the brain stem. This effect seems to result from a decreased sensitivity and responsiveness to increases in serum carbon dioxide tension (pCO_2). The narcotic analgesics also depress the pontine medullary centers responsible for regulation of the rate of respiration, thereby altering voluntary control of respiration. Initially, there is a depression of tidal volume followed by a decreased respiratory rate. Clinically, the narcotic-induced respiratory depression is characterized by slow, irregular, periodic respiration.

Since both primary and metastatic malignant involvement of the pulmonary system is common, the importance of determining the extent of any respiratory insufficiency prior to treatment becomes evident. The additional

Table 7-9
Side Effects of Narcotic Analgesics as Manifested in Terms of
End-Organ Function

Central Nervous System
euphoria (dysphoria)
sedation
lowering of seizure threshold
central depression of respiration, cough reflex, nausea, vomiting

GI Tract
decreased secretions
constipation
increased smooth muscle tone in biliary tract

Genitourinary System
urinary retention

Circulatory System
postural hypotension

Miscellaneous
anaphylactoid reaction
autonomic reactions
(diaphoresis, hyperglycemia, miosis, dry mouth)
antidiuresis
adverse interaction with monoamineoxidase inhibitors (especially meperidine)

From Houde RW: Systemic analgesics and related drugs: narcotic analgesics, in Bonica JJ,
Ventafridda V (Eds): Advances in Pain Research and Therapy, Vol. 2. New York, Raven Press,
1979, pp 263–273. Reprinted with permission.

carbon dioxide retention induced by the administration of opiates may be
sufficient to precipitate coma.

The diagnostic and treatment dilemma is further complicated when the
patient continues to breathe, despite the coma, through the hypoxic drive
mechanism regulated by the carotid and aortic chemoreceptors. If the
responsible physician is not aware of this situation, the instinct to support
the patient with administration of oxygen without assisted or controlled
ventilation will eliminate the hypoxic drive and rapidly produce apnea.
Additional problems relating to the hazards of the respiratory suppression
induced by opiates arise in the evaluation of patients with suspected
intracranial malignancies. The increased arterial pCo_2 will result in a
cerebrovascular dilatation with a consequent rise in cerebral blood flow and
cerebrospinal fluid pressure. In this case, administration of a narcotic
analgesic may cause what seems to be a paradoxical increase in pain.

A secondary action of the opiates on the respiratory system is worth
mentioning here, despite the fact it is not directly related to pain control.
This is the ability of opiates to suppress the cough reflex. The antitussive

action is a consequence of the direct effect of the cough centers in the medulla. This may occur with doses lower than those required for analgesia. Therapeutic suppression of the cough reflex has occurred with opiate congeners devoid of significant analgesic activity (i.e., dextromethorphan). In the treatment of pain this action could theoretically become an adverse effect that may need to be considered in the final choice of agents. The cough reflex is one of the body's natural defense mechanisms against invasion by foreign substances via the respiratory tract. Administration of certain narcotics nullifies this mechanism. Considering that malignant disease may produce a compromised host response system and a patient may receive immunosuppressive agents as part of therapy, suppression of cough mechanisms may be an undesirable effect.

Gastrointestinal Effects

Therapeutic doses of narcotic agonists produce a variety of effects on the gastrointestinal system as a result of both direct and centrally mediated mechanisms. Gastric, biliary, and pancreatic secretions are decreased by opiates, causing delay in digestion. Smooth muscle tone of the bowel is decreased in intensity and frequency of propulsive contractions. The ultimate result is constipation. Usually, the morphine congeners, meperidine and its congeners, and methadone are less constipating than morphine. The smooth muscle tone in the biliary tract, especially at the sphincter of Oddi, is increased. This may cause a rise in the common bile duct pressure from 20 ml to as high as 200–300 ml of water and precipitate biliary colic. Such spasm may result in plasma amylase and lipase levels as much as 2 to 15 times the normal values. Because of this effect, plasma amylase and lipase determinations are not reliable within 24 hours after a narcotic analgesic has been given.

Nausea and vomiting are a common occurrence with the initial administration of a narcotic analgesic. This effect may indirectly result from a central stimulation of the chemoreceptor trigger zone in the medulla oblongata. However, with continued administration, the narcotic analgesics depress the vomiting center; therefore, subsequent doses of these agents are unlikely to produce vomiting by this mechanism. Ambulatory patients and those patients not experiencing severe pain seem to have a higher incidence of nausea and vomiting than those who are in a supine position due to an enhanced vestibular sensitivity induced by narcotic analgesics.

Urinary Tract Effects

Narcotic analgesics increase muscle tone in the urinary tract and may induce spasms. Although the response of the ureters is quite variable, these drugs may increase tone and amplitude of contractions, especially of the lower third of the ureter. In the urinary bladder, tone of the detrusor muscle is increased, possibly resulting in urinary urgency. There is also an increase in the tone of the vesical sphincter, which may make urination difficult. Patients with prostatic hypertrophy or urethral stricture may be prone to urinary retention and oliguria when narcotic analgesics are used.

The initial decrease in urinary excretion usually seen following administration of narcotics may be an indirect effect of a central action causing an increased secretion of the antidiuretic hormone (ADH). However, results of one study[50] suggest that decreased urine output may occur without any apparent release of excess ADH and may be attributed to decreased renal plasma flow or increased reabsorption from the renal tubules.

Cardiovascular Effects

The circulatory effects of narcotics are caused by their central action with depression of the vasomotor center and stimulation of medullary vagal nuclei or by a histamine release and a direct effect on peripheral effector cells. When therapeutic doses are given to supine patients, narcotic analgesics have little cardiovascular effect. When the supine patient assumes a head-up position, however, orthostatic hypotension and fainting may occur as a result of peripheral vasodilation. The myocardial tone and contractility is usually increased by small doses and decreased by large doses of narcotics.

The adverse circulatory effects of opiates are increased in the presence of reduced circulatory blood volume and with the concomitant use of drugs that have alpha-adrenergic blocking activity (e.g., phenothiazines).

With the exception of meperidine, which has anticholinergic effects, narcotics usually decrease heart rate. They may also cause sinus bradyarrhythmias, which can be abolished by atropine.

Endocrine Effects

Opiates produce endocrinologic alterations, some of which may be related to central nervous system effects. In addition to the inappropriate ADH secretion previously mentioned, narcotic analgesics have been reported to inhibit the release of adrenocorticotropic and gonadotropic hormone from the pituitary. This results in decreased plasma and urinary 17-hydroxycorticosteroid and 17-ketosteroid levels. The secondary nature of the hypofunction has been demonstrated by the production of normal responses to administration of the appropriate tropic hormone.

Narcotic analgesics have also been associated with inhibition of release of thyroid-stimulating hormone, leading to a clinically detectable suppression of thyroid hormone production. Basal metabolism rates may be decreased by 10 to 20 percent in patients receiving narcotic analgesia.

Hyperglycemia may occur in patients receiving opiates. This response is thought to be secondary to a direct action on the paraventricular receptor sites near the foramen of Monro or as a result of stimulating release of epinephrine.

SPECIFIC PRINCIPLES OF ANALGESIC USE

Choice of Analgesic

Although most of the drugs classified as agonists produce a similar quality of analgesia in equianalgesic doses, factors such as oral effectiveness, duration of action, degree of action on smooth muscle, route of metabolism, and individual variation in patient response should be considered in the selection of a specific narcotic analgesic. No single drug or procedure is always or almost always best for every patient. The final criterion, as with any treatment of pain is patient comfort. General guidelines for the use of a systemic analgesics in cancer pain are presented in Table 7-10.

Table 7-10
Guidelines for Appropriate Use of Systemic Analgesics in
Chronic Cancer Pain

---

1. Establish a simple, practical analgesic schema (stepladder) to include a representative agent of each class.

    a. Non-narcotic—aspirin or acetaminophen.

    b. Weak narcotic—codeine.

    c. Strong narcotic—morphine.

2. Avoid pentazocine, and in patients with renal failure, meperidine.

3. If methadone is used, be familiar with its precautions for dosing and dose escalation.

4. The proper dose and schedule of a narcotic analgesic is dictated by the intensity of pain and not by the brevity of the prognosis. "Morphine exists to be given not merely withheld."

5. Diversional therapy is of great value.

6. Properly used and monitored, addiction *does not* occur with narcotic analgesics.

7. Physical dependence (not to be confused with addiction) does not prevent a downward adjustment of dose should pain ameliorate.

The most effective analgesics thus far tested have been the morphine surrogates but, even though the range of relative potency of these drugs extends up to several hundredfold, well controlled studies to date have failed to show appreciable differences in their "ceiling" effects. Relative potency is, of course, merely an expression of the ratio of doses to produce a given effect, and a more potent drug is not necessarily a more effective drug.

Among drugs of the same class, differences in side effect liability at equianalgesic doses tend to be insignificant. However, among drugs of different classes, the spectra of side effects can be quite different and may be important considerations. With increasing doses, higher degrees of pain relief can be obtained before encountering limiting toxic effects with drugs of the morphine type than with the narcotic agonist-antagonist type, methotrimeprazine (a phenothiazine), drugs of the antipyretic analgesic type such as the salicylates, acetaminophen, and the nonsteroidal anti-inflammatory agents. Thus, differences do exist among different classes of drugs as to their relative analgesic potentials that do not necessarily correlate with their relative analgesic potencies, or any demonstrable decrease in increment of analgesic effect with dose. The most severe complaints of pain can generally be controlled only by drugs with high analgesic potentials, although other undesirable side effect considerations (such as drug dependence liability) often dictate the choice of a drug with a lower potential in individual situations.

The determination of equivalent analgesic doses is usually based on a comparison of one drug with another, the most frequently used standard drugs being morphine and aspirin. Commonly the relative potencies or equianalgesic doses are expressed either as peak effect or as the area under the time-effect curve. When the time-effect curves are not the same for two drugs, neither the peak nor the total effect parameters adequately express the equivalent analgesic doses. The peak effects of a short-acting drug such as alphaprodine or hydromorphone may be underestimated when compared in terms of equivalent total effect to a longer acting drug such as morphine or methadone, and vice versa. Virtually all drugs are less potent and more variable in their analgesic effects when given orally than when given parenterally. When a drug is given orally, its time-effect curve also tends to be flatter and more extended than when it is administered parenterally, so that greater differences in potency are noted in peak than total effects. Appreciable differences exist in the relative oral-parenteral analgesic potencies of various narcotic drugs. Drugs such as morphine and oxymorphone have relatively low oral to parenteral potency ratios, whereas other drugs such as codeine, oxycodone, and methadone have relatively high oral to parenteral potency ratios. Selecting the appropriate drug dose and route of administration can make the difference between effective and ineffective use of analgesics (Table 7-10).

Tolerance, Physical Dependence, and Psychological Dependence

Tolerance, physical dependence, and psychological dependence are distinctly different phenomena that are often confused. Such misunderstandings have contributed greatly to the mismanagement of chronic pain.

Tolerance

Tolerance to opioid effects develops when repeated administrations produce less analgesia or when higher doses are required to provide the initial effectiveness. Tolerance is a shift to the right in the dose-response curve. Tolerance to opioids is not related to changes in metabolism; rather, it is related to undefined changes in the opiate receptors. There is no limit to the extent to which tolerance to the analgesic effect of opioids can develop.

The rate of tolerance development is dependent upon dose, route, frequency, and duration of repeated administrations. Tolerance does not necessarily accompany the repeated use of opioids. There is a minimum effective receptor concentration necessary to trigger development of tolerance, and this concentration is likely to be higher than that required for analgesia. When tolerance does develop, it can usually be overcome merely by increasing the dose.

Tolerance to the most threatening side effects develops at a rate comparable to tolerance to analgesia. Smooth muscle effects, however, are particularly slow in their rate of tolerance development. Problems arise when tolerance develops more rapidly to analgesic effects than to side effects. Continuous re-evaluation of the balance between analgesic and side effects, with occasional changes in dose, drug, and/or adjuvant medications, is required. Nonetheless, patients with chronic pain can often take a given dose of oral drugs for extended periods with only minor alterations.

A second problem related to tolerance arises when the volume of intramuscularly injectable drug required for adequate pain relief becomes unacceptably large; in this situation a more concentrated preparation should be used. Some drugs, such as salts of hydromorphone, are considerably more soluble than others, such as salts of morphine. This difference can be exploited in tolerant individuals who require intramuscular injections. One of the main arguments for the legalization of heroin relates to this specific point of concentration and dose. The availability of the salts of hydromorphone negate this argument; this issue is discussed by Howard-Ruben in Chapter 4 of this monograph.

Tolerance can be minimized by the use of several strategies. The obvious one being to initiate treatment with a non-narcotic analgesic that is not associated with tolerance development and to administer non-narcotics in combination with lower than usual doses of opiates. The lack of complete cross-tolerance between narcotic analgesics may be exploited by switching from one to another in lower than equianalgesic doses.[14] It has been reported that patients require less opiates if they are dosed at fixed intervals to prevent pain rather than on an as-needed basis. This concept is also discussed in more detail in Chapter 4.

Physical Dependence

Like tolerance, physical dependence is a pharmacologic phenomenon rather than a physiologic one, dependent on the same variables. Physical dependence on opiates is characterized by a withdrawal syndrome that develops following cessation of administration or that is precipitated by the administration of antagonists. The withdrawal syndrome is characterized by early purposive behavior signs and later nonpurposive, primarily autonomic symptoms. The entire syndrome has a variable time course in days that is particular to the drug involved. In contrast, precipitated withdrawal, or abstinence, results in an immediate, fullblown, considerably shorter, withdrawal syndrome.

Clinically recognizable physical dependence does not usually develop unless repeated doses of an agonist have been administered for approximately two weeks. Problems arise when the dose is reduced less than one-fourth of the previous dose, or a drug with narcotic antagonist activity is administered. It is not appropriate to use the agonist-antagonist agents in individuals who have been receiving narcotic agonists nor to abruptly stop the administration of a narcotic analgesic in a physically dependent patient once the source of pain is removed or when an analgesic procedure has been performed.

Withdrawal symptoms can differ quantitatively according to which opiate the patient is physically dependent upon. A general rule is that opiates with a shorter duration of action (e.g., meperidine, anileridine, etc.) tend to produce more intense symptoms over a shorter period.

Drugs that have a longer duration of action (e.g., methadone) produce a milder but a more prolonged period of withdrawal symptoms. This general rule holds true only when the drugs are stopped abruptly, not if a narcotic antagonist is administered. For example, if naloxone were administered to a patient physically dependent on methadone, the withdrawal symptoms may be extremely severe.

Psychological Dependence

The development of psychological dependence is a criterion for characterizing an individual as an addict. Psychological dependence is an overwhelming preoccupation with the procurement and use of a drug for other than a medical indication. Unlike tolerance and physical dependence, it is not a pharmacologic phenomenon; its cause lies within the individual. Psychological dependence can arise in the absence of tolerance and physical dependence.

The fear of producing drug addiction should never prevent the administration of morphine or other analgesics in patients with terminal disease.

Unfortunately, this fear is a major cause of underprescribing, even for terminal patients with severe pain. Results of a study on narcotic use in two hospitals showed that 32 percent of the patients remained in severe distress and 41 percent were in moderate distress, despite the administration of a narcotic.[59] A review of the medication records showed that the dosage ordered for these patients was lower than usually recommended, and the amount they received was substantially less than ordered.

A survey of the physicians determined that the principal reasons for underprescribing were a misunderstanding of optimal effective dosages, the duration of the drug's action, and potential side effects, especially dependence-liability and withdrawal symptoms. These physicians underestimated the dosage requirements and overestimated the drug's duration of action. Because of their misconceptions concerning the danger of addiction, they indicated a reluctance to increase the dosage or the frequency, even for patients with severe pain caused by a malignant disease.[59]

Experience has demonstrated that the likelihood of a hospitalized patient becoming "addicted" to meperidine is very slight. The report[59] points out that, "Ironically, under-treatment with analgesic medication may also encourage craving of the drug." This might be misinterpreted to suggest that the patient is developing a degree of dependence, which, in turn, may cause the physician to reduce the dose when it actually may need to be increased. Moreover, severe pain can best be relieved by morphine or its potent congeners, and it may be necessary to prescribe a more potent agent in place of an intermediate acting one to provide adequate relief. Most patients who receive a morphine-like drug for relief of pain, especially in a hospital, are able to discontinue its use without difficulty. Although some may develop mild degrees of dependence, only a small percentage become compulsive abusers.

Addiction and tolerance may possibly be delayed with the use of a dose adequate to control the pain. Narcotics should be administered at regular intervals. This recommendation is based on principles of operant conditioning.[14] The traditional method of giving narcotics when the patient complains of pain makes the administration of the drug contingent on the patient's complaint of pain. Thus, the pharmacologic and psychologic effects of the drug administration become a positive reinforcer for chronic pain behavior and may facilitate addiction. Using the operant conditioning strategy, it is first necessary to determine the average duration of pain relief produced by the drug given in response to a patient's request during a period of several days. Once the time duration of relief is ascertained, the drug is given at fixed intervals that are short of the predetermined period of relief. This strategy makes the administration of the narcotic not contingent on pain, but on "nonpain" or well behavior (Fig. 7-2.)

Combining the narcotic with barbiturates, chlorpromazine, or amphetamine may also help reduce the patient's fear of the pain. Fear may escalate pain and lead to an increased need for the narcotic.

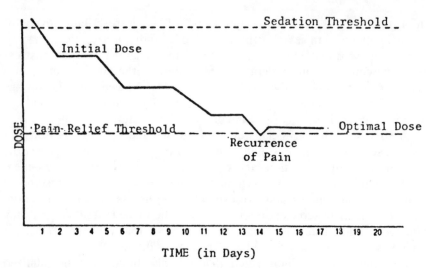

TIME (in Days)

Fig. 7-2. Narcotic dose titration in chronic pain.

NEW METHODS OF MORPHINE ADMINISTRATION

There are a wide variety of drugs and routes of administration that can be used in the treatment of cancer pain. This section reviews controlled release morphine, rectal administration, continuous infusion of morphine, and intraspinal administration of narcotics. Continuous subcutaneous infusion of morphine and patient-controlled analgesia are reviewed by Sheidler in Chapter 8 of this monograph, and intraventricular and intraspinal administration of narcotics is discussed by Carson in Chapter 9.

Controlled Release Morphine

Whenever possible, the majority of patients should have their pain controlled with the oral administration of narcotics, allowing a greater sense of independence and control. To date, no narcotic agent has proven more effective or less expensive than morphine.[102] Recently, two new morphine formulations have been introduced in the United States that may have significant advantages over existing narcotic preparations, although researchers are still addressing this issue. These new oral preparations are morphine sulfate intensified oral solution, (Roxanol, Roxane Labs Inc, P.O. Box 16532, Columbus, OH 43216) and a solid dosage form providing a sustained released preparation morphine sulfate (MS Contin, The Purdue Frederick Co, 100 Connecticut Avenue, Norwalk, CT 06856).

Roxanol is a high potency liquid preparation with a concentration of 20 mg of morphine per ml of solution. It is supplied in an easy to carry and easy to titrate plastic dropper bottle that obviates some of the inconvenience of lower potency morphine solutions for ambulatory patients or patients unable to swallow large volumes of fluid. The concentrated preparation has a bland taste and low alcohol content, which patients prefer. Roxanol SR is a sustained release tablet with an 8–12 hour duration.

MS Contin was released in the United States in October 1984, having accumulated four years of success in Europe under the name MST Continus.[6,39,42,104] Due to a wax matrix-controlled release system, the morphine is slowly released, resulting in a prolonged therapeutic blood level. This provides an advantage to patients requiring regular narcotic administration in that it may be given on a 12-hour rather than a 4-hour administration schedule. Methadone had been the only narcotic used successfully on a 6–8-hour basis. Unfortunately, because of the complex pharmacology of methadone, including high lipid solubility and long half-life, accumulation resulting in potential toxicity has been commonly found by those who do not understand the unique properties of methadone.[27]

When using MS Contin, one should begin with the appropriate calculated 12-hour dose and provide a 4-hour narcotic for breakthrough pain. The MS Contin dose can then be increased daily until supplements are no longer required. On occasion, a return to a 4-hour narcotic may be necessary during a intercurrent crisis, with resumption of the MS Contin scheduling once the patient is stable.

Rectal Administration

Despite the preferability of the oral route for morphine administration, sometimes it cannot be utilized due to severe confusion, nausea, vomiting, or dysphagia. Before resorting to the parenteral route of administration, one should consider rectal administration. Clinical trials have reported analgesic effectiveness of rectally administered narcotics such as morphine and hydromorphone using standard clinical methods of evaluation. Until recently, however, there were no data documenting what the obtainable plasma concentrations of this method of administration were and, more importantly, how they correlated with comparable doses given orally to allow some means of accurate conversion should changes in the route of administration be nessessary.

Ellison and Lewis[24] recently provided this valuable comparison in reporting their results of a single-dose study of oral versus rectally administered morphine sulfate. The pharmacokinetic data demonstrated that the rectally administered dose had a peak plasma concentration obtained at 1.5 hours as compared to a 1-hour peak for an orally administered dose. Surprisingly, the rectally administered dose of morphine achieved a significantly higher overall plasma morphine concentration as compared with the oral solution. It must be stressed that this was a single-dose comparison and did not address the more important issue of the clinical comparison of these dosage forms under steady-state conditions of chronic use. However, it did provide the first scientific evidence of the clinical efficacy of rectal administration of narcotic analgesics at a probable conversion ratio of 1:1.[24]

Continuous Infusion of Morphine

Indications for Use

In the majority of patients, oral narcotics may provide effective analgesia for moderate to severe pain. As the disease progresses, however, oral medications may become ineffective or poorly tolerated at the dosage or schedule required to maintain a pain-free state. Patients with progressive disease may also become refractory to parenteral forms of narcotics or may require frequent intramuscular injection. Currently, a growing body of literature indicates that continuous intravenous infusion of morphine is a safe and effective treatment for severe cancer pain.[20,26,44,55,64,90]

Continuous intravenous infusions of morphine are reserved for relief of severe, intractable pain of terminal patients who are unable to tolerate oral or intermittent parenteral medications due to (1) uncontrollable vomiting, (2) severe pain in which intermittent oral or parenteral medications give insufficient pain relief, (3) patients who have insufficient muscle mass to tolerate repeated intramuscular or subcutaneous injections, and (4) coagulopathies resulting in severe bruising following intramuscular or subcutaneous injections. This procedure is generally not done on a routine basis, but is reserved for use when more conventional methods of pain control have failed. The safety and efficacy of this route of administration are discussed in Chapter 4.

Guidelines for Use

The guidelines for proper initiation of a morphine infusion in a patient already receiving a more standard method of narcotic administration are as follows. Previous narcotics and sedatives should be discontinued and baseline respiratory rate, pulse, blood pressure, and sedation recorded. Sedation can be evaluated as (0) none (patient alert), (1) mild (patient drowsy on occasion but easily aroused), (2) moderate (patient often drowsy but easily aroused), and (3) severe (patient somnolent and difficult to arouse). Intravenous injections of 2 to 5 mg of morphine should be administered every 15 minutes until pain is relieved. Vital signs should be checked before each IV dose, although the typical hierarchy of response to narcotic analgesics would indicate that analgesia must be demonstrated before sedation and other toxicities would be detectable. After IV loading is completed, the patient should be started on an hourly infusion of morphine that is equal to the cumulative bolus doses required to achieve the initial analgesia. For example, if 5 mg IV of morphine were given to a patient every 15 minutes and four injections were required to obtain analgesia, then a 20 mg loading dose is required. Therefore, the patient would be started on a morphine infusion at 20 mg/hour, using an infusion pump to ensure correct dosing. After the infusion has started, vital signs and sedation should be recorded every 15 minutes for the first hour, every hour for the next four hours, every four hours for the next 24 hours, and every six to eight hours thereafter. If pain is not significantly relieved, the morphine dose should be escalated, although not by more than one-third of the previous hourly morphine dose. After each dose escalation, vital signs and sedation should be assessed as outlined above. Finally, the dose of morphine infusions generally ranges from 10 to 350 mg/hour. To accommodate these different doses, a variety of concentrations of morphine in IV solutions will have to be prepared.

Morphine doses should be initially adjusted to relieve pain while the patient is in bed. After the first day of infusion, the dose can be escalated as the patient's activity increases. However, the patient may become tolerant to the drug's analgesic action, necessitating further dose increments. Fortunately, the development of tolerance to the analgesic effect of morphine is paralleled by the development of tachyphylaxis to its respiratory and central nervous system effects. In contrast, morphine-induced constipation is dose-dependent and, unless properly treated, may be a discomforting side effect.

Toxicity

The major toxicity from continuous infusion of morphine is manifested clinically by changes in mental status and respiratory rate. Generally, bradycardia without a change in mental status is well tolerated. Severe toxicity is marked by a 40 percent or more reduction in respiratory rate and increasing somnolence. This may be heralded by incoherent and garbled speech. In patients who develop these signs, the morphine infusion should be discontinued and arterial blood gases obtained. The patient should be observed continuously until mental status and respiratory rate return to normal.

If the patient's mental status and respiratory rate improve, the use of a narcotic antagonist such as naloxone is not necessary and should be avoided. In cases of life-threatening toxicity, however, naloxone should be given by an infusion or by repeated intravenous injections. Care should be taken to anticipate an acute withdrawal syndrome, including vomiting, and an endotracheal tube should be inserted in comatose patients.

Administration of morphine by a constant infusion avoids the peaks and troughs in morphine blood levels. The result is that a patient does not fluctuate between toxic and subtherapeutic levels of the agent. Not only does the constant infusion eliminate the peaks and troughs, it also decreases the anxiety level in these patients caused by the anticipation of their next pain injection.[32,34,62] It allows for easily adjustable dosages simply by changing the infusion rate. Nursing time and effort in preparing and charting the medication is actually reduced over the course of treatment.

Intraspinal Administration of Narcotics

The discovery of the opiate receptors in the brain and spinal cord has led to the clinical use of narcotic analgesics intraspinally (epidural and subarachnoid) to control both acute and chronic pain.[56,73,74,80,85] It has been demonstrated that the endogenous opioids (Methionine-enkephalin and Leucine-enkephalin) play a role in pain perception.[97,108] The unique finding from these discoveries was that analgesia could be produced at the first level of sensory integration, that is, at the level of the spinal cord, simply by injection of the opioids into or near the receptors of the spinal cord. A thorough understanding of the material contained within Yaksh's[108] extensive review should precede attempts at this form of analgesic administration.

Patients with metastatic cancer often require large doses of narcotics, resulting in clouding of the sensorium, not to mention the added financial burden of large doses of drug. In the last several years, experience has accumulated with the use of a surgically placed epidural catheter connected to an implanted morphine infusion pump similar to the type currently used for chronic infusion of cytotoxic chemotherapy. This permits delivery of the analgesic directly to the central nervous system, thereby producing pain relief with minimal side effects. Good to excellent pain relief is achieved in 90 percent of patients.[74] Several studies have confirmed the effectiveness of endogenous opioids[73] and commercially available opiates.[36,73,74,80] Table 7-11 outlines reports of successful intraspinal narcotic analgesia.

The options available for intraspinal drug administration are epidural or intrathecal (IT). Epidural drugs are usually administered by intermittent bolus injections, while intrathecal opioid drugs are usually administered via an implanted catheter and subcutaneous reservoir by continuous infusion. The decision as to which route to employ is arbitrary. However, some factors do favor the IT route. The major advantage of the IT route is that the required dose is about 10 percent of the equianalgesic dose given by the epidural route.

Since patients being considered for this method of treatment are often very tolerant to systemic narcotics, the initial dose can vary tremendously. A relatively safe way to determine this initial dose for intrathecal morphine is to administer via lumbar puncture 1 mg for each 10 mg IM every four hours given systemically.[67] If the patient is taking a different opiate analgesic, the equivalent dose of morphine can be calculated from a table of

Table 7-11
Intraspinal Administration of Analgesics

Investigators	Patient Population	Medications	Comments
Oyama et al.[73]	14 patients with advanced cancer	B-endorphin (synthetic)	100% relief in all patients with 3 mg IT dose. Mean duration = 33 hrs. Toxicity = mild disorientation ± euphoria in 3 patients.
Leavens et al.[56]	6 patients with advanced cancer	Lumbar intrathecal morphine (2 pts.) Intraventricular morphine (4 pts.)	1 mg IT produced relief for 10–14 hrs. 2.5–4.0 mg intraventricularly produced relief for 12–24 hours. Treated for 3–7 months with gradual increase dose, but no complication.
Poletti et al.[80]	2 patients with advanced cancer	Epidural morphine via indwelling Broviac catheter	2 mg dose = 8–12 hours pain relief for 6 months without tolerance developing.
Onofrio et al.[74]	1 patient with advanced cancer	Intrathecal morphine via continuous infusion using Infusaid (implanted pump)	Pain free on 1.8 mg/24 hours by continuous infusion

equianalgesic doses. This initial dose can be gradually titrated upwards until a significant analgesic response is obtained. This dose provides the basis for calculating the initial morphine infusion. Although pharmacokinetic data are insufficient to predict the precise infusion rate, clinical experience indicates that approximately 2 to 3 times the bolus dose of morphine should be delivered over 24 hours. Once this infusion dose is determined, a permanent indwelling catheter is inserted, with its tip as close as possible to the segment of the spinal cord responsible for pain transmission in the dorsal horn. The reason for this is that there is a significant concentration gradient both rostral and caudal to the site of drug administration, and one wants to maximize CSF drug levels at the appropriate spinal cord segment.[68] If the initial infusion rate provides inadequate analgesia, the dose can be increased by 50 to 100 percent. Since the CSF elimination half-life for morphine is approximately two hours and it takes 8 to 10 hours to reach steady state,[69] it is important to assess each infusion rate over at least 24 hours before dose escalation.

In the clinical setting tolerance to the dose of IT analgesic will develop, but it is often difficult to separate the phenomenon of tolerance from increasing analgesic demands due to progression of the underlying disease state. For either or both of these reasons, the dose of IT morphine can increase to 100 or 150 mg per day.[37] These doses are close to the maximum that can be infused by an infusion limited to a maximum volume of 2 to 3 ml per 24 hours,[21] given the solubility of morphine sulfate in saline is approximately 60 mg/ml. In any case, central side effects almost always occur as the dose is increased, so that analgesic efficacy is limited. Careful observation of a sudden development of apparent tolerance should always raise the suspicion that the catheter tip has slipped out of its intended compartment (i.e., IT to epidural space or epidural space to subcutaneous tissue). This can be easily investigated by injection of 1 to 2 ml of metrizamide under fluoroscopy to confirm catheter placement.

Two recent reports[56,80] have combined this method of intraspinal analgesia with some innovative surgically implanted delivery systems to produce a system that allows self-administration of epidural or intrathecal analgesia via a controlled system. Poletti et al.[80] electively implanted indwelling catheter systems into the spinal epidural space. Their first attempt employed a partially indwelling Broviac catheter, with the second attempt being a morphine reservoir connected to a shunt pump and on/off Hakim valve assembly, which permitted the patients to self-administer an epidural morphine solution and still remain at home in relatively pain-free states. Leavens et al.[56] attempted a similar method by inserting an Ommaya reservoir with its catheter tip in the lumbar subarachnoid space or lateral ventricle. The reservoir was then used for percutaneous administration of morphine. This system required the training of a responsible family member to give the injections of morphine.

Onofrio et al.[74] recently reviewed the literature and concluded that the merits of chronic intrathecal morphine infusion, compared with the standard destructive neurosurgical procedures, include the preservation of motor and sensory modalities while achieving a pain-free state. They noted that intrathecal morphine in the dosage range needed to achieve a clinical effect on pain, unlike parenteral narcotics, did not lead to suppression of supraspinal centers. They also noted that the use of spinal opiates for chronic pain had three major objections: (1) the necessity of multiple punctures, (2) the dangers associated with respiratory depression as a result of the redistribution of the opiate to supraspinal centers, and (3) the development of tolerance with repeated spinal administration.

In the same report, Onofrio and his colleagues[74] reported successful use of a continuous infusion of morphine delivered through an indwelling intrathecal catheter supplied by a subcutaneous implanted pump. An implanted system obviates repeated lumbar puncture and lowers the risk of infection. The long-term infusion of the low concentrations of morphine ensures that the absolute level of opiate in the intrathecal space at any moment will be low, compared with the concentrations that are achieved in the cerebrospinal fluid when the dose sufficient for long-term relief of pain is administered in a single injection.

In summary, this pharmacologic approach to the relief of pain has one great advantage. In accomplishing a pain-free state, this method does not depend on the creation of a sensory deficit by disruption of ascending spinal cord tracts. Attempts at pain control by the use of ablative surgical procedures will lead to an unavoidable percent of motor system disasters as well as failure to achieve a lasting satisfactory level of cephalad dermatomal analgesia in many patients. In contrast to the relief of pain produced by the use of opiates parenterally, the beneficial effects accruing from the intrathecal infusion occur in the absence of any evidence of central nervous system depression. Voluntary motor function is enhanced by virtue of the relief of pain, and no effects on autonomic function were observed. The success of this administration system should have an important clinical impact on the management of pain states of a malignant origin that are mediated by somatic and visceral input.

CO-ANALGESICS

Several drugs, while not thought of as true analgesics in the pharmacological sense, have been demonstrated to relieve pain, either when used alone, or in combination with the standard forms of analgesics. These so-called "co-analgesics" should be considered for the treatment of all types of cancer pain, but are particularly important for pain syndromes relatively unresponsive to morphine alone, and in which certain types of these agents

Table 7-12
Choice of Adjuvant Therapy

Type of Pain	Co-analgesic	Non-drug Measures
Bone pain	Aspirin 600 mg 4 hourly or Ibuprofen 400 mg qid	Irradiation
Raised intracranial pressure	Dexamethasone 2–4 mg tid; Diuretic(?)	Elevate head of bed, avoid lying flat
Post-herpetic neuralgia, superficial dysaesthetic pain	Amitriptyline 25–100 mg; HS L-dopa (?)	
Nerve pressure pain	Prednisolone 5–10 mg tid	Nerve block; irradiation
Intermittent stabbing pain	Valproate 200 mg B-tid or Carbamazepine 200 mg T-qid	
Gastric tenesmoid pain/ bladder tenesmoid pain	Chlorpromazine 10–25 mg 8–4 hourly	
Gastric distenstion pain	Metoclopromide 10 mg 4 hourly	
Muscle spasm pain	Diazepam 5 mg bid or baclofen 10 mg tid	Massage
Lymphedema	Diuretic & corticosteroid(?)	Elevate foot of bed, elastic stocking, compression cuff
Infected malignant ulcer	Metronidazole 400 mg tid or alternate antibiotic	
Activity precipitated pain		Modify way of life (if possible)

appear to produce a clinical benefit when employed. Even if a narcotic analgesic produces a desired level of pain relief when used alone, the addition of a co-analgesic may often result in better pain control with fewer side effects.

The pharmacologic classes of drugs included in most lists of co-analgesics employed in cancer-related pain syndromes include corticosteroids, tricyclic antidepressants, major tranquilizers (Phenothiazines), minor tranquilizers (Benzodiazepines), anticonvulsants (i.e., Phenytoin, Carbamazepine), and miscellaneous agents (Histamine-2 Blockers, aspirin, NSAIDs). Table 7-12 attempts to categorize the specific types of cancer-related pain syndromes with the co-analgesic that has demonstrated some level of benefit when employed. Non-drug measures are presented as well.

The intent of this table is to make health care professionals aware of the use of these additive methods of pain management.

SUMMARY

Every clinician must at some point manage pain associated with malignant disease. Despite its sometimes hopeless prognosis, the problem of pain deserves an intelligent appraisal and a systematic plan for relief to conserve the patient's physical, mental, and moral resources and social usefulness as long as possible. Since the major objective in treating cancer pain is to keep the patient both free of pain and fully alert, the selection of therapy from the array of available options demands study of the individual patient and careful consideration of appropriate measures, potential for success, limitations, benefits, and risks. With comprehensive attention to the physical and personal needs of the patient and family, pain can be managed within a total framework of care. It is, therefore, only the rare cancer patient who will require referral for neurosurgical procedures as the only means of controlling pain.

REFERENCES

1. Abels: Analgesic nephropathy. Clin Pharmacol Ther 12:583–587, 1971
2. Ameer B, Greenblatt DJ: Acetaminophen. Ann Intern Med 87:202–209, 1977
3. Anonymous: Enkephalins: The search for a functional role. Lancet 2:819–820, 1978
4. Anonymous: Aspirin after myocardial infarction. Lancet 1:1172, 1980
5. Anonymous: Ibuprofen (Motrin)—a new drug for arthritis. Med Lett Drugs Ther 16:109–110. 1974
6. Arkinstall WN: Double-blind crossover between sustained release morphine tablets and oral morphine solution in patients with severe pain. The 1984 International Symposium on Pain Control. Toronto, Purdue Frederick Co., 1984, p 9 (Abstract)
7. Beaver WT: Mild analgesics: a review of their clinical pharmacology. Part II. Am J Med Sci 251:576–599, 1966
8. Beaver WT, Wallenstein SL, Houde RW: A clinical comparison of the effects of oral and intramuscular administration of analgesics: Pentazocine and Phenazocine. Clin Pharmacol Ther 9:582–597, 1968
9. Beaver WT, Wallenstein SL, Houde RW: A comparison of the analgesic effects of pentazocine and morphine in patients with cancer. Clin Pharmacol Ther 7:740–751, 1966
10. Bellville JW, Green J: The respiratory and subjective effects of Pentazocine. Clin Pharmacol Ther 6:152, 1965
11. Berdon JK: The effectiveness of D-propoxyphene in the control of pain after periodontal surgery. J Periodont 39:106–111, 1964
12. Black P: Brain metastases: current status and recommended guidelines for management. Neurosurgery 5:617–631, 1979
13. Bonica JJ: Cancer pain: the importance of the problem, in Bonica JJ, Ventafridda V (Eds): Advances in Pain Research and Therapy, Vol. 2. New York, Raven Press, 1979, pp 1–11

14. Bonica JJ: The total management of the patient with chronic pain. Drug Ther 3:33–47, 1973
15. Cady B, Oberfield RA: Regional infusion chemotherapy of hepatic metastases from carcinoma of the colon. Am J Surg 127:220–226, 1974
16. Cass LJ, Fredrich WS: Clinical comparison of the analgesic effects of dextropropoxyphene and other analgesics. Antibiot Med Clin Ther 6:362–370, 1959
17. Catalano RB: Supportive care of the seriously ill cancer patient: Control of pain, in Yarbro JW, Bornstein RS (Eds): Oncologic Emergencies. Orlando FL, Grune and Stratton, 1981, pp 365–393
18. Chafee FH: Aspirin intolerance. I. Frequency in an allergic population. J Allergy Clin Immunol 53:193–199, 1974
19. Chilton NW: Double-blind evaluation of a new analgesic agent in post extraction pain. Am J Med Sci 242:702–706, 1961
20. Citron ML, Johnston-Early A, Fossieck B, et al.: The safety and efficacy of continuous intravenous morphine for severe cancer pain. Am J Med 77:199–204, 1984
21. Coombs DW, Saunders RL, Pageau MG: Continuous intraspinal narcotic analgesia. Technical aspects of an implantable infusion system. Reg Anesth 7:110–113, 1982
22. Cooper SH: Comparative analgesic efficacies of aspirin and acetaminophen. Arch Intern Med 141:282–285, 1981
23. Dawson DM, Fisher EG: Host effects of cancer: pain, in Holland JF, Frei E (Eds): Cancer Medicine (2nd ed.). Philadelphia, Lea & Febiger, 1982, pp 1205–1219
24. Ellison NM, Lewis GO: Plasma concentrations following single doses of morphine sulfate in oral solution and rectal suppository. Clin Pharm 3:614–617, 1984
25. Ensminger W, Neiderhuber J, Dakhel S, et al.: Totally implanted drug delivery system for hepatic arterial chemotherapy. Cancer Treat Rep 65:401–411, 1981
26. Ensworth S: Morphine IV infusion for chronic pain. Drug Intell Clin Pharm 13:297, 1979
27. Ettinger DS, Vitale PH, Trump DL: Important clinical pharmacologic considerations in the use of methadone in cancer patients. Cancer Treat Rep 63:457–459, 1979
28. Ferreira SH: Inflammatory pain, prostaglandin hyperalgesia and the development of peripheral analgesics. Trends Pharmacol Sci 2:183–187, 1981
29. Flower RJ, Moncada S, Vane JR: Analgesic-antipyretic and anti-inflammatory drugs, in Gilman AG, Goodman LS, Dilman A (Eds): Goodman and Gilman's The Pharmacological Basis of Therapeutics (6th ed.). New York, MacMillan 1980, pp 682–728
30. Foley KM: Pain syndromes in patients with cancer, in Bonica JJ, Ventafridda V (Eds): Advances in Pain Research and Therapy, Vol. 2. New York, Raven Press, 1979, pp 59–75
31. Fracchia AA, Farrow JH, Miller TR: Hypophysectomy as compared to adrenalectomy in treatment of advanced breast cancer. Surg Gynecol Obstet 133:241, 1971
32. Fraser DG: Intravenous morphine infusion for chronic pain. Ann Intern Med 93:781–782, 1980
33. Goldberg M, Murray TG: Analgesic-associated nephropathy: an important cause of renal disease in the United States. N Engl J Med 299:716–717, 1978
34. Goldstein A: Opioid peptides (Endorphins) in pituitary and brain. Science 193:1081–1086, 1976
35. Graber CM: The post-partum patients in evaluating analgesic drugs. Clin Pharmacol Ther 2:429–440, 1961
36. Graves DA, Foster TS, Batenhorst RL, et al.: Patient-controlled analgesia. Ann Intern Med 99:360–366, 1983
37. Greenberg HS, Taren J, Ensminger WD, et al.: Benefit from and tolerance to continuous intrathecal infusion of morphine for intractable cancer pain. J Neurosurg 57:360–364, 1982
38. Guillemin R: Endorphins, brain peptides that act like opiates. N Engl J Med 296:226–228, 1977

39. Hanks GW, Trueman T: Controlled-release morphine tablets are effective in twice daily dosage in chronic cancer pain, in Wilkes E (Ed): Advances in morphine therapy. The 1983 International Symposium on Pain Control. London, The Royal Society of Medicine, 1988, p 103

40. Harris WH, Salzman EW, Athanasoulis CA, et al.: Aspirin prophylaxis of venous thromboembolism after total hip replacement. N Engl J Med 297:1246–1249, 1977

41. Harter HR, Burch JW, Majerus PW, et al.: Prevention of thrombosis in patients on hemodialysis by low-dose aspirin. N Engl J Med 301:577–579, 1979

42. Henriksen H, Knudsen J: MST Continuous tablets in pain of advanced cancer: a controlled study, in Wilkes E (Ed): Advances in Morphine Therapy. The 1983 International Symposium on Pain Control. London, The Royal Society of Medicine, 1984, p 123

43. Higg GA: Arachidonic acid metabolism, pain and hyperalgesia: the mode of action of non-steroid mild analgesics. Br J Clin Pharmacol 120 (Suppl 2):2335–2353, 1980

44. Holmes AH: Morphine IV infusion for chronic pain. Drug Intell Clin Pharm 12:556–557, 1978

45. Hopkinson JH: Acetaminophen vs propoxyphene for relief of pain in episiotomy patients. J. Clin Pharm 7:251–263, 1973

46. Horton J, Barter OH, Olsen KB: The management of metastases to brain by irradiation and corticosteroids. Am J Roentgenol Radiat Ther Nucl Med 111:334–336, 1971

47. Houde RW: Pain and the patient with cancer, in Karnofsky DA, Rowson RW (Eds): The Medical Clinics of North America: Symposium on the Medical Aspects of Cancer. Philadelphia, WB Saunders, 1956, pp 687–703

48. Houde RW, Fink BR: Management of pain of advanced cancer: systemic analgesics and related drugs, in Bonica JJ, Ventafridda, V (Eds): Advances in Pain Research and Therapy, Vol. 2. New York, Raven Press, 1979, pp 301–302

49. Houde RW: Systemic analgesics and related drugs: narcotic analgesics, in Bonica JJ, Ventafridda V (eds): Advances in Pain Research and Therapy, Vol. 2. New York, Raven Press, 1979, pp 263–273

50. Houde RW, Wallenstein SL, Beaver WT: Clinical measurement of pain, in deStevens, G (Eds): Analgesics, Orlando FL, Academic Press, 1965, pp 75–122

51. Kaiko RF: Basics of opioid analgesic pharmacodynamics. J Pain Symp Management 1:103–105, 1986

52. Kantor TG: Ibuprofen. Ann Intern Med 91:877–882, 1979

53. Katz SM, Capaldo R, Everts EA, et al.: Tolmetin, association with reversible renal failure and acute interstitial nephritis. JAMA 246:243–245, 1981

54. Koch-Weser J: Acetaminophen. N Engl J Med 295:1297–1301, 1976

55. Kowolenko M: Morphine IV infusion. Drug Intell Clin Pharm 14:296–297, 1980

56. Leavens ME, Hill CS, Cech DA, et al.: Intrathecal and intraventricular morphine for pain in cancer patients: initial study. J Neurosurg 56:241–245, 1982

57. Lewis JR: Misprescribing analgesics. JAMA 228:1155–1156, 1974

58. Loh YP, Loriaux LL: Adrenocorticotropic hormone, B-Lipotropian, and endorphin-related peptides in health and disease. JAMA 247:1033–1034, 1982

59. Marks RM, Sachar EJ: Undertreatment of medical inpatients with narcotic analgesics. Ann Intern Med 78:173–181, 1973

60. Mawsey WH, Fletcher WS, Judkins MP, et al.: Hepatic artery infusion for metastatic malignancy using percutaneous-placed catheters. Am J Surg 121:160–164, 1971

61. McLeod DC: Analgesic nephropathy. N Engl J Med 300:319, 1979

62. Menard PJ: Use of continuous narcotic infusions. Am J Hosp Pharm 39:1459–1460, 1982

63. Mielke CH: Comparative effects of aspirin and acetaminophen on hemostasis. Arch Intern Med 141:305–310, 1981

64. Miser AW, Miser JS, Clark BS: Continuous IV infusion of morphine sulfate for control of severe pain in children with terminal malignancy. J Pediatr 96:930–932, 1980

65. Moertel CG, Ohmann DL, Taylor WF, et al.: A comparative evaluation of marketed analgesic drugs. N Engl J Med 286:813–815, 1972
66. Moertel CG, Ohmann DL, Taylor WF, et al.: Relief of pain by oral medications. JAMA 229:55–59, 1974
67. Moulin DE, Max MB, Kaiko RF, et al.: The analgesic efficacy of intrathecal D-Ala2-D-Leu5-Enkephalin in cancer patients with chronic pain. Pain 23:213–221, 1985
68. Moulin DE, Inturrisi CE, Foley KM: Epidural and intrathecal opioids. CSF and plasma pharmacokinetics in cancer pain patients, in Foley KM, Inturrisi CE (Eds): Advances in Pain Research and Therapy, Vol. 8. New York, Raven Press 1986
69. Moulin DE, Inturrisi CE, Foley KM: Cerebrospinal fluid pharmacokinetics of intrathecal morphine sulfate and D-Ala2-D-Leu5-Enkephalin. Ann Neurol (in press)
70. Mount BM, Ajemian I, Scott JF: Use of the Brompton mixture in treating chronic pain of malignant disease. Can Med Assoc J 115:122–124, 1976
71. Murphy TM: Cancer pain. Postgrad Med 53:187–194, 1973
72. Murphy GP, et al.: Hypophysectomy and adrenalectomy for disseminated prostatic carcinoma. J Urol 105:817–825, 1971
73. Oyama T, Jin T, Yamaya R, et al.: Profound analgesic effects of B-endorphin in man. Lancet 1:122–124, 1980
74. Onofrio BM, Yahsh TL, Arnold PG: Continuous low-dose intrathecal morphine administration in the treatment of chronic pain of malignant origin. Mayo Clin Proc 56:516–520, 1981
75. Papper S, Papper EM: The effects of preanesthetics, anesthetics and post-operative drugs on renal function. Clin Pharmacol Ther 5:205, 1964
76. Parker RG: Pain relief for cancer patients through selective radiation therapy. Northwest Med 69:1022–1025, 1968
77. Perry DJ, Wood PHN: Relationship between aspirin taking and gastrointestinal hemorrhage. Gut 8:301–308, 1967
78. Pert CB, Pasternak GW, Snyder SH: Opiate agonists and antagonists discriminated by receptor binding in brain. Science 182:1359–1361, 1975
79. Plotz PH, Kimberly RP: Acute effects of aspirin and acetaminophen on renal function. Arch Intern Med 141:343–348, 1981
80. Poletti CE, Cohen AM, Todd DP, et al.: Cancer pain relieved by long term epidural morphine with permanent indwelling systems for self-administration. J Neurosurg 55:581–584, 1981
81. Procko LD: Evaluation of D-propoxyphene, Codeine, and Aspirin. Obstet Gynec 16:113–118, 1960
82. Pruss AG: Evaluation of Zomepirac. J Clin Pharmacol 20:215–222, 1980
83. Ramwell PW: Biologic importance of arachidonic acid. Arch Intern Med 141:275–279, 1981
84. Reichenberg S, Pobers F: Severe respiratory depression following Talwin. Am Rev Resp Dis 107:280–282, 1973
85. Richelsen E: Spinal opiate administration for chronic pain: a major advance in therapy. Mayo Clin Proc 56:523, 1981
86. Richlin DM, Brand L: The use of oral analgesics for chronic pain. Hosp Formulary 17:32–41, 1982
87. Robertson CE, Ford KJ, Someran V: Mefenamic acid nephropathy. Lancet 2:232–233, 1980
88. Rogers DG: 21 problems in pain control and ways to solve them. Your Patient and Cancer 65–69 (Sept), 1981
89. Rubin P: Current concept in cancer: metastases and disseminated cancer. V: Bone. Int J Radiat Oncol Biol Phys 1:1199–1200, 1976

90. Rutter PC, Murphy F, Dudley HAF: Morphine: controlled trial of different methods of administration for postoperative pain relief. Br Med J 1:12–13, 1980
91. Saunders CM: The Management of Terminal Illness. London, Edward Arnold, 1967
92. Scott WW: Rationale and results of primary endocrine therapy in patients with prostatic cancer. Cancer 32:1119–1125, 1973
93. Shimm DS, Logue GL, Maltbie AA, et al.: Medical management of chronic cancer pain. JAMA 241:2408–2412, 1979
94. Silverberg E: Cancer statistics, 1982. CA: A Cancer Journal for Clinicians 32:15–31, 1982
95. Smith AP: Response of aspirin-allergic patients to challenge by some analgesics in common use. Br Med J 2:494–496, 1971
96. Smith VT: Anaphylactic shock, acute renal failure and disseminated intra-vascular coagulation, suspected complication of Zomepirac. JAMA 247:1172–1173, 1982
97. Snyder SH: Opiate receptors in the brain. N Engl J Med 296:266–271, 1977
98. Snyder SH, Pert CB, Pasternak GW: The opiate receptor. Ann Intern Med 81:534–540, 1974
99. Taylor F: Aspirin: America's favorite drug. FDA Consumer 14:12, 1980
100. Tong D, Gillick L, Hendrickson FR: The palliation of symptomatic osseous metastases. Cancer 50:893–899, 1982
101. Twycross RG: The Brompton cocktail, in Bonica JJ, Ventafridda V (Eds): Advances in Pain Research and Therapy, Vol. 2. New York, Raven Press, 1979, pp 291–300
102. Twycross RG, Lack SA: Symptom control in far advanced cancer. Pain Relief. London, Pitman Publ Ltd, 1983
103. Vandam LD: Analgetic drugs—the mild analgetics. N Engl J Med 286:249–252, 1972
104. Walsh TD: Controlled study of oral slow-release morphine in pain due to advanced cancer. Proc Am Soc Clin Oncol 4:266, 1985 (abstract)
105. Weinstein EA: The effects of dexamethasone on brain edema in patients with metastatic brain tumors. Neurology 23:121–129, 1973
106. Weiss HJ, Aledorf LM: Impaired platelet/connective tissue reaction in man after aspirin ingestion. Lancet 2:495–497, 1967
107. West AB: Understanding endorphins: our natural pain relief system. Nursing 81(11):50–53, 1981
108. Yaksh TL: Spinal opiate analgesia: characteristics and principles of action. Pain 11:293–346, 1981
109. Young DJ: Propoxyphene suicides. Arch Intern Med 129:62–66, 1972
110. Zimmerman HJ: Effects of aspirin or acetaminophen on the liver. Arch Intern Med 141:333–341, 1981.

Vivian R. Sheidler, M.S., R.N.

8

New Methods in Analgesic Delivery

Pharmacologic management of the cancer patient with severe pain will predictably involve the use of narcotic analgesics. The oral route is usually the preferred choice for administration if the patients find the side effects acceptable and tolerable, and more particularly with narcotics that are readily absorbed from the gastrointestinal (GI) tract. However, GI alterations such as nausea, vomiting, dysphagia, and lack of oral intake as a result of surgery, as well as inadequate relief of pain despite high doses of oral narcotics, may necessitate the initiation of parenteral narcotics. Two newer methods of parenteral narcotic administration for cancer patients with pain are continuous subcutaneous infusions and intravenous patient controlled analgesia.

CONTINUOUS SUBCUTANEOUS INFUSIONS (CSI)

Intermittent subcutaneous and intramuscular administration of narcotics are acceptable methods for providing patients with necessary pain medication. However, repeated injections for days, weeks, and perhaps months can become arduous for patients. A number of factors may make intermittent subcutaneous and intramuscular administration an unrealistic option for pain control including painful injections, fluctuations in narcotic blood levels, decreased muscle mass from atrophy, as well as inadequate nutrition and severe thrombocytopenia.

Narcotic analgesics, similar to insulin, can be administered on a continuous

CANCER PAIN MANAGEMENT
ISBN 0-8089-1868-0

basis into the subcutaneous tissue. After the skin is adequately cleaned, a small gauge butterfly needle is inserted into the subcutaneous tissue. The narcotic of choice is delivered continuously in small volumes using an infusion device with a syringe driver apparatus or a bag-filled ambulatory pump. Table 8-1 is a detailed summary of devices, drugs, needle sizes, location, site change schedules, and durations of the infusion used for CSI.

The same infusion devices that are available for the continuous infusion of chemotherapy are appropriate for CSI of narcotics. The most suitable devices deliver small volumes at low rates and are easy for patients and families to operate. Standard safety features on infusion devices that indicate occlusion, high flow, low battery, low volume, and motor or microprocessor malfunction are recommended as well.

Clinical Experience

The use of continuous narcotic infusions is not new, since the intravenous (IV) route has been used safely in this way since the late 1970s.[14,15,20,24,28,37,52,55,64] In subsequent years, however, published work on this delivery system for narcotics has been quite limited.

Continuous subcutaneous infusions have been studied primarily in patients who required postoperative management of pain and in cancer patients with severe pain. Waldmann et al.[83] compared CSI with continuous intravenous infusions by measuring serum morphine levels for 24 hours in postoperative patients. There were no significant differences in blood levels of morphine or in the need for supplemental morphine doses in patients receiving both routes of administration. Assessment of pain relief through verbal reports was not included in the study measures. Although the investigators concluded that the subcutaneous route was safe and effective, it is significant to note that the patients in the study were receiving mechanical ventilation during the 24-hour study period.

In a more recent randomized, double-blind study of postoperative patients, Goudie et al.[30] compared the efficacy of CSI of morphine to around-the-clock intramuscular morphine. For 48 hours one group of patients received continuous subcutaneous infusion of morphine with around-the-clock placebo injections, and the second group received continuous subcutaneous infusion of a placebo plus around-the-clock morphine injections. There were no differences on pain severity measures, but nausea and sedation were significantly worse in the group receiving morphine intramuscularly ($p < .05$). Two patients in each group were evaluated as having received overdoses, which are a possibility when continued dosing is used. Despite this problem CSI was considered a practical and effective means for achieving pain control.

Although there have been no controlled trials using CSI of narcotics in the cancer patient population, numerous anecdotal reports indicate that the

Table 8-1
Summary of Technical Aspects of Continuous Subcutaneous Infusions

Investigator	Population (No. Patients)	Device	Drug	Needle	Location	Site Change	Duration
Hutchinson et al. (1981)[40]	Cancer (23)	Syringe	Diamorphine & antiemetics	25 g	Abdomen	4–5 days when antiemetics used	?
Dickson & Russell (1982)[21]	Cancer (0)	Syringe	Diamorphine	?	?	≥ 3 weeks	?
Miser et al. (1983)[51]	Cancer (17)	Syringe	Morphine	25–27 g	Deltoid	24–48 hrs.	.25–36 days
Campbell et al. (1983)[10]	Cancer	Syringe	Morphine	27 g	Abdomen	48 hrs.	> 2 mos.
Dickson et al. (1983)[20]	Cancer (100)	Syringe	Diamorphine	?	Abdomen or anterior chest	3 weeks	24 hrs.–5 mos.
Waldmann et al. (1984)[83]	Post-op (9)	Syringe	Morphine	21 g	Deltoid	Not Relevant	24 hrs.

(continued)

Table 8-1

Summary of Technical Aspects of Continuous Subcutaneous Infusions

Investigator	Population (No. Patients)	Device	Drug	Needle	Location	Site Change	Duration
Goudie et al. (1985)[30]	Post-op (48)	Syringe	Morphine	23 g	Anterior chest	Not Relevant	48 hrs.
Coyle et al. (1986)[18]	Cancer (15)	Ambulatory pump	Morphine, levorphanol, hydromorphone, methadone	27 g	Suggest anterior chest & clavicular area	6 hrs.–5 days suggest weekly	3–76 days
Smith & Bulich (1986)[70]	Cancer (40)	Ambulatory pump with PCA mode	Morphine	27 g	Avoid waist or bony prominences, radiation sites; use sites that promote patient comfort & mobility	48 hrs.	24 hrs.–4 mos.
Moss (1986)[53]	Cancer (50)	Syringe	Specifics not stated	25 g	Abdomen	PRN	?
MacDonald et al. (1986)[48]	Cancer	Disposable ambulatory infusor	Morphine and hydromorphone	?	?	8 ± 6 days	× 15 ± 12 days

technique is generally safe and, more importantly, effective for pain control. Dickson et al.,[20] in their experience with approximately 100 patients, reported that pain relief was achieved in nearly all cases with the CSI of diamorphine (heroin). Hutchinson et al.[40] also used diamorphine and achieved analgesia without sedation in 14 of 16 patients, the remaining receiving only partial relief of pain. Campbell et al.[10] published a case report describing the successful transfer of a patient on continuous intravenous morphine drip to CSI at the same drip rate. In a larger, more recent report, 40 patients who used a device providing continuous subcutaneous morphine infusion with a patient-controlled mode achieved relief of pain.[70]

Coyle et al.[18] reported on 15 patients receiving a variety of narcotics. Thirteen patients obtained excellent relief with continuous subcutaneous infusions when this method was initiated. The duration of the infusions was 3 to 76 days. Prior to the institution of the continuous subcutaneous route, the patients had been receiving various combinations of parenteral and oral narcotics. The authors of this report also provided a comprehensive description of the CSI technique, procedures, and guidelines that were used.

MacDonald et al.[48] treated 28 patients with CSI of morphine and hydromorphone using a portable disposable infusion device and concluded that the delivery system was safe and effective for the administration of narcotics. In this study six patients were able to resume oral medications, two patients required volumes greater than the device could deliver, and the remaining 20 patients eventually needed IV administration of narcotics. Twelve of the 28 patients were discharged with the device in use, but no data were available regarding long-term follow-up.

A report of CSI of morphine with a pediatric population demonstrated that 17 cancer patients with severe pain obtained satisfactory relief of pain.[51] In a separate study, 3 of the 17 patients had plasma concentration levels of morphine analyzed when they reached stable levels. All the samples taken at various times showed therapeutic morphine concentrations.[54]

Complications

Since CSI is a relatively new technique, the complications are not completely delineated. The most frequently reported complication from CSI has been local skin irritation at the needle site.[18,40,48] Other reported problems have included an allergic response to the needle in one patient[20] and infections at the needle site in 2 of 40 patients.[70] Additionally, three patients had their needles fall out during an infusion.[40] All the infusions were successfully restarted. Bleeding at the needle site occurred with one patient who was on anticoagulation therapy.[48] To date, no authors have reported any mechanical difficulties with the different devices, nor exacerbation of the usual narcotic side effects.

Limitations

Standard narcotic concentrations may not provide the flexibility required for use of CSI in patients who need large doses of narcotics, since the volume of fluid that can be absorbed from the subcutaneous tissue is limited. Morphine and hydromorphone, however, can be reconstituted to achieve higher mg/ml concentrations than what pharmaceutical companies have commercially available. Problems such as edema, leakage of fluid from the site, as well as inadequate pain relief, may be indications that the volume of fluid is too large to be absorbed. Coyle et al.[18] reported local irritation when volumes greater than 1 cc/hour were used. When a patient's dose is increased, changing the narcotic concentration (e.g., making hydromorphone 50 mg/cc instead of the usual 10 mg/cc or morphine 60 mg/cc instead of the usual 15 mg/cc) can provide smaller volumes that are more readily absorbed.[50,82]

Benefits

Administration of parenteral narcotics using the subcutaneous route appears to be an effective method for controlling pain. The most obvious advantage is patient comfort. The avoidance of repeated injections with subsequent formation of ecchymoses and associated discomfort make the patients much more comfortable as well as less apprehensive.

For patients who have received previous chemotherapy and as a result may have limited venous access, CSI is a tremendous advantage. For patients who do not have indwelling, central catheters that could be used for intravenous administration of narcotics, the alternative of using CSI is very appealing. When patients receive narcotics continuously, the peaks and troughs in blood levels that usually occur with the intermittent administration of narcotics are avoided, resulting in better control of pain.

Home versus Hospital Use of CSI

The use of CSI with oncology patients occurs in a variety of settings. Several reports indicated that patients were started on CSI while they were in the hospital, and some patients were discharged with the system in place.[10,18,48,51] Several investigators initiated the system in an outpatient setting,[53,70] and one group reported that patients were begun on this modality at home.[20] An advantage for home use of this delivery system may be decreased health care costs resulting from home (outpatient) care as opposed to inpatient care.

Several prerequisites must be met for CSI to be initiated in an outpatient or home setting. Patients must be monitored and followed by a nurse and/or responsible physician. Education of the patient and family regarding technical management, potential complications, and side effects is required.

Finally, the patient and family need to know the appropriate people to contact when they have questions or need to report problems.

The most appropriate setting for the initiation of CSI must be determined by the patient's specific circumstances. Family support, financial situation, previous sensitivity to narcotics, current intensity of inadequate pain control, and concomitant medical problems are important considerations.

Implications for Future Research and Practice

CSI is an effective method for controlling pain. However, many questions remain concerning administration techniques and the optimal achievement of pain control. For example, what is the best fluid volume per hour to achieve effective absorption? Is there a difference in absorption depending on the diluent that is used? Are CSIs more effective than continuous intravenous infusions in cancer patients? Is relief of pain affected by infusions containing higher concentrations of narcotics than standard commercial concentrations? How do absorption and relief of pain vary in relation to the anatomical placement of the needle and to perfusion? Controlled clinical trials may provide the answer to these questions and improve the options for control of pain.

In summary, continuous subcutaneous infusions of narcotics provide patients with effective pain relief and minimal complications. Although further research is needed, it is clear that this method can be considered an option for patients who require parenteral narcotic administration.

PATIENT CONTROLLED ANALGESIA (PCA)

The development of PCA (also known as demand analgesia, self-administered analgesia, and patient-controlled analgesic therapy) as a method to provide effective pain control evolved from undertreatment of pain using standard procedures for administration of analgesics. Postoperative patients who requested pain medication often had to wait varying periods of time for their medication if the nurse was busy. Additionally, the patients had to wait for medication if the prescribed dosing interval did not coincide with the onset of their pain. The unrelieved pain often increased in intensity because of these delays.

The medical and nursing literature contain numerous reports of patients receiving inadequate relief of pain with analgesics. The reasons cited include lack of knowledge about pharmacology of analgesics, fear of addiction, fear of respiratory depression, and altered perception of the severity and intensity of patients' pain.[12,17,32,43,49,56,71] The use of PCA eliminates these reasons, which interfere with patients obtaining satisfactory pain relief.

An underlying belief regarding the use of PCA is that the patient is the best judge of the nature and amount of his or her pain, and as a result, knows the best time to take medication. Also inherent in this belief is that patients will only take as much medication as they need to diminish or control their pain. Indeed, PCA studies have clearly documented that individuals who self-administer pain medication receive effective control of pain without a concurrent increase in narcotic side effects.[7,9,46,62,68]

Clinical Experience

In contrast to the work on CSI, which has involved primarily cancer patients, the extensive reports on PCA have dealt primarily with postoperative patients. The earliest description of PCA was in a postoperative population of 20 patients who received morphine or meperidine in a blinded fashion.[66] Patients pressed an analgesic demand button when they experienced pain. The results of this study revealed tremendous variation in the number of times the patients pressed the button (1 to 67 times), and obviously in the amount of drug received.

During the last few years there have been increasing numbers of PCA studies done in the United States, but the majority of investigations have come from Europe, particularly England and Sweden. In addition to postoperative patients, several other groups have been studied, including obstetrical patients in labor and delivery,[25,26,34,61] emergency room patients,[74] and patients with myocardial infarctions.[23] Until recently, the use of PCA with cancer patients has been infrequent.[4,13,16,45] This area is addressed in detail later in the chapter.

Technological Aspects of PCA

The PCA devices that were used in the early 1970s were rather large, making ambulation extremely difficult. Although they were complicated devices, reports of mechanical malfunction were rare.[25,27,44,65]

These initial devices contained some basic features that are available in PCA devices used today. For example, a pre-set volume (the incremental dose) is delivered when the patient presses a button. The rate of infusion is pre-set depending on the volume. An adjustable "lock-out" period, usually in minutes, places safety limits on the amount of time between doses. And finally, mechanisms used to deliver the narcotic prevent retrograde flow into the maintenance line that keeps the IV patent.

The implementation of PCA is variable. The most common method is for patients to push a button when they have pain. This self-activation provides them with the only medicine they will receive. Another method is a verbal prompt from a pre-recorded tape asking the patient if he is in pain. The prompt occurs primarily at the beginning of the postoperative period and can be turned off. The patient can also administer doses between verbal prompts. Hull et al.[39] based this latter form of PCA implementation on the fact that patients may have short-term amnesia in the immediate postoperative period, which may interfere with recall of preoperative instructions and/or any immediate reinforcement. A number of investigators have used this interactive demand method when fentanyl was the narcotic of choice.[38,39,42,63,85] An additional component of this method is that patients receive a continuous intravenous infusion of low-dose fentanyl as well as the demand doses.

Evaluation Studies

Most PCA studies have primarily evaluated the efficacy, safety, and side effects of the delivery system alone or in comparison to other methods of pain relief. Investigators addressing these issues have conducted both controlled and uncontrolled studies.

Controlled Studies

Although PCA has been used for over 18 years, it has only been in the last few years that most prospective randomized trials have been done. Evans et al.[25] were among the first to do a randomized trial of PCA in labor and delivery patients. In addition to demonstrating the safety of PCA, they also found that patients reported significantly better pain relief using PCA when compared with intramuscularly administered pethidine. In another obstetrical study, patients' pain ratings with PCA were better than with IM injections, but there were no statistically significant differences with regard to satisfaction with one method over another.[61] These researchers also found satisfactory infant Apgar scores that did not differ from infants whose mothers received only IM pethidine. Bennett et al.[7] found that morbidly obese postoperative laparotomy patients who used PCA had adequate analgesia without sedation with significantly greater frequency than the conventional IM group. The PCA group also indicated a greater satisfaction with their method of analgesia.

In the only blinded, cross-over design, patients who were receiving PCA had significantly less discomfort than with scheduled IM injections.[9] There were no differences between the two systems in amount of narcotic used, side effects, sedation, and activity level. Welchew[84] found no difference in pain scores in an analgesic study using IM morphine around-the-clock compared to PCA fentanyl. It is significant to note that these two studies compared PCA to around-the-clock analgesia, and conventional postoperative narcotic orders are usually written on *pro re nata* or PRN basis. Other investigators reported similar findings; the PCA groups had significantly less pain and more adequate analgesia.[1,8] One group of researchers also examined nocturnal sleep patterns and found that the PCA group awakened less during the night than the IM group.[8] Finally, Bennett et al.[6] studied the pulmonary function of patients on PCA and reported higher forced vital capacity and peak expiratory flow in gastric bypass patients who used PCA than those using conventional analgesia.

Another area of research dealt with comparing routes of administration. In examining epidural, intercostal block, PCA, and intramuscular routes, Rosenberg et al.[63] indicated that none of the delivery systems had an advantage over the other. Ellis et al.[22] studied intramuscular, sublingual, and PCA methods of administration and reported no difference with respect to pain scores. In fact, since PCA was not better than the other systems, Ellis et al. concluded that the method would not "achieve a role in the routine management of postoperative pain on the grounds of expense . . . failure to achieve superior analgesia, and the necessity to maintain a patent IV infusion cannula" (p 427).

Uncontrolled Studies

There are a number of uncontrolled trials involving PCA. Of the 14 reviewed, 13 showed efficacy, safety of the delivery system, and/or general patient satisfaction with the self-administration method.[4,5,7,13,19,38,39,41,46,47,67,69,79] In the one study that was not supportive of PCA,[2] ketamine was used as the drug of choice. Half of the patients were too drowsy to deliver the dose, and the study was stopped after ten patients had participated. Six of the ten patients reported satisfactory relief of pain; thus, the problem was not the delivery system, but rather a poor choice of drug.

Other researchers have studied the use of self-administered analgesics in non-surgical patients. Stewart et al.[74] used inhalational analgesia (a 50:50 mixture of nitrous oxide and oxygen) in over 1200 patients with acute medical-surgical problems before they were seen in the emergency room, achieving complete relief in 29.1 percent (n = 350) of the patients and partial relief in 61.3 percent (n = 736). There were no significant hemodynamic changes, patients' airways remained patent, and they could follow directions when asked. Minor side effects included nausea, vomiting, dizziness or lightheadedness, excitement, and numbness. Eltringham et al.[23] used PCA in myocardial infarction patients with severe chest pain. Using morphine, 21 of 26 patients obtained complete pain relief and the remaining five patients obtained partial relief. There were no significant side effects, respiratory depression, or excessive self-administration.

In summary, it appears from all the evidence amassed in both controlled and uncontrolled studies that PCA is a safe and efficacious method for administering analgesics to a variety of patient populations. There have been some problems, however, in achieving standard dosing across populations.

Dose Variation

Variation in the amount of narcotic that patients take while using PCA has been frequently reported and/or observed in controlled as well as uncontrolled studies. In the controlled studies, PCA patients used both less

Table 8-2
Most Commonly Used Drugs and Initial Incremental Dosages
and/or Ranges Using Patient Controlled Analgesia

Drug	Initial Incremental Dosage/Range
Meperidine (Pethidine, Demerol)	.2mg/kg/2–30mg
Morphine sulfate	.lmg/kg/ .2–3mg, .3–.mg/m^2, 1–5mg
Fentanyl	7.2–28mcg
Buprenorphine	.09–.2mg
Hydromorphone	.05–.2mg

and more total narcotic than patients on comparison methods. In addition to variation in use, there has been wide variation in selection of drugs and initial incremental dosages (Table 8-2).

Several researchers have proposed explanations for such variation in use. Differences in the particular surgical procedure (i.e., abdominal versus thoracic surgery)[66] and in personality and perception of pain[9] have been suggested as reasons for individual variation in drug consumption. In addition, Keeri-Szanto[46] identified patients as responding not to a pharmacologic need for analgesics but rather to the passage of time. Taking a more scientific approach, Tamsen et al.[76] explained that, in addition to differences in drug distribution and elimination, patients may have differences in sensitivity at the opiate receptor level. The demand for various doses of pethidine may be related to endorphin and substance P levels in the cerebrospinal fluid.[81]

The wide variation in doses of narcotic with PCA has clear implications for patient care. For patients who are receiving conventional intermittent intramuscular dosing, there must be flexibility in the dosing schedule to accommodate such differences. For example, if an analgesic order is written for every four hours and the patient experiences pain at three hours, consideration should be given to decreasing the interval between doses rather than having the patient wait an additional hour. Nurses taking care of patients on PCA must also realize that patients will exhibit wide variation in narcotic dosing, which does not suggest excessive use of drugs but rather indicates individual differences.

Miscellaneous Studies

Another group of studies were conducted with the PCA method to answer other research questions. For example, pharmacokinetic studies examining ketobemidone and pethidine were done using the PCA technique.[35,75,77,78,80] Efficacy studies examining two different drugs or examining two different dose levels of one drug were carried out using PCA.[11,29,33,68] In a totally different design, Graves et al.[31] examined the influence of diurnal variation in narcotic use with morbidly obese patients and found a significant difference in narcotic dosing rates for day and night periods. The peak narcotic use was at 9:00AM and the lowest was at 3:00AM.

Application of PCA to Oncology Patients

Prior to 1986 PCA has been studied and used infrequently with cancer patients, as mentioned earlier. One may assume that a portion of the postoperative patients in other studies had oncologic diagnoses, but they are rarely identified separately.[41] The earliest report describing the use of PCA in cancer patients was from Keeri-Szanto,[45] who presented three case reports of patients with advanced cancer and severe pain. Their standard (pre-PCA) and demand (PCA) dosages of narcotic are shown in Table 8-3. In each case, the lower dosages for all three patients provided satisfactory pain relief without undue side effects or problems.

More recently, several investigators have reported on the use of PCA in cancer patients. Citron et al.[16] reported adequate pain relief in 12 patients who underwent 14 PCA trials lasting an average of 11 days using intravenous and subcutaneous PCA. In addition to reporting that the use of PCA was safe and effective, they also indicated that outpatient treatment is a reasonable option. Patients' mental status and respiratory rates remained near baseline for all PCA trials. Baumann et al.[4] studied PCA with eight patients who had responded poorly to oral narcotics. Using a minimum time period of 48 hours, they found that the system was safe and effective. They used the PCA narcotic requirements to convert three of the eight patients to oral regimens. In another study, Citron et al.[13] used PCA for 21 to 40 hours in 8 patients who had severe pain. They found that patients required more PCA doses during the first four hours of using the system than at any other time period. However, they reported no significant respiratory depression and sedation during the first four hours or at any other time period during the study.

Using PCA for patients experiencing severe acute pain related to toxicities from bone marrow transplantation, Hill et al.[36] reported that patients who remained on PCA until their pain disappeared were satisfied with this method of analgesic delivery. In this non-randomized pilot study,

Table 8-3

Standard (pre-PCA) and Demand (PCA) Narcotic Dosages for Three Cancer Patients[45]

Case No.	Pre-PCA Analgesia	PCA Analgesia
1.	Parenteral morphine 75 mg/day	Morphine 50, then 30 mg/day
2.	Parenteral meperidine 400 mg/day	Morphine 20 mg/day
3.	Parenteral meperidine 700 mg/day	Meperidine 100 mg/day

patients remained on PCA an average of 12 days (range 3–32). Sedation and respiratory depression were not significant problems, demonstrating that PCA is a safe alternative to continuous intravenous infusions for this patient population.

Keeri-Szanto[45] identified several benefits of using demand analgesia in the cancer population. Nutritional status of patients improved because of the relief of pain. Psychological state improved because less energy was wasted on the anticipation and experience of pain. And finally, there was an improved general well-being because the peaks and troughs in blood levels of narcotics were avoided.

Despite these observed benefits of PCA for the medical oncology population, its use has been rather limited for several reasons. Patient controlled analgesia was originally intended for the surgical population with acute pain of short duration. Frequent dosing occurs during the first 24 hours postoperatively, and then the frequency decreases as the recovery period progresses. In contrast, pain usually does not decrease with the passage of time in the cancer patient who requires parenteral administration of narcotics. Frequent dosing over time is inconvenient and impractical.

An optional mode on several PCA devices allows patients to receive a continuous intravenous infusion with intermittent PCA doses.[58,60] This method maintains constant blood levels in patients and provides them with a self-dosing mechanism for periods of severe pain.

The infusion devices that are currently available were designed with the postoperative patient as the target population. The design of these machines precludes flexibility in adjusting the infusion rates. Although one device can be programmed so that the patient receives narcotic for one hour immediately after the PCA dose (called a tail dose),[59] the standard narcotic doses will still be infused in several minutes or less. The doses of narcotics for cancer patients are often much higher than standard postoperative doses because of tolerance to narcotics and progressive disease. The administration of 50 mg of morphine over one minute using PCA, for example, predisposes the patient to a very large peak effect, and can potentially cause hypotension, excessive sedation, nausea, and respiratory depression. If the infusion rate were adjustable so that the same amount of drug could be delivered as a 10 to 15 minute infusion, perhaps the side effects could be avoided.

Another role for PCA in the oncology patient with pain would be the titration of narcotics to improve control of pain. If the patient received parenteral narcotics using PCA, a quick determination of total narcotic requirement and appropriate dosing interval could be made. Such information then could be used when converting a patient to an oral regimen of narcotics.

Surgical oncology patients comprise a subset of the larger surgical population in which most of the PCA work has been done. Providing patients control over their analgesic administration may help allay fear about pain, particularly with patients who are facing a new cancer diagnosis or patients who have had previous surgery with the routine PRN administration. A critical component for using PCA with the surgical population is adequate preoperative teaching. Knowledge regarding aspects of the administration procedure should be presented as early as possible.

Patient controlled analgesia can also be considered an alternative for procedure-related, acute pain if the use of parenteral narcotics was considered. For example, if patients require analgesics for bone marrow aspirates, biopsies, and lumbar punctures, and a patent IV already is in place, then perhaps PCA could be used.

Although PCA does appear to have a role in the management of pain related to cancer, certainly not all patients who have pain should be offered PCA. Factors to consider in the decision would include the patient's mental status; adequate renal, hepatic, and respiratory functions; demonstrated understanding of the procedures; and a desire to use the method.

Complications

Complications in patients using PCA are rare. Tamsen et al.[79] reported two cases of respiratory depression, but they were attributed to hypovolemia and were not narcotic induced. Gibbs et al.[29] also reported two patients who had respiratory depression as evidenced by an increase in carbon dioxide retention, but their respiratory rates did not fall below 14. In fact, one of the patients had inadvertently received a dose of narcotic from the staff instead of with PCA, so the additional dose may have contributed to the problem. The second patient took five doses in five hours, the long-acting nature of the drug (buprenorphine) probably contributed to the respiratory difficulty.

The PCA system may be problematic for some people. Sprigge et al.[72] reported that all of the 18 patients in their study needed help to self-administer the initial PCA dose. Even after four hours, three patients still lacked the necessary coordination to self-administer the medication.

Tamsen et al.,[79] concerned about a lack of reported information on problems and side effects (particularly late ones), reported common side effects such as dry mouth, nausea, and drowsiness. They also described "late respiratory complications" such as tachycardia, fever, pneumonia, and atelectasis. It is likely that none of the common or late side effects were related to use of PCA.

Limitations

A major consideration for using PCA in a clinical setting is cost for the institution. The available PCA devices cost several thousand dollars, so a sizable initial investment is required if a program is to be instituted.

Eventually, however, insurance reimbursement from each patient's use and time-saving benefits with nursing personnel may make the system cost-effective.

A more obvious limitation is that a patient using PCA requires venous access. However, if postoperative patients in particular require parenteral administration of narcotics, they most likely will have an IV in place for either fluids or antibiotics.

Benefits

Patients can effectively titrate their relief of pain if they can control administration of their own narcotics. PCA research documents the tremendous variation among patients' needs, thus this method successfully accommodates such differences. As mentioned earlier, drug abuse occurs rarely with this system.

One of the most important benefits of PCA is that patients do not have to wait to receive their pain medication. Even in the most well-staffed, highly efficient nursing units, there is always a "normal" delay because the nurse must find the narcotic keys, sign out the drug, prepare the medication, and then administer it to the patient. PCA avoids these steps and allows patients to maintain pain at a level they choose.

A more subtle advantage is that patients using PCA can control a very important aspect of their care. The loss of control a person encounters when entering a health care setting can be a most distressing problem for some people. The knowledge that they can exert control over their own comfort may be a contributing factor to the amount of narcotic patients require. A dramatic example of this was demonstrated in a postoperative study.[46] Thirty percent of patients who had satisfactory pain control with PCA were much less comfortable when they subsequently received conventional intramuscular administration of narcotics. In fact, some patients required more drug and were less comfortable.

Home versus Hospital Use of PCA

The most appropriate setting for using PCA needs to be evaluated on an individual patient basis. The currently available devices allow for both home and hospital use. Three of the currently available PCA devices are similar in size to most of the hospital based infusion devices.[57-59] There is also an ambulatory pump that can be used as a continuous infusion with or without PCA, or it can be used strictly as a PCA pump.[60] This pump can be used in inpatient and outpatient settings.

The goal for cancer patients with severe pain who require analgesics is to render them as pain-free as possible. A common guideline for narcotic administration is around-the-clock dosing to prevent pain from returning.

Since PCA is based on PRN administration, is the delivery system appropriate for cancer patients? One report of long-term home administration with PCA alone did not indicate dosing frequency or intervals, but did report adequate pain relief for patients who had received PCA from 1 to 40 days.[16] Using PCA in conjunction with continuous IV infusion for home use has been reported.[73] The administration of extra doses of narcotic by the patient and family in this manner rather than other parenteral routes would be efficient and relatively simple.

Implications for Future Research and Practice

The efficacy of PCA in the postoperative population has been demonstrated, while the utilization and efficacy of PCA in the oncology patient is in its infancy. There is clearly a role for PCA in the surgical oncology patient. There is also a role for PCA in the medical oncology patient who requires parenteral narcotics for relief of pain. A major problem is the current design of the available devices. Research is required to demonstrate whether current devices are suitable for the oncology patient. It may be that adjusting delivery rates uniformly makes a difference.

Cost analysis studies need to be done to determine if the initial investment of equipment, education of nursing and pharmacy personnel, and evaluation of patient outcomes are cost-effective when compared to standard analgesic administration.[3] If the costs are not at least equal to that of usual parenteral narcotic delivery, then the benefit of improved pain control would have to be compared to increased costs.

Different analgesics need to be studied as well. For example, can long-acting narcotics like methadone hydrochloride and levorphanol tartrate be studied with cancer patients if the reason for using PCA is to titrate amounts of narcotic so that an appropriate oral dose can be prescribed? In summary, randomized, controlled trials need to be conducted to document the effectiveness of this system with the medical oncology population.

SUMMARY

Continuous subcutaneous infusions and intravenous patient-controlled analgesia are two relatively new methods for delivering analgesics to cancer patients. Each system has unique benefits and limitations, and each affords medical and nursing staff additional flexibility and alternatives in providing analgesics to cancer patients. These procedures can be implemented in major cancer centers as well as in community hospitals. Future research is needed to identify the optimal and most efficient way to deliver narcotics using these methods, thus rendering them more useful and available to the general oncology population.

REFERENCES

1. Atwell JR, Flanigan RC, Bennett RL, et al.: The efficacy of patient-controlled analgesia in patients recovering from flank incisions. J Urol 132:701–703, 1984
2. Austin TR: Ketamine on demand for postoperative analgesia. Anaesthesia 36:214, 1981
3. Barbarash RA, Wellman GS: Considerations in the cost analysis of patient controlled analgesia. Postgrad Med (A Special Report) 47–50, August 28, 1986
4. Baumann TJ, Batenhorst RL, Graves DA, et al.: Patient-controlled analgesia in the terminally ill cancer patient. Drug Intell Clin Pharm 20:297–301, 1986
5. Bennett RL, Batenhorst RL, Bivins BA, et al.: Patient controlled analgesia. A new concept of postoperative pain relief. Ann Surg 195:700–705, 1982
6. Bennett R, Batenhorst RL, Foster TS, et al.: Postoperative pulmonary function with patient controlled analgesia. Anesth Analg 61:171, 1982
7. Bennett R, Batenhorst R, Graves D, et al.: Morphine titration in postoperative laparotomy patients using patient controlled analgesia. Curr Ther Res 32:45–52, 1982
8. Bennett RL, Griffen WO: Effect of patient controlled analgesia on nocturnal sleep and spontaneous activity following laparotomy. Anesthesiology 61:A205, 1984
9. Bollish SJ, Collins CL, Kirking DM, et al.: Efficacy of patient-controlled versus conventional analgesia for post-operative pain. Clin Pharm 4:48–52, 1985
10. Campbell CF, Mason JB, Weiler JM: Continuous subcutaneous infusion of morphine for the pain of terminal malignancy. Ann Intern Med 98:51–52, 1983
11. Chakravarty K, Tucker W, Rosen M, et al.: Comparison of buprenorphine and pethidine given intravenously on demand to relieve postoperative pain. Br Med J 2:895–897, 1979
12. Charap AD: The knowledge, attitudes, and experience of medical personnel treating pain in the terminally ill. Mt Sinai J Med 45:561–580, 1979
13. Citron ML, Johnson-Early A, Boyer M, et al.: Patient-controlled analgesia for severe cancer pain. Arch Intern Med 146:734–736, 1986
14. Citron ML, Johnston-Early A, Fossieck BE, et al.: The safety of continuous intravenous morphine (CIVM) for intractable cancer pain or dyspnea. Proc Am Soc Clin Oncol 2:C353, 1983 (Abstr)
15. Citron ML, Johnston-Early A, Fossieck BE, et al.: Safety and efficacy of continuous intravenous morphine for severe cancer pain. Am J Med 77:199–204, 1984
16. Citron M, Walczak M, Seltzer V, et al.: The safety and efficacy of patient-controlled analgesia (PCA) for severe cancer pain: a long term study of inpatient and outpatient use. Proc Am Soc Clin Oncol 5:260, 1986 (Abstr)
17. Cohen FL: Postsurgical pain relief: patients' status and nurses' medication choices. Pain 9:265–274, 1980
18. Coyle N, Mauskop A, Maggard J, et al.: Continuous subcutaneous infusions of opiates in cancer patients with pain. Oncol Nurs Forum 13:53–57, 1986
19. Dahlstrom B, Tamsen A, Paalzow L, et al.: Patient controlled analgesic therapy. IV. Pharmacokinetics and analgesic plasma concentrations of morphine. Clin Pharmacokinet 7:266–279, 1982
20. Dickson RJ, Howard B, Campbell J: The relief of pain by subcutaneous infusion of diamorphine, in Wilkes E (Ed): Advances in Morphine Therapy, The 1983 International Symposium on Pain Control, Royal Society of Medicine International Congress and Symposium Series #64. London, Royal Society of Medicine, 1983, pp 107–110
21. Dickson RJ, Russell PSB: Continuous subcutaneous analgesics for terminal care at home. Lancet 1(8264):165, 1982 (Letter)
22. Ellis R, Haines D, Shah R, et al.: Pain relief after abdominal surgery—a comparison of IM morphine, sublingual buprenorphine, and self-administered pethidine. Br J Anaesthesia 54:421–428, 1982

23. Eltringham RJ, Jones MBS, Burlingham AN, et al.: Patient controlled analgesia following myocardial infarction. Int Care Med 9:142–143, 1983
24. Ensworth S: Morphine IV infusion for chronic pain. Drug Intell Clin Pharm 13:297, 1979
25. Evans JM, David H, Rosen M, et al.: Patient activated intravenous narcotic. Anaesthesia 31:847–848, 1976
26. Evans JM, McCarthy J, Rosen M, et al.: Apparatus for patient-controlled administration of intravenous narcotics during labour. Lancet 1:17–18, 1976
27. Forrest WH Jr, Smethurst PWR, Kienitz ME: Self administration of intravenous analgesics. Anesthesiology 33:363–365, 1970
28. Fraser DG: Intravenous morphine infusion for chronic pain. Ann Intern Med 93:781–782, 1980
29. Gibbs JM, Johnson HD, Davis FM: Patient administration of IV buprenorphine for postoperative pain relief using the "Cardiff" demand analgesia apparatus. Br J Anaesth 54:279–284, 1982
30. Goudie TA, Allan MWB, Lonsdale M, et al.: Continuous subcutaneous infusion of morphine for postoperative pain relief. Anaesthesia 40:1086–1092, 1985
31. Graves DA, Batenhorst RL, Bennett RL, et al.: Morphine requirements using patient controlled analgesia: influence of diurnal variation and morbid obesity. Clin Pharm 2:49–53, 1983
32. Grossman SA, Sheidler VR: Skills of medical students and house officers in prescribing narcotic medications. J Med Ed 60:552–557, 1985
33. Harmer M, Slattery PJ, Rosen M, et al.: Comparison between buprenorphine and pentazocine given IV on demand in the control of postoperative pain. Br J Anaesth 55:21–25, 1983
34. Harper NJN, Thomson J, Brayshaw SA: Experience with self-administered pethidine with special reference to the general practitioner obstetric unit. Anaesthesia 38:52–55, 1983
35. Hartvig P, Tamsen A, Fagerlund C, et al.: Pharmacokinetics of pethidine during anaesthesia and patient controlled analgesic therapy. Acta Anaesth Scand Suppl 74:52–54, 1982
36. Hill HF, Saeger LC, Chapman CR: Patient controlled analgesia after bone marrow transplantation for cancer. Postgrad Med (A Special Report) 33–40, August 28, 1986
37. Holmes AH Jr: Morphine IV infusion for chronic pain. Drug Intell Clin Pharmacol 12:556–557, 1978
38. Hull CJ, Sibbald A: Control of postoperative pain by interactive demand analgesia. Br J Anaesth 53:385–391, 1981
39. Hull CJ, Sibbald A, Johnson MK: Demand analgesia for postoperative pain. Br J Anaesth 51:570P–571P, 1979
40. Hutchinson HT, Leedham GD, Knight AM: Continuous subcutaneous analgesics and antiemetics in domicilliary terminal care. Lancet 1(8258),1279, 1981 (Letter)
41. Kane N, Lehman M, Dugger R: Use of patient controlled analgesia (PCA) in the rehabilitation of the post operative cancer patient. Oncol Nurs Forum Suppl 13:124, 1986 (Abstr)
42. Kay B: Postoperative pain relief. Anaesthesia 36:949–951, 1981
43. Keats AS: Postoperative pain: research and treatment. J Chronic Dis 4:72–83, 1956
44. Keeri-Szanto, M: Apparatus for demand analgesia. Can Anaesth Soc J 18:581–582, 1971
45. Keeri-Szanto M: Demand analgesia for the relief of pain problems in "terminal" illness. Anesth Rev 19–21, 1976
46. Keeri-Szanto M: Drugs or drums: what relieves postoperative pain? Pain 6:217–230, 1979
47. Keeri-Szanto M, Heaman S: Postoperative demand analgesia. Surg Gynecol Obstet 134:647–651, 1972
48. MacDonald N, Bruera E, Chadwick S, et al.: Treatment of cancer pain with a portable disposal device. Proc Am Soc Clin Oncol 5:252, 1986 (Abstr)

49. Marks RM, Sachar EJ: Undertreatment of medical inpatients with narcotic analgesics. Ann Intern Med 78:173–181, 1973
50. The Merck Index (9th ed.). Rahway, New Jersey, Merck and Company, Inc, 1976
51. Miser AW, Davis DM, Hughes CS, et al.: Continuous subcutaneous infusion of morphine in children with cancer. Am J Dis Child 137:383–385, 1983
52. Miser AW, Miser JS, Clark BS: Continuous intravenous infusion of morphine sulfate for control of severe pain in children with terminal malignancy. J Pediatr 96:930–932, 1980
53. Moss H: Subcutaneous continuous infusion narcotics at home. Oncol Nurs Forum Suppl 13:128, 1986 (Abstr)
54. Nahata MC, Miser AW, Miser JS, et al.: Analgesic plasma concentrations of morphine in children with terminal malignancy receiving a continuous subcutaneous infusion of morphine sulfate to control severe pain. Pain 18:109–114, 1984
55. Portenoy RK: Continuous intravenous infusions of narcotics, in Management of Cancer Pain, Syllabus of the Post Graduate Course, Memorial Sloan-Kettering Cancer Center. New York, November 14–16, 1985, pp 205–214
56. Porter J, Jick H: Addiction rare in patients treated with narcotics. N Engl J Med 302:123, 1980
57. Product Information, Abbott Life Care PCA Infuser, Abbott Laboratories, Hospital Products Division, North Chicago, IL 60064
58. Product Information, Operations Manual, Harvard PCA™ Pump, Bard Electro Medical Systems Division of C.R. Bard, Inc., Englewood, CO 80112
59. Product Information, Operator's Manual, Prominject^R Programmable Infusion Pump, Pharmacia, Inc., Piscataway, NJ 08854
60. Product Information, Technical Manual, CADD-PCA TM Computerized Ambulatory Drug Delivery, Deltec Inc., Pharmacia, Inc., Piscataway, NJ 08854
61. Robinson JO, Rosen M, Evans JM, et al.: Self-administered intravenous and intramuscular pethidine. Anaesthesia 35:763–770, 1980
62. Rosen M: Patient controlled analgesia. Br Med J 289:640–641, 1984
63. Rosenberg PH, Heino A, Scheinin B: Comparison of intramuscular analgesia, intercostal block, epidural morphine, and on-demand IV fentanyl in the control of pain after abdominal surgery. Acta Anaesth Scand 28:603–607, 1984
64. Rutter PC, Murphy F, Dudley HAF: Morphine: controlled trial of different methods of administration for postoperative pain relief. Br Med J 1:12–13, 1980
65. Scott, JS: Obstetric analgesia. Am J Obstet Gynecol 106:959–978, 1970
66. Sechzer PH: Objective measurement of pain. Anesthesiology 29:209–210, 1968
67. Sechzer PH: Studies in pain with the analgesic demand system. Anesth Analg 50:1–10, 1971
68. Slattery PJ, Harmer M, Rosen M, et al.: Comparison of meptazinol and pethidine given IV on demand in the management of postoperative pain. Br J Anaesth 53:927–930, 1981
69. Slattery PJ, Harmer M, Rosen M, et al.: An open comparison between routine and self-administered postoperative pain relief. Ann Royal College Surg Eng 65:18–19, 1983
70. Smith JM, Bulich R: Continuous subcutaneous infusion morphine sulfate: a report of 40 patients. Oncol Nurs Forum Suppl 13:87, 1986 (Abstr)
71. Somerville MA: Inadequate treatment of pain in hospitalized patients. N Engl J Med 307:55, 1982 (Letter)
72. Sprigge JS, Otton PE: Nalbuphine versus meperidine for post operative analgesia: a double blind comparison using the patient controlled analgesic technique. Can Anaesth Soc J 30:517–521, 1983
73. Stephens SH: Continuous infusion morphine sulfate in the home: a nursing challenge. Oncol Nurs Forum Suppl 13:98, 1986 (Abstr)
74. Stewart RD, Paris PM, Stoy WA, et al.: Patient controlled inhalational analgesia in pre-hospital care: a study of side effects and feasibility. Crit Care Med 11:851–855, 1983

75. Tamsen A, Bondesson U, Dahlstrom B, et al.: Patient-controlled analgesic therapy, Pharmacokinetics and analgesic plasma concentrations of ketobemidone. III. Clin Pharmacokinet 7:252–265, 1982
76. Tamsen A, Hartvig P, Dahlstrom W, et al.: Endorphins and on-demand pain relief. Lancet 1:769–770, 1980
77. Tamsen A, Hartvig P, Fagerlund C, et al.: Patient controlled analgesic therapy, Pharmacokinetics of pethidine in the pre and postoperative periods. I. Clin Pharmacokinet 7:149–163, 1982
78. Tamsen A, Hartvig P, Dahlstrom B, et al.: Patient controlled analgesic therapy in the early postoperative period. Acta Anaesth Scand 23:462–470, 1979
79. Tamsen A, Hartvig P, Fagerlund C, et al.: Patient controlled analgesic therapy: clinical experience. Acta Anaesth Scand Suppl 74:157–160, 1982
80. Tamsen A, Hartvig P, Fagerlund C, et al.: Patient-controlled analgesic therapy, Individual analgesic demand and analgesic plasma concentrations of pethidine in postoperative pain. II. Clin Pharmacokinet 7:164–175, 1982
81. Tamsen A, Sakurda T, Wahlstrom A, et al.: Postoperative demand for analgesics in relation to individual levels of endorphins and substance P in cerebrospinal fluid. Pain 13:171–183, 1982
82. The United States Pharmacopeia, 21st Rev, The United States Pharmacopeial Convention. Rockville, MD, 1984
83. Waldmann CS, Eason JR, Rambohul E, et al.: Serum morphine levels: a comparison between continuous subcutaneous infusion and continuous intravenous infusion in postoperative patients. Anaesthesia 39:768–771, 1984
84. Welchew EA: On demand analgesia. A double-blind comparison of on-demand intravenous fentanyl with regular intramuscular morphine. Anesthesia 38:19–25, 1983
85. White WD, Pearce DJ, Norman J: Postoperative analgesia: a comparison of intravenous on-demand fentanyl with epidural bupivacaine. Br Med J 2:166–167, 1979

Benjamin S. Carson, M.D.

9

Neurologic and Neurosurgical
Approaches to Cancer Pain

PHILOSOPHICAL ISSUES

Fear, pain, suffering, and death are frequent companions of cancer, and each must be dealt with specifically in order to provide comprehensive treatment of the cancer patient. This chapter discusses the physical pain associated with cancer. Many other aspects of cancer are affected by physical pain—fear, for example, may frequently result more from anticipation of pain than anticipation of death.

The treatment of the pain associated with cancer is nothing new to medical practitioners, and a large number of medical therapeutic interventions are available. These include both non-narcotic and narcotic analgesics as well as steroids, mood altering drugs, Calcitonin, and drugs aimed at hormonal manipulation. The vast majority of cancer pain can be controlled through either oral or injectable forms of these drugs. Unfortunately, this first line of therapy does fail in a minority of cases, which can be frustrating both to the medical practitioner and the patient. Fortunately in some of the failed cases, the pain can be treated with some of the newer medical modalities such as epidural, intrathecal, and intraventricular narcotics, which are discussed later in this chapter. Additionally, in the resistant cases, pain can sometimes be controlled by a direct attack upon the malignancy causing the pain. This can be accomplished with radiation therapy, chemotherapy, or direct surgical attack upon the lesion.

In a very small minority of cases, none of the above are effective,

CANCER PAIN MANAGEMENT
ISBN 0-8089-1868-0

usually due to significant local compromise of neurovascular structures, and it is this group of patients that would be appropriately considered for neurosurgical intervention.

The various neurosurgical therapeutic interventions for the control of cancer pain must be carefully matched to the patients to be treated. In addition to having failed the more conservative first lines of therapy, they must be physically strong enough to withstand the procedure or associated anesthesia. Additionally, a patient whose life expectancy is only three or four weeks should not be subjected to a procedure whose recuperative period is two or three weeks.

There are also psychological reasons why some patients should not be considered as neurosurgical candidates. Patients with a history of narcotic abuse tend to respond poorly to pain-relieving surgery. This may be as much associated with alterations in neurotransmitter levels in the brain as it is with a primary personality defect. Certainly a cancer patient with a relatively short life expectancy who can be controlled medically would not be a strong candidate for an interventional procedure that entails risks and would potentially result in some degree of neurological deficit. In addition, patients with a history of drug abuse or those with certain personality traits associated with chronic pain behavior may be inappropriate candidates for surgical management of pain.[2] Basically, if a cancer patient is not a drug abuser and has failed all conservative medical attempts at pain control, is physically able to withstand a surgical procedure, and is willing to risk further impairment of neurological function, he should be referred for neurosurgical evaluation for a pain-alleviating procedure.

There are a large number of interventional procedures that may ameliorate cancer pain, and it is essential that the physician be familiar with the various techniques available. Since many initial attempts at control of cancer pain are unsuccessful, the physician must be committed to the idea of pain control and persistent in attempting interventional procedures. Some institutions are fortunate enough to have more than one person specializing in pain control techniques, thus providing opportunities for collaboration, since decisions about which techniques to use can sometimes be difficult.

The ability to communicate with the patient and family is almost as important as being able to perform the various pain-relieving procedures. It is important to convey the risks and benefits of interventional procedures to the patient and family so that they might make intelligent decisions about how to proceed. No one undergoing a potentially destructive process for the purpose of pain alleviation should be allowed to do so without a thorough understanding of the risks and potential complications as well as the potential benefits of the procedure. The short life expectancy in many cancer patients, however, can be a mitigating factor in deciding to perform a relatively dangerous and irreversible procedure, since failure of the procedure or significant impairment as a result of the procedure is not likely to be a long-term consequence.[9]

Finally, the amount of suffering endured by the patient and also by his family and/or friends is immense. In dealing with the problem of cancer pain, the health professional must be willing to invest time in the psychological well-being of the patient and family. Neurological and neurosurgical procedures should not be entered into lightly nor performed by individuals who are unwilling or unable to invest an appropriate amount of time in the patient's welfare.

NEUROSURGICAL PROCEDURES

Surgical Anatomy

There are a large number of places where interruption of pain-conducting pathways can be accomplished. Non-myelinated free nerve endings comprise the most distal aspect of the pain-conducting pathway. These are found throughout the entire body, but are most heavily distributed in areas where excessive noxious influences might produce harm to the body, such as skin surfaces, corneal surfaces, and periosteum. Impulses travel from these nerve endings through the peripheral nerve and subsequently through the dorsal root ganglion and into the spinal cord substance on the ipsilateral side of the body. After making several connections in the dorsal horn of the spinal cord on the ipsilateral side, most of the pain fibers cross the midline and enter the lateral spino-thalamic tract on the antero-lateral aspect of the contralateral spinal cord. They then ascend in this tract to the level of the lower medulla, where they begin to merge as they travel more cephalad with the medial lemniscus. These fibers continue along the dorso-lateral aspect of the medial lemniscus until they reach the thalamus, where again multiple connections are made. The final leg of the journey commences with offshoots to the appropriate parts of the post-central gyrus of the cerebral cortex. A simplified schematic diagram of the pain pathway can be seen in Figure 9-1. All the subsequent discussions of techniques used for alleviating pain will be directed at some portion of this pathway.

Peripheral Neurotomy

Perhaps the least sophisticated method of neurosurgical ablation of pain involves the peripheral sectioning, avulsion, freezing, coagulation, or chemical destruction of a peripheral nerve. There is a consequence of neurotomy, of course, in that those sensory modalities subserved by the destroyed nerve will be lost to the patient. In the extremities it is common for both the motor and sensory fibers to run together in a single nerve, thus sectioning of such

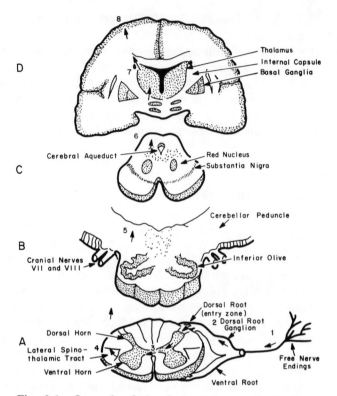

Fig. 9-1. In each of the four segments of this figure, important anatomical landmarks are illustrated. (A) Afferent pain pathway from the level of peripheral nerve endings to the contralateral lateral spinothalamic tract. (B) Continuation of ascending pain pathway in the lower brainstem. (C) Continuation of pain pathway in upper brainstem. (D) Continuation of pain pathway at and above the diencephalic level. In all four segments the short non-captioned arrows represent the afferent pain flow. Also, numbers are placed adjacent to portions of the pain pathway amenable to surgical intervention for pain relief as follows: 1—peripheral neurotomy, 2—rhizotomy, 3—myelotomy, 4—cordotomy, 5—medullary tractotomy, 6—mesencephalic tractotomy and deep brain stimulation, 7—thalamotomy, 8—gyrectomy.

nerves clearly produces not only sensory disturbances but motor deficits as well. For this reason, neurotomy is generally not recommended in extremities where useful function still exists. Even if sensory denervation is achieved and motor function left intact, the extremity could still be rendered useless, since the sensory information necessary to coordinate meaningful movement of the extremity might be lost. On the other hand, if the extremity is already useless from a functional standpoint, sectioning of major nerves can provide tremendous relief of pain to the patient.

A common setting for peripheral neurotomy is in the case of chest wall pain secondary to either breast or lung cancer. By doing a series of intercostal nerve blocks prior to destroying the nerve, it is possible to specifically delineate the area that should be denervated. The most reliable and safest method of proceeding with such denervation is actual intra-operative identification of the individual nerves and sectioning under direct vision. This technique frequently requires general anesthesia, but in those patients who cannot undergo major anesthesia, it is possible to perform a neurotomy with an electrical probe (thermocoagulation) or with a chemical such as phenol or alcohol.[34] Pain caused by head and neck cancer also lends itself well to control using these types of peripheral interventions.

It is wise whenever possible to perform nerve blocks with temporary anesthetic agents prior to actual neurotomy, since this gives the patient an opportunity to experience the sensory deficits on a temporary basis and determine whether such deficits would be tolerable. In equivocal cases, the nerve blocks should be repeated as many times as necessary to clarify the situation to the satisfaction of all parties. There is a phenomenon known as anesthesia dolorosa that can result from neurotomy, and consists of severe anesthesia, which the patient perceives as intolerable. Affected individuals will frequently state that they would prefer to have the original pain rather than suffer from the lack of feeling. In some cases of anesthesia dolorosa, despite an area of demonstrable anesthesia, some patients continue to feel pain, which is similar to a phantom limb type of phenomenon. Fortunately anesthesia dolorosa occurs in only approximately 10 percent or less of patients undergoing neurotomy. It seems particularly prevalent in cases of long-standing facial pain after neuroablative procedures are attempted. There is no effective treatment for anesthesia dolorosa, although some investigators working with deep brain stimulation have some promising results.

Finally, when considering a person as a candidate for a neurotomy, it is important to remember that with the exception of the face, areas of the body innervated by a single nerve are rare. There is much overlap of nerves on the trunk and the extremities, so it is unusual for a single neurotomy to alleviate pain in these areas. This means that several neurotomies are frequently necessary to achieve control of pain.

Rhizotomy

Dorsal rhizotomy, also known as radicotomy, was first performed in the late 19th century, and involves the sectioning of preganglionic sensory nerve root fibers (Fig. 9-2). This technique has the significant advantage of sparing the motor fibers. The traditional approach requires laminectomy and general

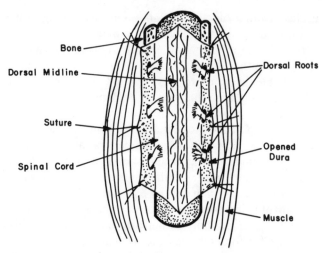

Fig. 9-2.   Surgical exposure for dorsal rhizotomy. Dotted
lines demonstrate level at which the dorsal roots are interrupted. Important anatomical landmarks are labelled.

anesthesia and has therefore been done only in reasonably healthy patients.
More recently, a technique has been developed for percutaneous rhizotomies using radio-frequency lesion techniques,[34] thus making the procedure
available to severely debilitated patients who might not be considered for
such a major procedure as an open rhizotomy. The percutaneous procedure
can be carried out with local anesthesia and is relatively safe in experienced
hands with good fluoroscopic support. The potential for producing motor
deficits, however, is greater with this method since the rootlets are not
visualized and minor mispositions of the probe can result in coagulation of
motor fibers.

   Like neurotomy, dorsal rhizotomy eliminates all forms of sensation
entering the dorsal spinal cord. For this reason, many of the same types of
restrictions discussed earlier have traditionally applied to this procedure. In
recent years surgeons have developed methods of performing super-selec-
tive rhizotomies that spare non-pain sensory fibers, thereby providing a
mechanism for the other sensations such as proprioception and vibration to
reach the spinal cord and participate in the feedback mechanisms that allow
useful coordination of muscles in an involved extremity. Due to sensory
overlap, more dorsal roots than corresponding dermatomes have to be
eliminated to ensure adequate coverage of the desired area. In fact, if one
performs a single-level rhizotomy in the thoracic region, for example, it is
unlikely that one would be able to observe any analgesia at all. Rhizotomies
appear to be the most practical method for the relief of pain associated with
pancoast tumors of the lungs, and head and neck tumors.[24] Rhizotomies are

easily performed and widely used, with success rates of greater than 80 percent. Percutaneous trigeminal or glossopharyngeal rhizotomy with thermal coagulation are examples that may be familiar to most health professionals.

Rhizotomies can be effective for visceral as well as somatic pain. There are several potential complications of rhizotomy. One must be particularly careful when performing sacral rhizotomies on males, since it is quite easy to cause impotence if any anesthesia of the penis occurs. It is equally easy to disturb the bowel and bladder function with sacral rhizotomies. Because of these dangers, it is usually wise to avoid the use of sacral rhizotomies unless the patient has already lost control of these organs.

Whenever an open rhizotomy is done along the spinal cord, the patient must be observed postoperatively for the development of progressive weakness below the level of the laminectomy. This complication is associated with a hematoma compressing the spinal cord. A partial or complete transverse myelitis can be induced if significant injury occurs to the important radicular arteries that accompany the nerve roots.

The success in terms of abolishing significant portions of cancer pain with rhizotomies or neurotomies depends on the accuracy and the extensiveness of the procedures. Clearly, if the involved area can be desensitized, pain relief should approach 100 percent in patients with a physiological pain pattern who lack psychological overlay. Unfortunately, anesthesia dolorosa and phantom limb-like deafferentation pain occur frequently enough to discourage many surgeons from using rhizotomy.

Cordotomy

Ever since the introduction of anterolateral cordotomy, also known as spinothalamic tractotomy, in the second decade of the 20th century, it has probably been the most popular neurosurgical method for relief of cancer pain.[25] It involves the interruption of ascending pain and temperature fibers within the substance of the anterolateral spinal cord (Fig. 9-3). One of the reasons that this technique enjoys significant popularity is that a successful cordotomy will produce anesthesia while preserving other major sensory functions. During the first 50 years of use, cordotomy required general anesthesia, cervical or thoracic laminectomy, and division of the contralateral spino-thalamic tract. In the early 1960s, however, a technique for percutaneous cervical cordotomy was developed that could be performed under local anesthesia.[25] In addition to making the procedure available to many more patients, the percutaneous approach allowed immediate assessment of the effects of the lesion, since the spinal cord could be stimulated and the neurological examination carried out while the lesion was created and incrementally increased with a thermocoagulating probe.

Cordotomy is ideally suited for unilateral pain, since only one anterior

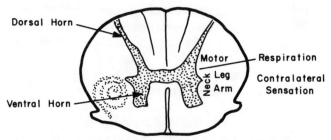

Fig. 9-3. Cross-section of the spinal cord demonstrating location of interruption of the lateral spinothalamic tract during percutaneous radiofrequency cordotomy. The same area is cut during open anterolateral cordotomy (dotted spiral). Important anatomical landmarks are indicated, including the relative positions of pain fibers serving the neck, leg, and arm. The corticospinal (motor) tract is in the dorsolateral spinal cord as seen.

quadrant of the spinal cord has to be disturbed. It is also possible to control bilateral or midline pain with bilateral cordotomies. The placement of the cordotomy lesion along the spinal axis is very important. Pain that is located below the level of the umbilicus can generally be controlled by cordotomy in the region of the upper thoracic spinal cord on up to the high cervical cord. In the case of pain above the level of umbilicus, the greatest success is achieved with high cervical cordotomy. The relief that is achieved is usually quite satisfactory to the patient and generally lasts for 6 to 12 months, although there have been reports of relief lasting beyond three years.

If one compiles all the series of cordotomy results, a general success rate in unilateral sections of 60 to 70 percent can be anticipated while a success rate of 70 to 80 percent can be anticipated with bilateral cordotomy (unpublished data, Long DM). The mortality rate with unilateral cordotomy is in the 5 to 10 percent range and is at least double that with bilateral cordotomy. The risks of the procedure are substantial and include hemiplegia and death.[26] Hemiplegia can occur if the corticospinal tract is injured or if damage to blood vessels supplying the pyramidal tract occurs. The risk of death is much greater with cervical cordotomy, since significant damage to the phrenic nucleus and outflow can occur in the cervical region. If after high bilateral cervical cordotomy, segmental loss of respiratory reflexes occurs, the patient may be incapable of mounting an appropriate respiratory response to hypercarbia and hypoxia when sleeping. This condition, known as Ondine's curse, can cause the patient to become apneic during sleep, with subsequent severe hypoxia and cardiac arrest. Of course, this problem is compounded in the patient with preexistent compromise of pulmonary capacity by carcinoma or pleural effusions. In light of these potential complications, if an open upper thoracic cordotomy can be carried out successfully, the patient has a much smaller chance of a life-threatening complication. The procedure is effective for both visceral and somatic pain and can be particularly helpful when tumor involves one of the neural plexuses.

It is sometimes distressing to find that once a unilateral cordotomy is done and successful resolution of pain is achieved, the patient begins to complain of pain on the opposite side of the body. In this situation a careful historical analysis generally reveals that the patient was already having some mild pain on the opposite side. Once the severe pain on the predominant side is alleviated, the residual lesser pain becomes increasingly significant. Since this situation can occur frequently, it is usually a good idea to plan a bilateral cordotomy in patients who have severe pain on one side and less severe pain on the other side. Bilateral cordotomies are not done simultaneously, but rather the patient is generally brought back after a couple of weeks for the second procedure.

In addition to the usual potential complications of cordotomy such as bleeding, infection, sensory disturbance, hemiplegia or hemiparesis, death, and risks from anesthesia, there is also a 15 to 30 percent risk of significant impairment of bladder function with unilateral cordotomy and a 30 to 60 percent risk in bilateral cordotomy. Thus, although cordotomy is an effective procedure, the risks are high and it should not be undertaken lightly. Its use is generally encouraged only in those patients whose life expectancy is relatively short.

Myelotomy

Mediolongitudinal myelotomy, also known as commissural myelotomy, was introduced in the 1920s and basically consists of division of the anterior white commissure in the spinal cord midline.[1] The operation requires general anesthesia as well as multilevel laminectomy and microsurgical techniques. The technique interrupts pain and temperature fibers that are in the process of crossing before they reach the opposite spino-thalamic tract. The cord is divided longitudinally along the midline from the dorsal midline through the anterior white commissure. This is done over several segments, since pain fibers cross the anterior commissure from the level of their entry into the spinal cord up to three or four segments above that level.

The procedure is particularly suitable for intractable bilateral pain involving the perineal region, the pelvis, the lower extremities, and the abdomen. It has been used higher in the spinal cord to attempt control of localized pain due to breast and lung cancer as well. When myelotomy is successful, the pain relief can be excellent, although frequently it is not permanent, generally lasting somewhere between three months and one year. For this reason, as in the case of cordotomy, it is probably most appropriately applied to those patients who have a relatively short life expectancy.

The success rates using this procedure vary so tremendously from one report to another that success appears to depend on the skill of the surgeon and the appropriate selection of patients. Assuming appropriate selection and good surgical skill, relief of perianal or pelvic pain can be anticipated in the range of 60 to 80 percent. Success begins to drop off when dealing with pain in the extremities, localized lung, and breast. Sometimes pelvic pain can be relieved using sacral rhizotomy rather than midline myelotomy. Disturbance of bowel and/or bladder function is a significant complication, occurring frequently enough that some surgeons are reluctant to perform midline myelotomies in patients who still retain good bowel and bladder function.

Stereotactic Variation of Myelotomy

"Stereotactic" means pertaining to or characterized by precise positioning in space. Stereotactic procedures involve the utilization of various apparatuses that allow the definition of specific points in space that can be reached with a probe, electrode, or needle with great precision and minimal interruption of surrounding structures. Stereotactic devices have been used for decades in neurosurgery to allow, for example, the creation of lesions in deep central structures of the brain (e.g., thalamus) for movement disorders. Although the stereotactic procedures are frequently quite elaborate, it is clear that they usually provide a less dangerous means of approaching otherwise inaccessible areas.

A stereotactic variation in the procedure has been described in which a small midline lesion of the anterior commissure is made at the cervicomedullary junction.[12] However, one would not want to create cervicomedullary lesions in patients whose pain was below the level of umbilicus, since a lower and safer lesion would suffice. In addition to bowel and bladder complications (which are not as great as with bilateral cordotomy), there can be disturbances of proprioception after myelotomy, although these are frequently transient.

Brainstem Procedures

Destructive procedures in the brainstem must clearly be reserved for those patients who did not obtain relief with the preceding and less dangerous modes of intervention. Brainstem procedures are potentially life-threatening and can be associated with significant morbidity. They should be performed only by those who are highly skilled in the necessary techniques. Three separate procedures are discussed below.

Medullary Tractotomy

Medullary tractotomy (trigeminal tractotomy) can be performed for ipsilateral facial pain of malignant origin. In this procedure, the sectioning is done in the descending spinal tract of the trigeminal nerve.[30] The fibers assume a segmental arrangement, with the mandibular fibers located most dorsomedially, the ophthalmic fibers most ventrally, and maxillary fibers between them. This anatomic arrangement makes it theoretically possible to be relatively selective in terms of lesion production and control of pain. Interestingly, fiber tracts from the sensory components of cranial nerves VII, IX, and X lie next to the trigeminal spinal tract and, with appropriate extension of the lesion, one can obtain relief of pain in the head and neck areas served by these nerves as well. These procedures can be done with the patient awake (provided the individual is cooperative), making it possible to actually assess the effect of the lesion as it is progressively extended. Medullary tractotomy can be done by way of an open operative procedure or stereotactically. The ability to perform medullary tractotomy stereotactically has greatly enhanced the popularity of this procedure since its introduction in the 1960s.

In situations where severe pain affects both head and neck and upper body, it is possible to combine high sections of the spinathalamic tract with sections of the descending tract of the fifth cranial nerve. Such procedures were first attempted by way of an open operative exposure in the late 1930s and there are many technical variations for accomplishing the sections. Complications include contralateral hemiparesis and decreased coordination of the ipsilateral arm and/or leg with proprioceptive disturbances, as well as vocal cord paralysis. Success rates vary greatly, but generally appear to be at least 50 percent in terms of alleviation of significant amount of the pain.

Mesencephalic Tractotomy

Mesencephalic tractotomy[31] is a procedure that was envisioned in the late 1940s, when it was discovered that pain-conducting pathways converged in the midbrain beneath the quadrigeminal plate. It was also discovered that the fibers in the pain tracts were somatotopically arranged with fibers from the lower portions of the body crossing dorsolaterally, while fibers from the head, neck, and upper body crossed ventromedially. The open tractotomy was carried out according to the area of the body in which anesthesia was desired. Although initially this procedure was met with enthusiasm, the development of severe painful dysesthesias by most of the patients subsequently limited its use and today it is used less frequently. The application of stereotactic techniques and improved understanding of the anatomy in this region have revived this operation and it is likely to increase in utility in the future.

Thalamotomy

Brainstem procedures such as the tractotomies described above and thalamotomy have become relatively uncommon. With the emergence of the magnetic resonance imaging scanner, the potential exists for performing stereotactic procedures in conjunction with this scanner, since it provides detailed anatomical information. Thus, it is likely that enthusiasm for these procedures will reemerge in the near future, as they will be able to be carried out more accurately and safely than in the past. Thalamotomies are done stereotactically with local anesthesia in cooperative patients. When they are used for cancer pain, the primary areas of concern are the head and neck. The targets are the specific somatosensory nuclei such as the ventroposterolateral and ventroposteromedial nuclei. Non-specific thalamic nuclei such as the intralaminar nucleus, centrum medianum, perivesicular nucleus, and nucleus limitans are also targeted at times, along with the frontothalamic system and the pulvinar nucleus. The most popular group of targets center around the intralaminar nuclear group and reticulothalamic tract, since optimal pain relief and minimal sensory disturbances are achieved here.

The initial relief of pain achieved with thalamotomy ranges from 70 to 80 percent or more. Unfortunately, pain usually recurs within 3 to 6 months in about one-third of patients, with more than two-thirds having recurrence of pain after one year. The complications other than bleeding and infection result from impaired function of compromised adjacent sensory nuclei. Ill-placed lesions can also affect motor tracts that are in close proximity to the outer portions of the thalamus. In addition, compromise of the anterior and dorso-medial nuclei can lead to confusion, memory impairment, and disorientation, which are usually transient but can be permanent. The mortality rate is relatively small, since this is a stereotactic procedure. Nevertheless, thalamotomy for cancer pain should not be undertaken lightly and again should be performed only by an extremely skillful surgeon in patients with relatively short life expectancy who have not responded to lesser procedures.[32,33]

Cortical Lesions

Cortical gyrectomy, frontal lobotomy, and cingulotomy are uncommon procedures but should be included in any complete discussion of neurosurgical modalities for relief of pain because the latter two have great historical significance and the former has future potential.

Cortical Gyrectomy

Cortical gyrectomy involves the resection of a portion of the postcentral gyrus that receives sensory projections from the area of the thalamus that processes pain impulses from the somatic area of concern. It has been used primarily for facial pain, but is a very extensive procedure, requiring a major craniotomy, and is thus not appropriate for many severely debilitated patients with cancer pain. The logic of the procedure, however, is unquestionable, and if the technical feasibility can be improved to make this procedure compatible with debilitated patients, its future use will grow.

Frontal Lobotomy

Frontal lobotomies, as is well known, have been used since the 1930s for psychiatric disorders, but subsequently became recognized as effective in controlling some forms of intractable pain. In the bifrontal lobotomy, the frontothalamic projection fibers are interrupted; this procedure actually does not control pain, but rather it affects the patient's concern regarding the pain. The procedure can be done by way of craniotomy or stereotactically with thermocoagulation, cryofixation, or injection of chemicals such as alcohol, glycerin, and phenol.

Besides the usual surgical complications, there is a high incidence of profound personality disturbance or alteration. In patients with significant depression, anxiety, or other emotional disturbances, however, this may be a desirable outcome. Although success rates can be over 70 percent, the success is generally quite transient, with pain returning within six months, but the personality alterations persist permanently.

Cingulotomy

Cingulotomy involves the interruption of the fiber tracts of the cingulate gyrus, which integrates fibers of the cortex, thalamic nuclei, and other components of the thalamic system. It works very much like frontal lobotomy in that it does not directly affect pain pathways but rather influences affective responses to pain. The procedure must be done bilaterally with a stereotactically placed radiofrequency probe. The procedure probably has its greatest application in cancer pain involving the head and neck areas.[10] It does not seem to be associated with as much disturbance of intellectual function as frontal lobotomy. There is not enough reported experience with these cases involving cancer pain to give meaningful statistics about success, but limited trials have been greeted with enthusiasm so far.[11,15] Again, this procedure requires a great deal of skill and will probably gain in popularity with the integration of magnetic resonance imaging and evolving stereotactic technologies.

Hypophysectomy

Hypophysectomy involves removal or destruction of the pituitary gland, which can be done transcranially or transphenoidally, and more recently is done stereotactically.[20] If the stereotactic approach is utilized, the gland can be destroyed with a radiofrequency probe, a cryoprobe, placement of radioactive implants, or injection of alcohol. These procedures are most successful when employed with pain caused by bony metastases from breast or prostate cancer, particularly when the cancers have been shown to respond favorably to previous endocrine therapy. Hypophysectomy results in alterations of the hormonal balance in the body and affects not only the pain but also the growth of metastatic lesions in the cancers previously mentioned.[6]

The results in hypophysectomy vary greatly, with effectiveness ranging anywhere from 42 to 92 percent. When the procedure is effective, it tends to produce long-term relief of pain and is associated with few complications. It is an extremely effective procedure that can be done in almost any medical center. When the procedure is done with alcohol there have been reports of pain relief in previously non-hormone responding carcinomas, which may be due to the diffusion of the alcohol into the hypothalamus.[19]

Chemical modulation of pituitary function with alpha-2-bromo-ergocryptine has been described as effective in controlling cancer pain resulting from prostate and cervical cancer. Experience with this drug is minimal thus far, but it is potentially quite promising as a modality for the control of pain.[16,17,29]

Sympathectomy

The term "sympathectomy" can be defined as interruption or removal of a portion of the sympathetic nervous pathway. Sympathectomy can be accomplished in the paravertebral sympathetic chain or in a more peripheral sympathetic ganglion such as the celiac ganglion.

Sympathectomy is not particularly useful in cancer pain, although in the occasional patient with purely visceral pain it can be of benefit. The recurrence rate of pain is high and relief is frequently incomplete because afferent fibers from a particular visceral organ do not necessarily all cross through the same sympathetic ganglion. A diagnostic block performed with an anesthestic agent before the procedure allows one to assess the effects. Subsequent sympathectomy can be carried out surgically or chemically (percutaneous route), and can include peripheral ganglia such as the celiac ganglion in addition to the paravertebral plexi.[37]

NEUROLOGIC PROCEDURES

The techniques described in the remainder of the chapter frequently involve surgery, but only as a means of implantation or access or neurologic and anesthetic modalities of pain control. Some of these procedures, such as epidural, intrathecal, and intraventricular administration of narcotic agents, have become very popular in recent years and probably warrant a whole chapter for adequate discussion. There is no clear line of demarcation to indicate when these neurologic and anesthetic techniques should be employed as opposed to some of the previously discussed more invasive neurosurgical procedures. Clearly, many decisions as to which modality will be employed will depend upon patient and physician preference.

Neurostimulation

The use of neurostimulation as a method to eliminate pain is based on the gate control theory of pain that was advanced by Melzack and Wall.[23] One of the basic premises of this theory is that a certain amount of sensory stimulation enters the dorsal horn of the spinal cord before sensory overload occurs. If benign stimulation such as vibratory impulses can be used to overload the system, then the pain impulses may not be perceived because the sensory gate theoretically closes after sensory overload occurs. Pain impulses are conducted by lightly myelinated or non-myelinated afferent fibers, and travel at much slower speeds than vibratory stimulation, which is transmitted on heavily myelinated fibers of large caliber. These latter faster impulses reach the gate first and can theoretically close it before the slower pain impulses arrive. In addition to the gate control theory, a number of other theories have been advanced to explain why neurostimulation is sometimes effective in control of pain. The important point is that neurostimulation can be effective in controlling pain.

Neurostimulation can be applied transcutaneously (such as in the commonly known transcutaneous electrical nerve stimulator, or TENS) or electrodes can be placed directly on the meningeal coverings of the spinal cord, producing dorsal column stimulation. The latter procedure requires invasive techniques such as percutaneous placement of epidural wires, or laminectomy with direct placement of a dorsal column electrode plate. The degree of success in control of pain is directly proportional to the skill and experience of the surgeon and his familiarity with electrical modulating devices.[22] In recent years a number of very sophisticated computer assisted stimulators have become available for use in conjunction with the dorsal column stimulator. The use of this technology can increase the success rate significantly.

Deep Brain Stimulation

In addition to neurostimulation of the spinal cord, recent advances have occurred in the area of deep brain stimulation. Electrodes can be implanted in the periaqueductal gray matter and with subsequent stimulation, be used to control chronic pain. The probable mechanism involves release of important neuropeptides such as beta endorphins by stimulation, which bind to appropriate sites, thus elevating the patient's pain threshold. Deep brain stimulation techniques are complex and require a great deal of expertise, and until recently were available only on a very limited basis.[13,14,28]

The risk of deep brain stimulation, which is done stereotactically, are intracranial hemorrhage, infection, failure of the mechanical devices, and eye movement abnormalities. Other than failure of the mechanical hardware, all of these risks are in the less than 5 percent range in the most recent series. These deep brain stimulatory techniques hold great promise for the present and even greater promise for the future.[38]

Anesthetic Procedures

For the purposes of this chapter, anesthetic procedures are defined as those procedures that depend upon local application of drugs and chemicals to achieve pain relief. In general, therapeutic anesthetic techniques such as alcohol and phenol rhizotomy for the control of cancer pain are reserved for those patients who are unsuitable for surgical intervention because of debilitation, unwillingness, or other surgical contraindications. On the other hand, diagnostic nerve blocks such as somatic blocks to outline dermatomal areas of pain involvement are an extremely useful and common component of cancer pain therapy.[5] Not only do such diagnostic blocks delineate and identify the nerve or nerves requiring intervention, but they also afford the patient an opportunity to experience the lack of sensation associated with a permanent neuroablative procedure. Additionally, chronic pain, including cancer pain, sometimes substantially dissipates or even disappears after one or more diagnostic nerve blocks. The reason for this phenomenon is not fully understood, although it may be related to breaking the pain cycle. Thus, a trial of neural blockade whenever feasible is indicated when considering possible modes of permanent analgesia for the control of cancer pain.

As was mentioned earlier, the autonomic nervous system can be involved in the sensation of pain in the visceral organs. Blockage of the autonomic system can be performed to control this pain. The most important autonomic plexi involved in such pain are the stellate and the celiac plexi. The former is frequently involved in head and neck cancer as well as regional lung and breast cancers, while the latter is usually involved with abdominal visceral organs such as the pancreas. In these autonomic plexi, a series of temporary blocks should be initiated first. If temporary but effective relief is achieved, then alcohol or phenol injection by an experienced practitioner can be contemplated as a means of obtaining more permanent relief.

Intrathecal blocks (in the subarachnoid space) can be performed to demonstrate segmental involvement in cancer pain of somatic origin. This is particularly important in situations where surgical procedures are contraindicated, since if temporary relief can be achieved with local anesthetic, then intrathecal phenol or alcohol injected at the appropriate dermatomal level can be utilized to achieve a permanent effect. In other words, the block with a local anesthetic agent is a diagnostic procedure that, if effective in bringing about temporary relief, is followed by the therapeutic procedure, which is the installation of the neurodestructive chemical. This technique requires a very cooperative patient, because positioning is critical to success and must sometimes be maintained for up to an hour.

These chemical intrathecal neurolytic procedures carry a high incidence of loss of bowel or bladder function, especially if the sacral roots are targeted. Additionally, care givers must keep in mind that the chemicals used have specific properties that can help to increase their effectiveness. The alcohol solution is hypobaric and tends to admix with cerebrospinal fluid or rise to the uppermost area of the intrathecal space. Phenol, which is usually mixed with glycerol, is hyperbaric and thus has a tendency to migrate to the lowest portion of the intrathecal space. Patients must be positioned in such a way as to take advantage of these chemical properties.[7]

The placement of an indwelling epidural catheter with a subcutaneous reservoir provides an excellent avenue for multiple trials of epidural neural blockade. This technique can be quite useful in determining whether an individual is a candidate for subsequent chemical neurolysis. The placement of epidural anesthetic agents is not entirely without risks. High blood levels of local anesthetics can occur secondary to absorption via the epidural venous plexi. Accidental intravenous injection can also occur with severe effects involving the cardiovascular or central nervous systems. For these reasons the first few trials of epidural anesthesia should be performed with appropriate cardiopulmonary resuscitation equipment and personnel available. If after several epidural blocks with local anesthestic agents, the physicians and patient agree that effects are satisfactory (and the patient is not a surgical candidate), a neurolytic agent can be placed in the epidural space to achieve neurolysis. The preferred location is the thoracic region in order to limit the effects of thoracic and abdominal segments, and to avoid loss of motor function in the extremities. Accidental intrathecal injection must be avoided, particularly at the thoracic level, since this would result in a transverse myelitis. It is frequently worthwhile to inject a contrast material preceding the neurolytic agent to be absolutely certain of the placement of the catheter. Finally, these neurolytic procedures are frequently complicated by painful dysesthesias, which can be worse than the pain one is attempting to abolish.[35] There is no way to avoid these dysesthesias, and sometimes it is difficult to distinguish dysesthesias from residual pain. Fortunately, severe dysesthesias occur in less than 20 percent of patients.

Epidural and Intrathecal Medications

In addition to anesthetic agents and neurolytic agents, some clinical experience has been gained with the administration of epidural narcotics. These can be quite effective in achieving analgesia on a short-term basis. As with systemic narcotics, however, relatively rapid tolerance may develop. A newer technique is the use of intrathecal narcotics via a catheter placed in the subarachnoid space and connected to a reservoir or a motorized subcutaneous pump. There have been data supporting the claim that a continuous infusion of intrathecal narcotic perhaps diminishes the development of tolerance and is an acceptable mode of therapy for patients with cancer pain.[3,4,36] On the other hand, other investigators have not found this to be true and it is an issue of controversy presently. Even in situations where tolerance to intrathecal narcotic doses does develop, the use of the technique seems to diminish the need for systemic narcotic supplements.

One of the major problems with epidural narcotics has been respiratory depression, which can sometimes progress to respiratory arrest.[8] This may be because when epidural narcotics are instilled, a relatively high plasma level of narcotic develops quickly. On the other hand, low plasma levels are found with infusion of intrathecal narcotics even though it is still recommended that very small dosages be administered initially, with gradual increases to the point of effectiveness.[27,36]

Intraventricular Narcotics for Cancer Pain Therapy

Painful syndromes induced by cancer of the cervical and facial regions have been treated successfully through the use of intraventricular morphine. This technique takes advantage of the specific opiate receptors that have been discovered in the human brain and spinal cord in recent years.[18] By instilling the morphine directly into the ventricle, the blood phase can be bypassed and theoretically much smaller dosages of drug will be needed to control pain and fewer side effects will be encountered.

This of course requires the operative placement of a ventricular catheter connected to a subcutaneous reservoir that can be percutaneously filled with the narcotic agent as needed. One major advantage of this technique is that it can be performed on an outpatient basis. Although most patients develop tolerance, this does not require withdrawal from this mode of therapy, and usually some simple manipulations in the drug dosage and schedule can be quite effective in helping combat this problem. The major risks of the procedure include bleeding and infection, with the first complication occurring at the time of surgery and the second complication occurring anywhere along the course of treatment. Both of these risks are quite small and even smaller is the risk of neurological impairment on the basis of the placement of the catheter through brain substance. The results for neoplastic pain arising in the cervical and craniofacial regions appear to be quite excellent in the majority of patients. There are several reports of patients actually experiencing a lack of pain rather than a feeling of indifference toward the pain as frequently happens with systemic morphine administration.[19,21]

The whole area of neuroaugmentation and central nervous system chemical manipulation is in its infancy. Much more sophisticated and effective techniques are on the horizon. It is clearly only a matter of time before pain mechanisms and pain control are understood thoroughly enough to apply the rapidly advancing technology to solving completely and safely the problem of cancer pain control.

CONCLUSION

Many of the techniques for the alleviation of cancer pain are complex and not fully understood. Technological advances such as the merging of compatible stereotactic devices and magnetic resonance imaging will greatly reduce the danger and technical difficulty of some procedures. Presently cordotomy, both open and stereotactic, and intrathecal and epidural narcotic administration enjoy the most popularity of all the procedures mentioned. It is likely, however, that as our technical capabilities improve and our knowledge increases, techniques for the one-time permanent ablation of the involved sensory area of the central nervous system will increase in popularity.

In summary, cancer pain is among the consequences of this unfortunate disease process. Our arsenal for dealing with cancer pain has increased dramatically in recent decades and most patients can be kept comfortable with currently available techniques. Complete control frequently requires a multi-disciplinary approach by experienced professionals. This is being recognized by more practitioners and appropriate referrals are being made. As our clinical approaches to cancer pain become based on more scientific knowledge, and our technological capabilities increase, there is no doubt that the future promises effective resolution of this feared complication of cancer.

REFERENCES

1. Armour D: Surgery of the spinal cord: Lancet 2:691–697, 1927
2. Bond MR: Personality studies in patients with pain secondary to organic disease. J Psychosom Res 17:257–263, 1973
3. Coombs DW, Maurer HL, Saunders RL: Outcomes and complications of continuous intraspinal narcotic analgesia for cancer pain control. J Clin Oncol 2:1414–1420, 1984
4. Cousins MJ, Mather LE: Intrathecal and epidural administration of opiates. Anesthesiology 61:276–310, 1984
5. Doyle D: Nerve blocks in advanced cancer. Practitioner 226(1365):539–544, 1982
6. Evans PJ, Lloyd JW, Moore RA, et al.: Pituitary function following hypophysectomy for pain relief. Br J Anesth 54:921–925, 1982
7. Flanigan S, Boop WC: Spinal intrathecal injection procedures in the management of pain. Clin Neurosurg 21:229–238, 1974
8. Florez J, McCarthy LE, Borison HL: A comparative study in the cat of the respiratory

effects of morphine injected intravenously and into the cerebrospinal fluid. J Pharmacol Exp Therap 163:448–455, 1968

9. Foley KM: The treatment of cancer pain. N Engl J Med 313:84–95, 1985
10. Foltz EL, White LE Jr: Rostral cingulotomotomy and pain "relief," in Knighton RE, Dumke PR (Eds): Pain. Boston, Little, Brown, 1966, pp 469–491
11. Foltz EL, White LE, Jr: Pain relief by frontal cingulotomy. J Neurosurg 19:89–93, 1962
12. Hitchcock E: Stereotactic cervical myelotomy. J Neurol Neurosurg Psychiatry 33:224–230, 1970
13. Hosobuchi Y: Subcortical electrical stimulation for control of intractable pain in humans. Report of 122 cases. J Neurosurg 64:543–553, 1986
14. Hosobuchi Y, Adams JE, Linchitz R: Pain relief by electrical stimulation of the central gray matter in humans and its reversal by naloxone. Science 197:183–186, 1977
15. Hurt RW, Ballantine HT Jr: Stereotactic anterior cingulate lesions for persistent pain: a report of 68 cases. Clin Neurosurg 21:334–351, 1974
16. Jacobi GH, Altwein JE, Hohenfellner R: Adjunct bromocriptine treatment as palliation for prostate cancer: experimental and clinical evaluation. Scan J Urol Nephrol 55:107–12, 1980
17. Jacobi GH, Altwein JE: Bromocryptin, a new therapeutic principle in adenoma and carcinoma of the prostate. Presuppositions, possibilities and limitations. Minerva Urol 32:167–173, 1980
18. Kuhar MJ, Pert CB, Snyder SH: Regional distribution of opiate receptor binding in monkey and human brain. Nature 245:447–450, 1973
19. Lenyi A, Galli G, Gandolfini, et al.: Intraventricular morphine in paraneoplastic painful syndrome of the cervicofacial region: experience in thirty-eight cases. Neurosurgery 17:6–11, 1985
20. Levin AB, Katz J, Benson RC, et al.: Treatment of pain of diffuse metastatic cancer by stereotactic chemical hypophysectomy: long term results and observations on mechanism of action. Neurosurg 6:258–262, 1980
21. Lobato RD, Madrid JL, Fatela LV: Intraventricular morphine for control of pain in terminal cancer patients. J Neurosurg 59:627–633, 1983
22. Long, DM, Hagfors H: Electrical stimulation of the nervous system for relief of pain. Pain 1:109–123, 1975
23. Melzack R, Wall PD: Pain mechanisms: a new theory. Science 150:971–979, 1965
24. Mracek Z: Surgical treatment in intractable pain in advanced malignant tumors of the face, oral cavity, pharynx and larynx. Cesk Otolaryngol 29(27):104–109, 1980
25. Mullan S: Percutaneous cordotomy (RF). Adv Neurol 4:677–682, 1974
26. Nathan PW: Results of antero-lateral cordotomy for pain in cancer. J Neurol Neurosurg Psychiatry 26:353–363, 1963
27. Poletti CE, Schmidek HH, Sweet WH, et al.: Pain control with implantable systems for the long term infusion of intraspinal opioids in man, in Schmidek H, Sweet W (Eds): Operative Neurosurgical Techniques: Indications, Methods and Results, Vol. 2. Orlando FL, Grune and Stratton, 1982, pp 1199–1210
28. Richardson DE, Akil H: Pain reduction by electrical brain stimulation in man. II. Chronic self-administration in the periventricular gray matter. J Neurosurg 47:184–194, 1977
29. Ruge S: Bromocriptin in the treatment of carcinoma of the cervix: a phase II trial. Gynecol Oncol 21:356–358, 1985
30. Schvarcz JR: Spinal cord steotactic techniques re trigeminal nucleotomy and extralemniscal myelotomy. Appl Neurophysiol 41:99–112, 1978
31. Spiegel EA Wycis HT, Szekely EG, et al.: Medial and basal thalamotomy in so-called intractable pain, in Knighton RS, Dumke PR (Eds): Pain. Boston, Little, Brown, 1966, pp 503–517

32. Spiegel EA, Sycis HT: Mesencephalotomy in the treatment of "intractable" facial pain. Arch Neurol 69:1–13, 1953
33. Spiegel EA, Wycis HT, Szekely, EG, et al.: Combined dorsomedial, intralaminar and basal thalamotomy for relief of so-called intractable pain. J Int Coll Surg 42:160–168, 1964
34. Uematsu S: Percutaneous electrothermocoagulation of spinal nerve trunk, ganglion, and rootlets, in Schmidek H, Sweet W (Eds): Operative Neurosurgical Techniques: Indications, Methods and Results, Vol. 2. Orlando, Grune and Stratton, 1982, pp 1177–1198
35. Ventafridda V, Martino G: Clinical evaluation of subarachnoid neurolytic blocks in intractable cancer pain, in Bonica JJ, Albe-Fessard DG (Eds): Advances in Pain Research and Therapy. New York, Raven Press, 1976, pp 699–703
36. Wang JK: Analgesic effect of intrathecally administered morphine. Regional Anesthesia 4:2–3, 1977
37. White JC: Role of sympathectomy in relief of pain. Progr Neurol Surg 7:131–152, 1975
38. Young RF, Brechner T: Electrical stimulation of the brain for relief of intractable pain due to cancer. Cancer 57:1266–1272, 1986

Tim A. Ahles, Ph.D.

10

Psychological Techniques for the Management of Cancer-Related Pain

Although psychological techniques have been used for the management of cancer-related pain for many years, systematic research examining the efficacy of these techniques has only begun in the last few years. A recent review of this literature[1] concluded that a tremendous amount of research is necessary to clearly establish the utility of psychological techniques in the management of cancer-related pain. Noyes[46] reached a similar conclusion and proposed that the study of the efficacy of psychological techniques has been largely neglected.

The magnitude of the problem certainly justifies the research effort required to develop techniques for the improved management of cancer-related pain. Several studies have indicated that cancer-related pain (pain secondary to the disease and/or its treatment) afflicts 50 to 80 percent of patients with metastatic disease.[5,26,28] However, cancer-related pain has been managed primarily with somatic treatments including (1) pharmacologic approaches, e.g., non-narcotics, narcotics, antidepressants; (2) neurosurgical, neuroablative, and neurostimulatory approaches; (3) anesthetic approaches, e.g., epidural infusion of local anesthetics, nitrous oxide etc.; and (4) radiation approaches.[18,48] Although great advances in the somatic treatments of cancer-related pain have been made, numerous difficulties remain: (1) no treatment is consistently effective; (2) the effects of pharmacological treatments diminish over time as tolerance develops, thereby requiring dosage escalation; (3) pharmacological treatments often produce negative side effects including nausea and vomiting, constipation, respiratory depression, and sedation[11]; (4) surgical procedures often provide only temporary relief, with pain recurring within several weeks[11]; and (5) complications of surgical procedures include weakness or paralysis, orthostatic hypotension, and sexual dysfunction.[45] The recognition of the problems inherent in the somatic treatments has stimulated the search for alternative treatment approaches including psychological techniques.

THE MULTIDIMENSIONAL NATURE
OF CANCER-RELATED PAIN

Since the original publication of Melzack and Wall's[43] Gate Control Theory, researchers and clinicians have recognized the need for a multidimensional approach to the treatment of chronic, benign pain syndromes. Recently, Ahles, Blanchard and Ruckdeschel[3] proposed that a multidimensional model is appropriate for understanding cancer-related pain. These authors identified five components of cancer-related pain: (1) physiological (the organic etiology of the pain); (2) sensory (attributes such as intensity, location, and the quality of the pain); (3) affective (affective variables such as depression and anxiety associated with the pain); (4) cognitive (the manner in which the pain influences a person's thought processes or the meaning the person attaches to the pain); and (5) behavioral (pain behaviors such as activity level and analgesic intake). Evidence for the relevance of the physiological,[11,18] sensory,[3] affective,[3,15,17,42,57,67] cognitive,[3,57] and behavioral[3,37] components to cancer-related pain has been reported in the literature (see Chapter 1 of this book for a further discussion of the multidimensional nature of cancer-related pain[41]).

The multidimensional conceptualization of pain has contributed to the development of psychological techniques for the management of chronic pain. Techniques such as biofeedback, relaxation training, and hypnosis have been effective in alleviating or reducing the pain associated with chronic pain syndromes such as migraine and muscle contraction headaches, low back pain, etc.[12,63,64] This chapter reviews the application of psychological techniques to the management of cancer-related pain.

HYPNOSIS

Hypnosis has long been used for pain control; however, the recent scientific study of hypnosis has elevated the technique from the shroud of mysticism to the status of a useful clinical tool in the control of pain.[33] Although numerous techniques have been used, Barber and Gitelson[7] have described six hypnotic strategies used for the control of cancer-related pain:

(1) direct blocking of pain from awareness through the suggestion of anesthesia or analgesia; (2) substitution of another sensation (e.g., pressure) for pain; (3) moving the pain to a smaller or less important part of the body; (4) changing the meaning of the pain so that it becomes less threatening; (5) increasing pain tolerance; and (6) dissociating part of the body from the patient's awareness.

Spiegel[58] recently described three basic principles for teaching any hypnotic technique:

1. "Filter the hurt out of the pain." Patients are taught that there is not a one-to-one correlation between the amount of physical damage and the perceived intensity of the pain. By separating the affective component (which amplifies the pain) from the somatic component of the pain, the suffering experienced can be reduced.
2. "Do not fight the pain." Patients are taught that struggling with the pain can cause an exacerbation of it either through increasing reactive muscle tension or the affective component of the pain.
3. "Use self-hypnosis." Finally, the patients are taught self-hypnosis so that they can utilize the techniques apart from the therapist.

One of the earliest descriptions of the use of hypnosis for pain relief in cancer was provided in a series of papers by Butler[19–22] written in the 1950s. Since that time, several additional case reports have appeared that suggest that hypnosis is effective for approximately 50 percent of the patients so treated.[6,7,23,33,38,50,51] A close examination of the case reports presented suggests that a significant number of patients treated with hypnosis were experiencing psychological difficulties such as anxiety and depression. Therefore, hypnosis may reduce the self-report of pain by influencing the affective component of the pain experience as well as by directly altering the sensory component of the pain.

Support for this hypothesis was provided in the only control-group outcome study of hypnosis found in the literature. Spiegel and Bloom[56] studied a group of women with metastatic breast carcinoma. These women were randomly assigned to one of three groups: (1) psychological support group only; (2) psychological support group plus self-hypnotic training; and (3) a no-treatment control group. Their results demonstrated that the two treatments produced reduced reports of pain and suffering post-treatment as compared to the control group. Additionally, patients who received self-hypnosis training reported significantly less pain than patients who were treated with the support group alone. Finally, patients in the treatment group reported an improvement in mood as measured on the Profile of Mood States, and this improvement was inversely correlated with reports of pain.

These data support the hypotheses that hypnosis is effective in managing cancer-related pain and that reductions in pain are associated with elevations in mood. However, caution must be taken in interpreting this correlation since, as the authors point out, it is equally plausible to assume that decreased pain caused the elevation in mood as to assume that the elevation in mood caused the decrease in reported pain. Further caution must be taken in interpreting the results of the study because 41 percent of the patients reported no pain at baseline and only six patients in the entire sample were taking prescription analgesics. Therefore, the patients in this sample appear to have been experiencing a relatively low level of pain. It is unclear how effective these techniques would be for patients with more intense pain.

Hypnosis has a long history of use in the treatment of cancer-related pain (hypnosis has also been used to reduce pain associated with medical procedures such as bone marrow transplantation, e.g., Bayuk[8]). Unfortunately, most of the studies reported in the literature are anecdotal case reports. However, Spiegel and Bloom,[56] the one control group outcome study, supported the utility of self-hypnosis in reducing reports of pain and elevating mood. Additional research of this caliber is clearly necessary.

RELAXATION TRAINING AND BIOFEEDBACK

Relaxation Training

Relaxation training is a procedure designed to produce physiological and mental relaxation.[59] Although several methods for relaxation training have been proposed,[9,35,53,66] progressive and autogenic relaxation procedures are the most commonly used. Progressive relaxation, as described by Bernstein and Borkovec,[10] consists of systematically tensing and relaxing 16 muscle groups. Patients are also instructed in deep breathing exercises and taught to associate expiration with calming words such as "relax." Autogenic relaxation,[53] by contrast, is a relatively passive technique. Patients are instructed to adopt a quiet attitude and repeat "autogenic phrases" such as "my arms are warm and heavy" and "my legs feel heavy and relaxed." In many ways, autogenic relaxation training is analogous to many self-hypnotic techniques.

For both techniques, training is typically completed in 6 to 10 sessions. Initially, live relaxation training sessions with a therapist present are preferable to simply providing audio tapes.[47] However, audio tapes of the relaxation exercises are typically provided for home practice and patients are encouraged to practice the technique for 15 to 30 minutes twice per day. Regular home practice is crucial in order to receive the maximal benefit from the technique. Although the initial training procedures are relatively lengthy, the ultimate goal is to teach the person to relax quickly. To this end, cue-controlled relaxation is taught; this consists of repeatedly pairing a cue word such as "relax" with a deep breath. The cue-controlled relaxation provides the patient with a portable technique for relaxing in every day situations.

Biofeedback

Biofeedback has been defined as "a process in which a person learns to reliably influence physiological responses of two kinds: either responses that are not ordinarily under voluntary control or responses that ordinarily are easy to regulate but regulation has broken down because of trauma or disease.[14] Biofeedback training occurs in a special electronic environment with devices that detect and amplify various biological responses and convert these amplified responses to signals that are easily processed by the patient. A typical signal is a tone where the pitch varies proportionately with the level of the biological response.

One of the most common types of biofeedback is electromyographic (EMG) biofeedback-feedback. EMG electrodes are attached to major muscles, e.g., frontalis or trapezius muscles. Patients are taught to reduce EMG activity, which is indicated by a reduction in the biofeedback signal (e.g., the pitch of the tone). Other types of biofeedback include (1) temperature biofeedback (teaching patients to raise hand temperature); (2) skin conductance level (SCL) biofeedback (teaching patients to reduce SCL); and (3) electroencephalographic (EEG) biofeedback (theta, teaching a person to produce 4 to 8 HZ activity, and alpha, teaching the person to produce 8 to 13 HZ activity). Similar to the relaxation training, biofeedback training is typically completed in 6 to 10 sessions.

Relaxation techniques are often combined with biofeedback to facilitate training. Direct comparisons of the two techniques have typically found them equally efficacious[55]; therefore, the purchase of expensive biofeedback equipment may be unnecessary. However, this hypothesis requires empirical validation within a cancer population. The primary purpose of both techniques is to (1) reduce muscular tension and/or sympathetically mediated responses such as vasoconstriction, which may produce pain or exacerbate an existing pain problem and (2) reduce affective variables such as anxiety, which may amplify the pain.

Applications to Cancer-Related Pain

Although relaxation and biofeedback techniques have been suggested for use with cancer patients,[25,46,48] only one study utilizing relaxation exercises[27] and two studies utilizing biofeedback[29,30] have examined the application of these techniques to the management of cancer-related pain. Fleming[27] reported that 36 of 58 patients with far-advanced cancer reported a reduction in several symptoms including pain. Unfortunately, no statistical analysis was reported that would allow an evaluation of the efficacy of the relaxation training in the control of pain specifically.

Fotopoulos et al.[29,30] examined the utility of biofeedback techniques in the reduction of cancer-related pain. In their first study,[29] these authors examined the influence of a combination of EMG and theta EEG biofeedback on the pain reports of seven cancer patients. All seven patients showed significant reductions in reported pain during biofeedback sessions; however, only two patients were able to obtain significant relief at home. In a similar study,[30] these authors treated 12 patients with a combination of EMG and SCL biofeedback. Unfortunately, complete data was available on only five of the patients (two patients died, three became too ill to participate, and one moved from the area). Two of the five patients were able to reliably reduce their pain outside the biofeedback laboratory and three of five reduced their use of analgesic medications.

The patients seen by Fleming had far-advanced cancer and were being cared for in a hospice. Additionally, the patients seen by Fotopoulos et al.[29,30] had failed to respond to all other pain management modalities. Therefore, their pain was difficult to control and many of them saw biofeedback as their last resort. Despite this, the results suggest that relaxation and biofeedback may hold promise for reducing the suffering of cancer-related pain. Control group outcome studies, particularly with patients who have not failed all other pain management attempts, are clearly necessary.

A potential disadvantage of relaxation training and biofeedback is that both procedures are relatively labor-intensive for the therapist and time-consuming for the patient, particularly outpatients who may need to make extra weekly appointments. However, recent work with the treatment of vascular[36] and muscle contraction[60] headaches have shown that minimal-therapist-contact, home-based treatments using both relaxation and biofeedback are equally efficacious as a traditional clinic-based treatment. This type of home-based treatment approach may be ideal for the cancer patient.

OPERANT TECHNIQUES

Fordyce[31] demonstrated that pain behaviors (e.g., analgesic intake, pain complaints, grimacing, limping, etc.) can be influenced by factors other than pain intensity. Working from an operant conditioning model, he has proposed that pain behaviors can be influenced by environmental factors or reinforcers such as attention, social support, or the avoidance of unpleasant tasks (e.g., job, housework, etc.).

Although the influence of environmental reinforcement on pain behaviors has been discussed in relation to numerous pain syndromes, only a few authors have discussed this issue with regard to patients with cancer-related pain.[32,52] A possible reason is that cancer-related pain is typically associated with terminal stages of the disease, whereas back pain, headaches, etc. can be life-long problems. Therefore, the cancer patient may not have the opportunity to adopt a chronic pain "career." However, Ahles et al.[3] reported that cancer patients experienced pain for an average of 16 months, with a range of 1 month to 18 years. These data suggest that pain can be a long-standing problem for a certain proportion of cancer patients. Additionally, advances in cancer treatment are producing longer life expectancies for many patients. Unfortunately, a subpopulation of these patients may continue to experience pain.

The same investigators[3] found that the majority of patients felt that significant others in their environment could identify when the patient was in pain or experiencing an exacerbation of the pain. Typical responses of the significant others were expressions of concern and offers to retrieve medications and assume responsibilities for the patient (e.g., doing housework). When family members can identify the presence or escalation of pain and the typical responses reported, the potential for the operant reinforcement of pain behaviors appears possible for certain patients.

Recently, Keefe et al.[37] reported the development of a methodology for the behavioral assessment of patients with head and neck cancer. Six areas are evaluated through direct observation and a structured interview: (1) motor pain behaviors (e.g., guarded movement, grimacing, rubbing, and sighing); (2) specific activities that are painful; (3) general activity level; (4) pain-relieving methods utilized by the patients; (5) pain medication intake; and (6) weight loss. These authors have also developed a Behavioral Dysfunction Index based on a combination of the above factors that is correlated with self-report measures of pain intensity. The development of this type of methodology will greatly enhance the ability of researchers to measure changes in behavior associated with various treatments.

One area that has been discussed in relation to the cancer patient is *pro re nata* (PRN) versus fixed time schedule of analgesic administration.[32,65] Fordyce[31] has proposed that within a PRN regimen the analgesic becomes a contingent reinforcer for pain behaviors and/or the patient feels obligated to emit pain behaviors in order to justify his request for analgesics. Either situation leads to an increase in pain behaviors. Most physicians working with chronic pain patients prefer a fixed time schedule (e.g., every four hours) so that analgesics no longer serve as contingent reinforcers for pain behavior.[32,65]

The operant approach to cancer-related pain has largely been ignored except with regard to the administration of analgesics. Although operant variables may have little relevance for patients in the terminal stages of the disease, they may play a role in the behavior of patients who experience pain for extended periods. The methodological advances proposed by Keefe et al.[37] should greatly enhance the ability of investigators to study this area.

A COGNITIVE-SOCIAL LEARNING APPROACH

Recently, theorists have developed cognitive-social learning models of pain.[61,62] According to these models, pain can be described in terms of its objective qualities (e.g., location, intensity, etc.) and in terms of its psychological significance for the patient. This appraisal is based on the person's evaluation of the pain and of their coping resources, which is based on beliefs and attitudes acquired throughout one's social learning history. The goal of the cognitive-social learning approach is to help patients modify thoughts, beliefs, or behaviors that may exacerbate pain, depression, or anxiety, as well as provide them with specific skills to aid in coping with episodes of pain. Both laboratory studies[2,39] and studies with clinical populations[34,49] have supported the utility of cognitive approaches in producing reductions in various measures of pain.

Turk and Rennert[62] have described a cognitive-social learning approach designed for the treatment of cancer-related pain. The treatment package consists of four components: (1) pre-treatment preparation; (2) conceptualization-translation; (3) coping skills training; and (4) rehearsal.

The purpose of the pre-treatment preparation phase is twofold. First, patients are provided with a brief overview of the program that emphasizes the notion that pain can be influenced by multiple factors including beliefs, attitudes, and emotions. Therefore, since these are factors that can be influenced by the patient, there are skills they may have or can learn that will aid them in controlling their pain and discomfort. Second, patients often fear that the referral to such a program implies that they are having "psychological problems" or that the pain is "all in their heads." This issue is dealt with directly by explaining that cancer patients experience a large number of stressors and negative emotions (e.g., anxiety and depression), which is normal. However, developing skills to aid in coping more effectively with stress and affective responses will lead to improved pain management.

During the conceptualization–translation phase, the multidimensional model of pain, similar to the one outlined earlier, is described to provide a framework for understanding the interrelationships among the sensory, affective, and cognitive components of pain and the logic of the various aspects of treatment. Patients are also taught problem-solving skills that enable them to translate vague, seemingly overwhelming problems into specific difficulties with potential solutions.

Within the coping-skills training phase, the patients are taught a variety of skills designed to aid in managing their pain. Relaxation techniques (see above) are taught to reduce the sensory (e.g., muscle tension) and affective (e.g., anxiety) components of pain. Cognitive techniques such as attention diversion are also presented. Attention diversion techniques can be divided into two categories: (1) environmental stimulation techniques (e.g., social events, reading, watching television) and (2) cognitive coping strategies (e.g., focusing attention on aspects of the environment, non-painful sensations, or positive thoughts and imaging pleasant scenes). The latter techniques are particularly useful for patients who are too ill or weak to be physically active.

Since the use of imagery is integral to some of these techniques, training in the use of imagery is provided. Through a guided imagery technique, patients are encouraged to include as many senses as possible in their imagery. Laboratory studies have demonstrated that vividness and involvement in the imagery serve as potent distractors from noxious stimuli.[62]

The final phase, rehearsal, provides the patient with the opportunity to practice the skills acquired. Patients either describe methods for coping with a hypothetical episode of pain or engage in a role-reversal exercise where they explain the techniques to the counselor, who pretends to be a patient. Homework assignments (e.g., home practice of the relaxation exercises) are also given. The patients describe their progress at the next session, and solutions for problems encountered are developed.

Unfortunately, Turk and Rennert[62] provide no data relative to the efficacy of the cognitive-social learning approach with cancer patients. However, Moore and Mitchell-Altmaier[44] described a similar program designed to aid nine patients in coping with the stress of cancer and chemotherapy. Their data suggest that the skills taught were effective in reducing stress and anxiety.

The cognitive-social learning treatment package provides a comprehensive approach to the psychological management of cancer-related pain. Although the Moore and Mitchell-Altmaier data are encouraging, control group outcome research is necessary to evaluate the efficacy of this package in the management of cancer-related pain.

QUALIFICATIONS OF PROFESSIONALS PROVIDING PSYCHOLOGICAL TREATMENTS

The qualifications/training necessary for the effective use of the procedures described varies with each technique. Relaxation training is a relatively simple technique that can be taught by nearly any professional following adequate training. Within the cancer pain area, the discussion of the use of relaxation training is predominantly in the nursing literature.

However, Levy and Morrow[40] warn that the simplicity of behavioral techniques such as relaxation can lull people into the mistaken belief that handing a patient a relaxation tape and instructing him to listen to it at home is providing adequate relaxation training. Training in the use of relaxation requires (1) a thorough explanation of the technique and the rationale for its use in pain management; (2) adequate training in the technique, preferably at least initially by a therapist; (3) specification of problems the patient may encounter; (4) monitoring the patient to ensure sufficient home practice; and (5) the identification of activities or situations that cause exacerbations of the pain and the development of strategies for utilizing the relaxation techniques during these times.

Other techniques described in this chapter require a higher level of training than the relaxation procedures. Within the cancer pain literature, the majority of professionals utilizing hypnosis are psychiatrists or psychologists. Training in the use of hypnotic techniques is typically obtained during formal education for the degree or by attending seminars and workshops.

Biofeedback not only requires specialized training but specialized equipment. Although the equipment may appear complicated, recent advances have made most biofeedback equipment relatively easy to use. Most clinics have biofeedback therapists who provide the training. For example, in our own clinic we have a Master's level psychologist who conducts the biofeedback training under the supervision of a doctoral level clinical psychologist.

The development and implementation of cognitive-social learning approaches is done primarily by clinical psychologists. In many ways, this approach is the most comprehensive, requiring a broad knowledge of various pain management techniques and sophisticated therapy skills.

Finally, as stated earlier, no clinical treatment studies utilizing operant techniques are available in the cancer pain literature. However, these techniques are traditionally used by clinical psychologists and nurses, typically on inpatient pain wards, who have received specialized training in these techniques.

Perhaps the most relevant issue is the need for specialized training rather than the degree held (although this is a controversial area cutting across issues of the level and type of training necessary to perform certain treatments, licensing laws, third party payment, etc.). However, it is obvious that a large number of professionals have expertise relevant for the multidimensional management of cancer-related pain.

Another issue with regard to the appropriate providers of psychologically based pain management techniques is whether patients should be referred to a specialized pain clinic or treated by professionals who are part of the oncology team. While some complicated pain management cases (e.g., a patient with a significant psychiatric problem, the presence of secondary gain, etc.) may need a referral to a pain clinic, many of the techniques could be implemented in outpatient oncology clinics and inpatient wards. Generally patients are more accepting of professionals who are part of the oncology staff. Many of these techniques can be presented as a normal component of treatment with an emphasis on their use in the management of pain. De-emphasis of the ''psychological'' nature of these treatments may reduce the fears that the pain is ''all in my head'' or ''the doctor thinks I have psychological problems.''

TARGETING PATIENTS AND
TIMING INTERVENTIONS

Psychological treatments require time, energy, and concentration on the part of the patient. Spiegel[58] noted several impediments to the success of hypnosis: (1) the presence of constant, intense pain; (2) extreme fatigue secondary to treatment of the cancer or sedation from narcotics; and (3) brain metastases or hepatic decomposition. These conditions decrease the patient's ability to concentrate and actively participate in psychological types of treatment. In addition, since psychological techniques take time to learn before noticeable affects are produced, patients whose condition is deteriorating rapidly are typically not good candidates.[27] Finally, two recent studies, one on cancer pain[27] and one on headache,[13] reported that older patients (over 60) tend to receive less benefit from techniques such as biofeedback and relaxation training. Although the reason for this observation is unclear, it is an important area for future research, since many patients who experience cancer-related pain are above 60 years of age.

Bond[16] has suggested that most of the psychological problems experienced by cancer patients (e.g., depression and anxiety) are reactive in nature. He proposed that carefully designed education programs that describe the causes and significance of pain and potential treatment options will help alleviate distress and fear for the patients and their families. This type of program seems particularly relevant, since patients often have misconceptions about cancer and the possibility of experiencing extreme pain. In addition, several studies have demonstrated that patients who believe that their pain is an indication of disease progression experience greater distress and disability.[3,26,57] These education programs could be implemented immediately following diagnosis or the onset of pain.

The identification of patients in need of pain management is a problem that has received little attention. Cleeland[24] has proposed that the development and routine use of relatively simple tools for the assessment of pain and psychosocial distress would greatly improve the identification of patients in need of a multidisciplinary approach to the management of their pain.

Finally, no studies have examined the role of spouses or family members in the treatment of the patient's pain. However, studies with other pain syndromes (e.g., ref. 54) have indicated that emotional distress of spouses and marital discord are common problems.

FUTURE DIRECTIONS

Psychological approaches to the management of cancer-related pain appear to hold promise for reducing pain and suffering for the cancer patient. However, a great deal of research is necessary to validate the efficacy of these techniques despite the many difficulties encountered in conducting psychological/behavioral research with cancer patients.[4]

Another major issue that needs examination is the interaction between psychological and somatic treatments. As Cleeland[24] noted, none of the psychological approaches described are inherently incompatible with somatic treatments such as the use of analgesics. In fact, a likely advantage of psychological approaches is the reduction of analgesics needed for pain management and a reduction in the negative side effects associated with high doses of analgesics. Therefore, the purpose of the development of psychological approaches is not to replace somatic treatments; rather, they are designed to treat the affective, cognitive, and behavioral aspects of cancer-related pain.

Finally, another issue that requires examination is the time necessary to implement psychological interventions. Approaches such as relaxation, biofeedback, and cognitive-social learning treatment packages require much more effort on the part of the patient as well as the oncology staff. Therefore cost-benefit analysis research that identifies which techniques will most effectively treat which group of patients at what point in their disease will be very important. If this level of information can be established, the challenge of implementing psychological treatment approaches into the time-consuming and exhaustive therapeutic regimen of cancer patients will be well worth the time and effort required.

REFERENCES

1. Ahles TA: Psychological approaches to the management of cancer-related pain. Semin Oncol Nurs 1:141–146, 1985
2. Ahles TA, Blanchard EB, Leventhal H: Cognitive control of pain: attention to the sensory aspects of the cold pressor stimulus. Cognitive Ther Res 7:159–178, 1983
3. Ahles TA, Blanchard EB, Ruckdeschel JC: The multidimensional nature of cancer-related pain. Pain 17:277–288, 1983
4. Ahles TA, Cohen RE, Blanchard EB: Difficulties inherent in conducting behavioral research with cancer patients. Behav Ther 7:69–70, 1984
5. Ahles TA, Ruckdeschel JC, Blanchard EB: Cancer-related pain. I. Prevalence in an outpatient setting as a function of stage of disease and type of cancer. J Psychosom Res 28:115–119, 1984
6. Barber J: Hypnosis as a psychological technique in the management of cancer pain. Cancer Nurs 11:361–363, 1978
7. Barber J, Gitelson J: Cancer pain: psychological management using hypnosis. CA 30:130–136, 1980
8. Bayuk L: Pain management through hypnosis and relaxation of patients undergoing bone marrow transplantation. Semin Oncol Nurs 1:147–150, 1985
9. Benson H: The Relaxation Response. New York, Avon Books, 1976
10. Bernstein DA, Borkovec TD: Progressive Relaxation Training. Champaign, IL, Research Press, 1973
11. Black P: Management of cancer pain: an overview. Neurosurgery 5:507–518, 1979
12. Blanchard EB, Ahles TA: Biofeedback therapy for pain, in Bonica JJ, Chapman, CR, Fordyce WW, Loeser JD (Ed): Management of Pain in Clinical Practice. Philadelphia, Lea & Febiger, in press
13. Blanchard EB, Andrasik F, Evans DD, Hillhouse J: Biofeedback and relaxation treat-

ments for headache in the elderly: a caution and a challenge. Biofeed Self-Regul 10:69–73, 1985

14. Blanchard EB, Epstein LH: A Biofeedback Primer. Reading, MA, Addison-Wesley Publishing Co., 1978

15. Bond MR: The relation of pain to the Eysenck Personality Inventory, Cornell Medical Index, and Whiteley Index of Hypochondriasis. Br J Psychiatry 119:671–678, 1971

16. Bond MR: Cancer pain: psychological substrates and therapy. Clin J Pain 1:99–104, 1985

17. Bond MR, Pearson IB: Psychological aspects of pain in women with advanced cancer of the cervix. J Psychosom Res 13:13–19, 1969

18. Bonica JJ, Ventafridda V: Advances in Pain Research and Therapy, Vol 2. New York, Raven Press, 1979

19. Butler B: The use of hypnosis in the care of the cancer patient. Cancer 7:1–14, 1954

20. Butler B: The use of hypnosis in the care of the cancer patient. (Part I). Br J Med Hypnotism 6:2:2–12, 1954

21. Butler B: The use of hypnosis in the care of the cancer patient. (Part II). Br J Med Hypnotism 6:3:2–12, 1955

22. Butler B: The use of hypnosis in the care of the cancer patient. (Part III). Br J Med Hypnotism 6:4:9–17, 1955

23. Cangello VW: Hypnosis for the patient with cancer. Am J Clin Hypn 4:215–226, 1962

24. Cleeland CS: The impact of pain on the patient with cancer. Cancer 54:2635–2641, 1984

25. Copley Cobb S: Teaching relaxation techniques to cancer patients. Cancer Nurs 7:157–161, 1984

26. Daut RL, Cleeland CS: The prevalence and severity of pain in cancer. Cancer 50:1913–1918, 1982

27. Fleming U: Relaxation therapy for far-advanced cancer. The Practitioner 229:471–475, 1985

28. Foley KM: Pain syndromes in patients with cancer, in Bonica JJ Ventafridda V (Eds): Advances in Pain Research and Therapy, Vol. 2. New York, Raven Press, 1979, p 59

29. Fotopoulos SS, Graham C, Cook MR: Psychophysiologic control of cancer pain, in Bonica JJ, Ventafridda V (Eds): Advances in Pain Research and Therapy, Vol. 2. New York, Raven Press, 1979, p 231

30. Fotopoulos SS, Cook MR, Graham C, Cohen H, Gerkovich M, Bond SS, Knapp T: Cancer pain: evaluation of electromyographic and electrodermal feedback. Prog Clin Biol Res 132D:33–53, 1983

31. Fordyce WE: Behavioral Methods for Chronic Pain and Illness. St. Louis, The C.V. Mosby Co., 1976

32. Gybels J, Adriaensen H, Cosyns P: Treatment of pain in patients with advanced cancer. Europ J Cancer 12:341–351, 1976

33. Hilgard ER, Hilgard JR: Hypnosis in the Relief of Pain. Los Altos, CA, William Kaufmann, Inc. 1975

34. Holroyd KA, Andrasik F, Westbrook T: Cognitive control of tension headache. Cognitive Ther Res 1:121–133, 1977

35. Jacobson E: Progressive Relaxation. Chicago, University of Chicago Press, 1938

36. Jurish SE, Blanchard EB, Andrasik F, et al.: Home-versus clinic-based treatment of vascular headache. J Consult Clin Psychol 51:743–751, 1983

37. Keefe FJ, Brantley A, Manuel G, Crisson JE: Behavioral assessment of head and neck cancer pain. Pain 23:327–336, 1985

38. LaBaw W, Holton C, Tewell K, Eccles D: The use of self-hypnosis by children with cancer. Am J Clin Hypn 17:233–238, 1975

39. Leventhal H, Brown D, Schaham S, Enquist G: The effects of preparatory information about sensations, threat of pain, and attention on cold pressor pain. J Pers Soc Psychol 37:688–714, 1979

40. Levy SM, Morrow GR: Behavioral interventions in behavioral medicine. Cancer 50 (Suppl):1936–1938, 1982
41. McGuire D: The multidimensional phenomenon of cancer pain, in McGuire DB Yarbro CH, (Eds): Cancer Pain Management. Orlando, FL, Grune & Stratton, pp 1–21
42. McKegney FP, Bailey LR, Yates JW: Prediction and management of pain in patients with advanced cancer. Gen Hosp Psychiatry 3:95–101, 1981
43. Melzack R, Wall P: Pain mechanisms: a theory. Science 150:971–979, 1965
44. Moore K, Mitchell-Altmaier E: Stress inoculation training with cancer patients. Cancer Nurs 4:389–393, 1981
45. Murphy T: Cancer pain. Postgrad Med 53:187–194, 1973
46. Noyes R: Treatment of cancer pain. Psychosom Med 43:57–70, 1981
47. Paul GL, Trimble RW: Recorded versus "live" relaxation training and hypnotic sugges-tion: comparative effectiveness for reducing physiological arousal and inhibiting stress response. Behav Ther 1:285–302, 1970
48. Payne R, Foley KM: Advances in the management of cancer pain. Cancer Treat Rep 68:173–183, 1984
49. Rybstein-Blinchik E: Effects of different strategies on chronic pain experience. J Behav Med 2:93–101, 1979
50. Sacerdote P: Additional contributions to the hypnotherapy of the advanced cancer patient. Am J Clin Hypn 7:308–319, 1965
51. Sacerdote P: Theory and practice of pain control in malignancy and other protracted or recurring painful illnesses. Int J Clin Exp Hypn 18:16–180, 1970
52. Schafer DW: Pain, emotions, and the cancer patient. Surg Annu 16:57–67, 1984
53. Schultz JH, Luthe W: Autogenic Training. New York, Grune and Stratton, Inc., 1959
54. Shanfield SB, Heiman EM, Cope N, Jones JR: Pain and the marital relationship: psychiatric distress. Pain 7:343–351, 1979
55. Silver BV, Blanchard EB: Biofeedback and relaxation training in the treatment of psychophysiological disorders: or, are the machines really necessary? J Behav Med 1:217–239, 1978
56. Spiegel D, Bloom JR: Group therapy and hypnosis reduce metastatic breast carcinoma pain. Psychosom Med 45:333–339, 1983
57. Spiegel D, Bloom JR: Pain in metastatic cancer. Cancer 52:341–345, 1983
58. Spiegel D: The use of hypnosis in controlling cancer pain. CA 35:221–231, 1985
59. Taylor BC: Relaxation training and related techniques, in Agras S (Ed): Behavior Modification: Principles and Clinical Applications. Boston, Little, Brown and Co., 1978
60. Teders SJ, Blanchard EB, Andrasik F, et al.: Relaxation training for tension headache: comparative efficacy and cost-effectiveness of a minimal therapist contact versus a therapist-delivered procedure. Behav Ther 15:59–70, 1984
61. Turk DC, Meichenbaum D, Genest M: Pain and Behavioral Medicine. New York, Guilford Press, 1983
62. Turk DC, Rennert K: Pain and the terminally ill cancer patient: a cognitive-social learning perspective, in Sobel HJ (Ed): Behavior Therapy in Terminal Care: A Humanistic Approach. Cambridge, MA, Ballinger Publishing Co., 1981
63. Turner JA, Chapman CR: Psychological interventions for chronic pain: a critical review. I. Relaxation training and biofeedback. Pain 12:1–21, 1982
64. Turner JA, Chapman CR: Psychological interventions for chronic pain: a critical review. II. Operant conditioning, hypnosis, and cognitive behavioral therapy. Pain 12:23–46, 1982
65. Wetchler BV: The management of cancer pain. The Stress/Pain Manager 5:6–7, 14, 1984
66. Wolpe J: Psychotherapy by Reciprocal Inhibition. Stanford, Stanford University Press, 1958
67. Woodforde JM, Fielding JR: Pain and cancer. J Psychosom Res 14:365–370, 1970

Katherine L. Patterson, B.S.N., R.N. and
Patricia M. Klopovich, M.N., R.N.

11

Pain in the Pediatric Oncology Patient

Patients with cancer frequently experience pain, as either a symptom of their underlying disease or as a result of treatment for that disease. Though recent literature has explored the assessment and treatment of pain in general, only a fraction has been devoted to this problem in the pediatric cancer patient. The available literature also fails to document the incidence, prevalence, and natural history of pain in children with cancer. This chapter reviews problems surrounding the detection and control of pain in children with cancer. It includes assessment strategies for pain, children's reactions to and descriptions of pain, and a variety of behavioral and pharmacological treatments used in children. The special contributions that nurses have made and can continue to make toward controlling pain in the child with cancer are also emphasized.

PAIN IN CHILDREN

Many definitions of pain have been developed. The International Association for the Study of Pain defines pain as "an unpleasant sensory and emotional experience associated with actual or potential tissue damage, or described in terms of such damage (p. 250)."[8] Margo McCaffery defines pain as "whatever the experiencing person says it is, existing whenever he says it does (p. 11)."[28]

These and other definitions describe pain as a multidimensional experience, with the assumption that the person in pain can explain or verbalize the physical and psychological dimensions of the experience. But what of the person who is too young to describe these perceptions? Because children's cognitive abilities are limited by their developmental level, they present a unique challenge to the health care provider attempting to assess and alleviate their pain. Theories of pain[32,56] present a global understanding of the phenomenon of pain but have not successfully included pain occurring in the early phases of human development, especially during the preverbal phase. Therefore, when the patient in pain is a child, developmental level and cognitive abilities of that child, as well as interactions between parent and child, must be considered in the overall assessment of pain.

Developmental and Cognitive Considerations

Children perceive and react to pain based on their developmental level. Infants display primarily reflex behaviors. They react to a painful stimulus with a generalized response and diffuse body movements. They communicate by crying and rely on the practitioner or their parent to distinguish the meaning of their cries. Infants are easily distracted when the pain ceases.[1,25] This fact is perhaps the rationale behind the performance of minor surgical procedures on neonates without the use of anesthesia (i.e., circumcision). In a recent study, however, Dale[9] identified many responses of infants to pain, such as wrinkling of the forehead, withdrawing the affected extremity, and moving the arms and legs.

Toddlers and pre-school children react to a painful stimulus both locally, by withdrawing the affected body part, as well as with generalized body movement and other nonverbal behaviors. Egocentricity and magical thinking, characteristic of this age group, lead the toddler to see himself as the cause of his pain (e.g., punishment for a misdeed). In addition, children in this age group have a poor concept of temporal relationships. They cannot conceive that a discomfort will have an end, nor can they understand that a painful procedure is related to future healing. The presence of a parent during painful experiences is very comforting to children in this age group.[1,25,51,54]

School-aged children begin to have an increased understanding of pain and can usually describe their pain to the health care provider. Several studies have been conducted with school-aged children to elicit their unique interpretation of pain and painful experiences. In an early study, Schultz[48] asked 74 10 to 11 year-old children questions about the meaning pain had for them. She found that fears of bodily injury and death were universal among the subjects. In addition, 64 of the 74 children who were questioned also related pain to being afraid or nervous.

Scott[49] interviewed 58 children aged 4 to 10 years regarding the color, texture, shape, pattern, and continuous-versus-intermittent quality of pain. She found that younger children (4 to 6 years old) tended to differentiate pain sensations in terms of color, shape, and texture more often than did the older children. This finding is consistent with Piaget's description of the child in the pre-operational stage of development. Children at this stage of development are more intuitive and sensory oriented according to Piaget. Scott's findings can be useful in the development of assessment tools for young children.

A group of investigators[47,55] studied 214 hospitalized and non-hospitalized children aged 9 to 12 years. Findings of one study indicated that these children could adequately describe pain.[47] In the other study,[55] hospitalized children were unable to identify coping strategies that could help them with painful situations as often as were non-hospitalized children.

Ross and Ross[43,45] undertook a large study (n = 994) of school-aged children 5 to 12 years old to further explore what they knew about pain. The majority of children equated pain with discomfort only, and could not identify anything positive associated with pain. Seventy percent of these children used a large repertoire of descriptions showing that, if asked in an age-appropriate manner, they could adequately describe their pain. Only a small number (n = 213) identified any self-initiated coping techniques used to deal with pain. Ross and Ross offered several recommendations for interviewing children about pain. The use of open-ended statements or questions designed to generate responses are superior to a supplied standardized format in eliciting descriptions of pain. The interviewer must make the session appear to be a conversation rather than a test, and the interviews should be taped. Finally, the interviewer should utilize warm-up questions to help the children understand exactly what is expected of them.

In a follow-up study, Ross and Ross[46] tested the ability of third and fourth grade children to learn about pain. Twenty-eight children participated in an instruction program about pain that discussed a variety of topics such as the early warning value of pain, hospitalization, maladaptive use of pain, procedures with needles, and training in cognitive coping strategies. Pre-test/post-test score differences indicated that these children were able to learn about pain. Unfortunately, a test for long-term retention was unable to be administered to these children. Currently Ross and Ross are conducting further studies to test the efficacy of these programs.

Based on the data described above, it can be concluded that school-aged children do have the ability to describe pain adequately, although Ross and Ross[43] show that their understanding of the meaning of pain is poor. Inadequate cognitive abilities and possibly a reluctance on the part of parents and educators to discuss pain may account for this lack of understanding. However, as demonstrated by the second Ross and Ross[46] study, these children can learn coping strategies that may be useful to them in health care settings.

Adolescents share the same concerns as school-aged children (e.g., the inability to describe pain and fears of bodily injury). In addition, they also experience the psychological pain of isolation from their peer group during hospitalization or long-term treatment for cancer or other chronic illnesses. Such isolation can interfere with the establishment of identity, an important developmental task of adolescents. Furthermore, the loss of control over their lives may increase anxiety for this age group.

Treatment for cancer places children in a variety of painful situations. The practitioner should take into consideration the developmental differences discussed above when assessing the child's pain and his adaptation to his disease and treatment. Anxiety and fear may be a large component of responses to pain in children. Whereas adult cancer patients may have fears related to the disease itself, children's difficulties may be a result of fear of needles and the specific procedures, fear of having to be restrained during intrusive procedures or anxiety if the parent is absent.

CHILDREN'S RESPONSE TO PAIN

Children respond to pain both physiologically and behaviorally. In children too young to explain their pain (usually four years and younger), behavioral indicators of pain may be more reliable than verbal indicators. In addition, the practitioner must include parents in the assessment process. Often the parent can tell if the child is in pain, although in some situations, the parents' own anxiety level may prevent them from adequately assessing their child. In some instances, the parents may never have observed their child in pain and therefore may not be able to identify pain as the cause of a particular change in behavior.

Physiological manifestations of pain are those controlled by the sympathetic nervous sytem. Heart rate, respiratory rate, temperature, and blood pressure may increase. Pupils may be dilated and/or the child may be diaphoretic or pale. Usually, these changes are responses to acute pain. If the pain becomes prolonged or chronic, physiologic adaptation occurs and these signs may not be evident.

Children respond to pain with a variety of verbalizations including an acknowledgement or description of the pain, protests, or anger and accusations. Specific verbal response may be more difficult for younger children. For them, vocalizations such as sighing, moaning, screaming, and crying may be their most important means of communication in expressing pain.

Behavioral indicators of pain include facial expressions and body movements. Facial expressions that might indicate pain include widely open or tightly shut eyes, clenched teeth, tightly shut lips or biting of the lower lip, or a wrinkled forehead or frown. Escape movements and protective body movements, such as splinting or touching an abdominal incision, may indicate that a child has pain. Purposeless movements such as thrashing about or moving rhythmically can also mean pain is present. Some children

Table 11-1
Behavior Scales Used to Study Pain in Children with
Categories Used to Rate Pain Behaviors

Behavior Rating Scale adapted from Johnson by Hester[14]	Observation Scale of Behavioral Distress (OSBD)[19]	Procedure Behavioral Rating Scale (PBRS)[21]
Vocal	Cry	Cry
Verbal	Scream	Cling
Facial parameters	Physical restraint	Fear verbal
Eyes	Verbal resistance	Pain verbal
	Requests emotional support	Scream
Forehead	Muscular rigidity	Stall
Jaw	Verbal fear	Carry
Motor parameters	Verbal pain	Flail
Movement	Flail	Refusal position
Tone	Nervous behavior	Restrain
	Information seeking	Muscular rigidity
		Emotional support
		Requests termination

will remain completely immobile, afraid to move, while others may rub the affected area. Children may also reach out to loved ones in a help-seeking contact to show that they are in pain.

The behavioral responses to pain discussed above have been reported extensively in the literature.[26,30,51,54] A number of researchers have used these observations to develop behavioral checklists that can be used to measure pain in children undergoing either surgery or other painful procedures. Another use of such behavioral checklists is the validation of tools for assessing pediatric pain (Table 11-1).[2,3,14,19,20,21]

As mentioned above, behavioral observations can be more accurate than verbal statements in assessing pain, especially in younger children and infants. In addition to the specific behavioral indicators discussed previously, some children may exhibit more subtle behaviors that could indicate the presence of pain. Such behaviors might include irritability, restlessness, lowered tolerance for frustration, or decreased appetite. Cessation of play may be a subtle indicator that the child is not well, while clinging or whining behaviors can also be indicators of discomfort. Pain-induced fatigue that leads to sleep is a frequent occurrence in children. Although many practitioners erroneously think that if a child is sleeping he is not having pain, in actuality, the child is exhausted from the pain. Additionally, children in pain have altered patterns of sleep. They may sleep for short periods and wake up crying. A change in activity level, either increased or decreased, can also be indicative of pain. Some children utilize activity to distract them from their pain.[12]

As children mature their response to pain changes. Developmental changes that occur during childhood best explain the complexity of children's pain behavior. For this reason, assessment of pain in children is not an easy task. Assessment tools must be adapted to the changing cognitive abilities of children as they mature.

Tools to Assess Pain in Children

Health care professionals who work with children must utilize many techniques to determine if a child is hurting. Developmental stages, subtle behavioral changes, and physiological parameters should all be considered when assessing pain in children. Recently a number of researchers have developed pain rating scales and assessment tools for use in children.

Hester[14] developed the Poker Chip assessment tool and validated it in children aged four to six years receiving immunizations. This tool incorporates the use of four white poker chips that are equated as pieces of hurt. For example, one chip is a little bit of hurt and four chips are the most hurt. The child is asked if he hurts. If he says no, the score is 0; if he says yes, he is then asked to take the number of chips that equal his hurt. Hester found that the tool correlated well with behavioral observations.

Molsberry[37] designed the Hurt Thermometer to assess pain. This tool was tested on 21 children aged four to eight years undergoing surgery. The children moved the elastic sleeve of the thermometer until it corresponded to the amount of pain they felt. Low temperature readings corresponded with little pain, while high thermometer readings corresponded with increased levels of pain. This investigation found mean responses of the Hurt Thermometer and a modified version of the Hester poker chip tool to be similar.

Abu-Saad[2,3] developed a ten-centimeter scale on which children rated the intensity of their pain. The investigator used a convenience sample of 10 children aged 9 to 15 years admitted for surgical procedures. Their ratings were compared to physiologic and behavioral parameters as well as verbal descriptions of pain. Based on chi square analysis of medication effects by pain response indicators on the ten-centimeter scale, this investigator found the scale to be a reliable indicator of pain in this sample.

Beyer[6] has developed a scale called the Oucher to measure pain intensity as rated by children aged 3 to 15 years. The Oucher is a poster card with a series of photographs of a young child in various degrees of discomfort. The photographs are rank ordered and assigned a numerical value of 1 to 6 on one side of the card. A 100-point visual analogue scale is placed opposite the photographs for use by older children (i.e., those who can count to 100). Beyer[6] conducted initial studies to determine validity and reliability, including comparisons of the numeric and photographic scales, measures of Oucher scores postoperatively to measure changes over time, and a comparison with the Hester Poker Chip tool. Initial statistical analysis revealed encouraging reliability and validity measures for the Oucher tool. Beyer is currently completing a battery of studies to further examine the validity and reliability of Oucher ratings (personal communication, 1985).

Eland developed a color tool that has evolved from years of research on children's pain.[10,11,12] The instrument uses crayons and body outlines for children to indicate how much and where they hurt. A child is asked to rank order four colors (red, green, blue, yellow) according to which color represents the *least* and which the *most* hurt. The child is then asked to draw on the outline of the body (using the color corresponding to the amount of hurt he is experiencing) exactly where the pain is located. Eland found this tool to be useful in younger children, but she recommended the use of a numeric or visual analogue scale to assess pain in older children.

With the exception of Hester's Poker Chip Tool, each of the scales described above is an adaptation of the classic visual analogue scale. Visual analogue scales have been tested widely in the adult population,[4,17,18,29,52,53] and found to be very reliable and valid indicators of pain intensity. In addition, researchers have developed and tested various methods of statistical analyses using these types of scales.

In children as well as adults, however, it is difficult to separate the psychological from the physiological aspects of pain. Furthermore, it is difficult to determine how much anxiety or fear is measured by visual analogue scales, in addition to pain, especially the Beyer Oucher. Shacham and Daut[50] have asked this question of behavioral checklists: How much of the scale is measuring pain rather than associated distress or anxiety? It is these authors' opinion that researchers should attempt to assess the degree of fear and anxiety measured by their particular tool. This is especially important because the most painful experiences that children undergo elicit both fear and anxiety as well as pain.

Tools for the assessment of pain in children that appear most useful from those reviewed here include the Oucher and the Eland Color Tool.[6,11] The Oucher can be used for a wide range of ages and is currently the only scale that has been tested in children as young as three years. A smaller version of the poster card could be easily pocketed by staff nurses and used quite readily on a busy pediatric unit both to assess pain and evaluate the effectiveness of pain control interventions. However, the ability of Eland's Color Tool to localize pain as well as assess its intensity can also be very useful for practitioners. Additionally, the Color Tool can be administered very quickly and is an interesting task for children.

Pediatric clinicians must be very creative in their approach to assessing children's pain. The development of the tools described above and the attempts to establish reliability and validity measures have been a great help to these clinicians. Not only do they enable them to objectively assess the pain children are experiencing, but also to carefully evaluate the success of pain control measures. In addition, researchers are able to use these tools to measure pain in children as they conduct their various studies.

CONTROL OF PAIN IN THE PEDIATRIC ONCOLOGY PATIENT

Upon diagnosis of a malignancy, a child is immediately faced with a multitude of potentially painful experiences. Acute pain may stem from a number of sources, including the disease itself. Operative interventions for either diagnostic biopsy or excision of the primary tumor may result in acute pain. Finally, certain diagnostic procedures, (e.g., spinal tap and bone marrow aspiration) may also be quite painful. This latter group of procedures is particularly problematic for children, as they universally dislike needles. Eland[11,12] asked 242 chronically ill hospitalized children, "of all the things that have ever hurt you, what has been the worst?" Nearly half replied "shot" or "needles." Recent interviews of children with cancer conducted by Eland revealed that venipuncture was the worst source of pain, even more than bone marrows and spinal taps. The children who were interviewed rationalized that venipunctures were a more commonplace occurrence than the other procedures and therefore caused more pain more frequently.[11]

Chronic progressive pain occurs in children during the terminal phases of treatment and/or disease, and is often associated with progressive disease. The treatment of this type of pain differs from that for chronic non-malignant pain syndromes seen in children. Administration of narcotics is the treatment of choice for pain of malignant origin as compared to behavioral interventions, which are often used to treat other chronic pain syndromes in children.

Treatment of Acute Illness/Postoperative Pain

All of the principles involved in the optimal treatment of adult cancer pain, including giving medicines around the clock as opposed to when needed to control pain, are applicable to children. Historically, children have been grossly undermedicated for acute postoperative pain.[7,13,24] A number of factors have contributed to this practice, including lack of formal assessment of pain as well as unfounded concerns of addiction and respiratory depression. Use of the assessment tools described earlier to assess level of pain both before and after administration of medication is essential in order to determine the success or failure of treatment.

Children metabolize narcotics faster than adults do. Consequently, doses may need to be given more frequently.[41] Since children interpret shots as being the worst aspect of hospitalization or surgery, narcotics should be given intravenously in the immediate postoperative period until oral medications can be used. Many staff nurses and physicians fear this method of administration, but the fact is that drugs can be given as a 10- to 15-minute infusion very safely and effectively. The use of this route of administration for narcotics will help children to more readily accept medication for pain. Many pediatric nurses may remember the frustrations of caring for a child who refused pain medication or denied that he was in pain because he did not want an injection.

Parents need to be reassured about the use of pain medication. Some parents may fear addiction if their child receives narcotics. Parents, and in some cases adolescent patients, require education about the need for the medication, as well as reassurance that addiction is virtually nonexistent in patients who require narcotics for short-term relief of acute pain.

Treatment of Acute Pain Related to Procedures

The treatment of childhood cancer includes many painful procedures. Treatment for acute lymphocytic leukemia, the most common of childhood malignancies, usually requires frequent bone marrow aspirations, spinal taps, and parenteral medications. The management of pain associated with procedures can be approached utilizing a variety of methods. Pre-procedural preparation of patient and parents, pre-procedural sedation, support of parents and care givers during the procedure, and distraction have all been employed to treat the pain and anxiety related to these procedures. In a recent survey, Hockenberry and Bologna-Vaughan[16] asked nurses from 29 Pediatric Oncology Group institutions active in the care of children with cancer to complete a questionnaire regarding preparation for procedures. Categories of preparation methods used most frequently included drugs or sedatives, relaxation techniques, and hypnosis.

The use of sedative medications prior to invasive procedures is frequently unsuccessful in decreasing pain and anxiety in children. Many times sedation is used for the initial diagnostic bone marrow and spinal tap, as there is little time for adequate preparation or behavioral training in the newly diagnosed patient. Frequently the use of sedation is the only way to assure the cooperation necessary to obtain the multiple samples required for accurate diagnosis and staging. Parents and children need to be cautioned that these medications will not make the child sleep through the procedure. During the painful parts of the procedure, the child will be awake and will still feel pain. In these authors' experience, young children (aged two to five) are cooperative during the initial diagnostic period and then actually become more distressed and less cooperative with subsequent procedures.

The ideal approach to procedural preparation in children should include pre-medication for procedures performed during diagnosis and staging, followed by behavioral interventions as treatment progresses. In addition, both the child and the parents should have adequate instructions about any procedure before it is undertaken.[23,31]

Recently, the increased use of behavioral techniques, such as hypnosis, guided imagery, relaxation, self-talk, and thought-stopping have also been shown to be beneficial. Behavioral techniques used to treat the pain associated wth painful procedures have been reported by many authors.[15,16,22,23,27,38–40,42,44,57] Distraction is a very effective tool for children during painful procedures. This technique utilizes methods that may include watching a picture on the wall, counting, singing, listening to music, and telling or reading a story during the procedure. In essence, one must employ methods that distract the child's attention from the activity causing the pain. Distraction can be used by either practitioners or parents, since less preparation is required than for some other behavioral techniques.

Thought-stopping, recently reported by Ross,[42] can be used as a coping strategy for reducing the anticipatory anxiety that may occur prior to painful procedures. The child prepares a set of positive thoughts about the feared procedure and then memorizes them. Each time the child begins to think about the impending procedure, he is instructed to stop and immediately repeat the set of cognitions aloud or to himself. Examples of such cognitions include, 'A needle in my arm is quick. I have good veins. The girl who does it is nice. The doctor has to know how my blood is. It won't hurt much if I think hard about something nice (p. 394).''[44] Although this procedure has not been systematically tested in pediatric cancer patients, anecdotal reports have indicated that the technique is effective in controlling anxiety as well as helping the child attain self-control.[42,44]

Positive self-talk[38] is similar to thought-stopping. The child uses statements such as "I can make it" or "I am doing terrific" during the procedure. This approach can be combined very effectively with relaxation techniques during painful procedures.

Progressive muscle relaxation[5] is another technique that can help to decrease pain and anxiety during a painful procedure. It must be taught by a trained individual and practiced regularly to be effective. The technique involves alternating contraction and relaxation of all muscle groups in the body. With practice the patient can eventually relax muscle groups on command. Children are encouraged to use this method to relax before a painful procedure.

Guided imagery consists of concentrated focusing on mental images. It is the focusing on the imagination rather than existing external stimuli that distinguishes imagery from distraction. Hypnosis, to which many young children are especially susceptible, is closely linked to guided imagery. Hypnosis can be performed on children by a trained psychologist or health professional before painful procedures. Often progressive muscle relaxation and guided imagery are used to induce hypnosis in children.

Each of the behavioral techniques discussed above has been found to be effective in treating the pain and anxiety related to painful procedures in children with cancer. Techniques such as distraction, thought-stopping, and positive self-talk are easily instituted before the procedure. Relaxation, imagery, and hypnosis require more preparation time for both the professional and the patient. Advanced training and practice are necessary for the techniques to be effective. Investigation is needed to identify children who may have increased difficulties with painful procedures. If children who are at risk can be identified early, training for techniques such as progressive muscle relaxation and hypnosis can begin early in the course of treatment.

In summary, painful procedures are commonplace for children with cancer and the treatment of the pain and anxiety related to them is an integral part of the overall care of these children. In dealing with pain and anxiety, children can learn coping strategies that they then can employ in other treatment-related activities that are distressing or difficult for them.

Treatment of Chronic Progressive Pain in the Terminal Phase

The treatment of pain in children with terminal cancer presents a unique challenge to the practitioner. The ultimate goal is pain relief without over-sedation, a goal that can be realized by using oral analgesics around the clock. With the advent of the new longer acting narcotic preparations, pain management has greatly improved. On occasion oral pain medications may not be sufficient to control pain in the final stages of disease. In such cases, continuous intravenous administration of narcotics is used. The safety and efficacy of this method in children has been documented by Miser et al.[34,35]

Parents need education and support in order to participate in the pain management of their child in the final phase of disease. Educational efforts should center on prevention and management of narcotic side effects such as constipation, gastrointestinal upset, and pruritis, as well as proper administration of the drugs. Parents also need to be able to assess when titrations (increases or decreases) in the dosage need to be made. When their child is hospitalized, parents should be encouraged to take part in pain management. At the University of Kansas Medical Center, parents of children who have been on long-term pain medications continue to administer these drugs during hospitalization. This practice allows the parents to assume an important role in the care of their child and also prevents any delays in the administration of medication due to nurses' time constraints. Parents maintain records of the medications administered during hospitalization that are transcribed onto the medical record. The authors have found that most parents welcome this opportunity to become involved in their child's care during hospitalization and are quite capable of administering the drugs safely and effectively.

The control of pain in the terminal phases of disease requires careful management. Childrens Hospice International has developed two excellent publications for both parents and professionals regarding many aspects of pain control in the terminal phase of treatment.[33,36] Use of the material in these documents should assist parents and professionals in providing the best pain relief possible for children in the final stages of their disease.

CONCLUSION

General interest in the assessment and control of pain in adults has developed rapidly over the past 20 years. The same level of interest in children's pain, however, has been slower to emerge. The early literature on pain in children, the development of assessment tools, and studies of children's pain has been published for the most part by pediatric nurses. These authors applaud the creative research that has been conducted to adequately study pain in children.

Although much work has been accomplished in the past decade, many studies of pain in children still need to be done. Research should focus on a number of areas. There is a need for the continued development of valid and reliable pain assessment tools for use with children, especially infants and young children. Further documentation of the pharmacokinetics of analgesics in children needs to be made, as well as determination of the most effective and acceptable routes of administration. More coping strategies for children undergoing painful procedures need to be developed and tested. Finally, the identification of optimal drug regimens for the control of the chronic progressive pain in end-stage disease needs to be accomplished.

In summary, children, because of their varied cognitive abilities and developmental levels, present a challenge to pediatric oncology nurses who wish to provide optimal pain management. The adequate control of pain is especially important, since childhood experiences of pain may be the most critical determinant of future responses to pain. Whenever possible, nurses need to empower children to recognize the importance of pain, particularly its warning nature; to learn how to alleviate their pain; and to identify strategies for coping with pain.

REFERENCES

1. Abu-Saad H: The assessment of pain in children. Issues Compr Pediatr Nurs 5:327–335, 1981
2. Abu-Saad H, Holzemer W: Measuring children's self-assessment of pain. Issues Compr Pediatr Nurs 5:337–349, 1981

3. Abu-Saad H: Assessing children's response to pain. Pain 19:163–171, 1984
4. Aitken R: Measurement of feelings using visual analogue scales. Proc Roy Soc Med 62:989–993, 1969
5. Bernstein D, Borkovec T: Progressive Relaxation Training: A Manual for the Helping Professions. Champaign, IL, Research Press, 1973
6. Beyer J: The Oucher: A User's Manual and Technical Report. Available with purchase of Beyer Oucher from Hospital Play Equipment Co., P.O. Box 6011, Evanston, Illinois 60606
7. Beyer J, DeGood D, Ashley L, Russel G: Patterns of post-operative analgesic use with adults and children following cardiac surgery. Pain 17:71–81, 1983
8. Bonica J: The need of a taxonomy. Pain 6:250, 1979
9. Dale J: A multidimensional study of infant's responses to painful stimuli. Pediatr Nurs 12:27–31, 1986
10. Eland J: Children's Communication of Pain. Ames, Iowa, University of Iowa, 1974 (unpublished master's thesis)
11. Eland J: The child who is hurting. Semin Oncol Nurs 1:116–122, 1985
12. Eland J, Anderson J: The experience of pain in children, in Jacox A (Ed): Pain: A Source Book For Nurses and Other Health Professionals. Boston, Little, Brown, & Co, 1977, pp 453–476
13. Hawley D: Postoperative pain in children: misconceptions, descriptions and interventions. Pediatr Nurs 10:20–23, 1984
14. Hester N: The preoperational child's reaction to immunization. Nurs Res 28:250–254, 1979
15. Hilgard J, LeBaron S: Relief of anxiety and pain in children and adolescents with cancer: quantitative measures and clinical observations. Int J Clin Exp Hypn 30:417–442, 1982
16. Hockenberry M, Bologna-Vaughan S: Preparation for intrusive procedures using noninvasive techniques in children with cancer: state of the art vs. new trends. Cancer Nurs 8:97–102, 1985
17. Huskisson E: Measurement of pain. Lancet 2:1127–1131, 1974
18. Huskisson E: Visual analogue scales, in Melzack R (Ed): Pain Measurement and Assessment. New York, Raven Press, 1983, pp 33–37
19. Jay S, Ozolins M, Elliott C, Caldwell S: Assessment of children's distress during painful medical procedures. Health Psychol 2:133–147, 1983
20. Johnson M: Assessment of clinical pain, in Jacox A (Ed): Pain: A Source Book for Nurses and Other Health Professionals. Boston, Little, Brown & Co, 1977, pp 139–166
21. Katz E, Kellerman J, Siegel S: Behavioral distress in children with cancer undergoing medical procedures: developmental considerations. J Consult Clin Psychol 3:356–365, 1980
22. LaBaw W, Holton C, Tewell K, Eccles D: The use of self-hypnosis by children with cancer. Am J Clin Hypn 17:233–238, 1975
23. Lutz W: Helping hospitalized children and their parents cope with painful procedures. J Pediatr Nurs 1:24–32, 1986
24. Mather L, Mackie J: The incidence of post-operative pain in children. Pain 15:271–282, 1983
25. McBride M: Assessing children with pain: can you tell me where it hurts? Pediatr Nurs 3:7–8, 1977
26. McCaffery M: Brief episodes of pain in children, in Bergusen B (Ed): Current Concepts in Clinical Nursing. St Louis, CV Mosby Co, 1969, pp 178–191
27. McCaffery M: Pain relief for the child: problems areas and selected nonpharmacological methods. Pediatr Nurs 3:11–16, 1977
28. McCaffery M: Nursing Management of the Patient With Pain. Philadelphia, Lippincott, 1979
29. McGuire D: The measurement of clinical pain. Nurs Res 33:152–156, 1984
30. McGuire L, Dizard S: Managing Pain . . . in the young patient. Nurs 82 12:52–55, 1982
31. Melamed B, Robbins R, Graves S: Preparation for surgery and medical procedures, in Russo D, Varni J (Eds): Behavioral Pediatrics: Research and Practice. New York, Plenum Press, 1982, pp 225–267

32. Melzack R, Wall P: Pain mechanisms: a new theory. Science 150:971–979, 1965
33. Milch R, Freeman A, Clark E: Palliative Pain and Symptom Management for Children and Adolescents. Alexandria, VA, Childrens Hospice International, 1800 Diagonal Road, Suite 600, Alexandria, Virginia 22314, 1985
34. Miser A, Miser J, Clark B: Continuous intravenous infusion of morphine for control of severe pain in children with terminal malignancy. J Pediatr 96:930–932, 1980
35. Miser A, Davis D, Hughes C, et al.: Continuous subcutaneous infusion of morphine in children with cancer. Am J Dis Child 137:383–385, 1983
36. Moldow D, Martinson I: Home care for seriously ill children: a manual for parents. Alexandria, VA, Children's Hospice International, 1800 Diagonal Road, Suite 600, Alexandria, Virginia 22314, 1984
37. Molsberry D: Young Children's Subjective Quantification of Pain Following Surgery. Ames, Iowa, University of Iowa, 1979 (unpublished master's thesis)
38. Nocella J, Kaplan R: Training children to cope with dental treatment. J Pediatr Psychol 7:175–179, 1982
39. Olness K: Imagery (self-hypnosis) as adjunct therapy in childhood cancer. Am J Pediatr Hematol Oncol 3:313–321, 1981
40. Poster E: Stress immunization: techniques to help children cope with hospitalization. Matern Child Nurs J 12:119–131, 1983
41. Rogers A: Pharmacology of analgesics. J Neurosurg Nurs 10:180–184, 1978
42. Ross D: Thought-stopping: a coping strategy for impending feared events. Issues Compr Pediatr Nurs 7:83–89, 1984
43. Ross D, Ross S: Childhood pain: the school-aged child's viewpoint. Pain 20:179–191, 1984
44. Ross D, Ross S: Stress reduction procedures for the school-age hospitalization leukemic child. Pediatr Nurs 10:393–395, 1984
45. Ross D, Ross S: The importance of type of question, psychological climate and subject set in interviewing children about pain. Pain 19:71–79, 1984
46. Ross D, Ross S: Pain instruction with third and fourth grade children: a pilot study. J Pediatr Psychol 10:55–63, 1985
47. Savedra M, Tesler M, Ward J, et al.: Description of the pain experience: A study of school-age children. Issues Compr Pediatr Nurs 5:373–380, 1981
48. Schultz N: How children perceive pain. Nurs Outlook 19:670–673, 1971
49. Scott R: "It hurts red:" a preliminary study of children's perception of pain. Percept Mot Skills 47:787–791, 1978
50. Shacham S, Daut R: Anxiety or pain: what does the scale measure? J Consult Clin Psychol 49:468–469, 1981
51. Smith M: The preschooler and pain, in Brandt P, Chinn P, Smith M (Eds): Current Practice in Pediatric Nursing. St Louis, CV Mosby Co, 1976, pp 198–209
52. Sriwatanakul K, Kelvie W, Lasagna L, et al.: Studies with different types of visual analogue scales for measurement of pain. Clin Pharmacol Ther 34:234–239, 1983
53. Stewart M: Measurement of clinical pain, in Jacox A (Ed): Pain: A Source Book for Nurses and Other Health Professionals. Boston, Little, Brown, & Co, 1977, pp 107–137
54. Taylor P: Post-operative pain in toddler and preschool age children. Matern Child Nurs J 12:35–50, 1983
55. Tesler M, Wegner C, Savedra M, et al.: Coping strategies of children in pain. Issues Compr Pediatr Nurs 5:351–359, 1981
56. Wachter N: Pain theories and their relevance to the pediatric population. Issues Compr Pediatr Nurs 5:321–326, 1981
57. Zeltzer L, LeBaron S: Hypnosis and nonhypnotic techniques for reduction of pain and anxiety during painful procedures in children and adolescents with cancer. J Pediatr 101:1032–1035, 1982

Index